The Mental Status
Examination Handbook

THE MENTAL STATUS EXAMINATION HANDBOOK

Mario F. Mendez, MD, PhD

Director, Behavioral Neurology Program,
David Geffen School of Medicine at UCLA;
Director, Neurobehavior Unit,
V.A. Greater Los Angeles Healthcare, Los Angeles, California

ELSEVIER

Elsevier

1600 John F. Kennedy Blvd. Ste 1800
Philadelphia, PA 19103-2899

THE MENTAL STATUS EXAMINATION HANDBOOK   ISBN: 978-0-323-69489-6

Notice

Practitioners and researchers must always rely on their own experience and knowledge in evaluating and using any information, methods, compounds or experiments described herein. Because of rapid advances in the medical sciences, in particular, independent verification of diagnoses and drug dosages should be made. To the fullest extent of the law, no responsibility is assumed by Elsevier, authors, editors or contributors for any injury and/or damage to persons or property as a matter of products liability, negligence or otherwise, or from any use or operation of any methods, products, instructions, or ideas contained in the material herein.

Library of Congress Control Number: 2020947895

Senior Acquisitions Editor: Melanie Tucker
Content Development Manager: Meghan Andress
Senior Content Development Specialist: Angie Breckon
Publishing Services Manager: Shereen Jameel
Project Manager: Manikandan Chandrasekaran
Cover Design and Design Direction: Patrick Ferguson

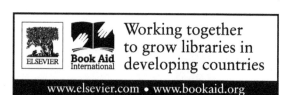

Printed in the United States of America
Last digit is the print number: 9 8 7 6 5 4 3 2 1

To Mary, Paul, and Mark

Preface

This book is meant as a practical handbook of mental status assessment for clinicians. It is about the mental status testing of cognitive functions as part of the neurological examination, rather than the mental status assessment involved in the psychiatric interview or neuropsychological testing. A clinician's ability to disclose alterations in neurocognitive or related behavioral functions can prove as valuable as the general neurological examination or other aspects of a physical examination. In fact, the mental status examination is critical in evaluating behavioral disorders from brain dysfunction, and it is particularly indispensable for documenting delirium and characterizing dementia. Moreover, there are many different types of dementia, and the pattern of deficits on mental status examination offers clues to whether it is Alzheimer disease, one of the vascular dementias, dementia with Lewy bodies, or a frontotemporal degeneration syndrome. Mental status testing is also essential for diagnosing focal disorders of cognition, for example, a low-grade glioma in the frontal lobes with changes in executive functions, a prior stroke in the right parietal region with spatial deficits, or a neurodegenerative process in the left anterior temporal lobe with loss of semantic concepts. In addition to diagnosis, clinicians use the mental status evaluation to establish the severity of deficits and to follow the patient's course over time.

This handbook is devoted to mental status testing in the clinic, at the "bedside," or via telephone or videoconferencing ("tele-neurobehavior"). It aims to help the busy clinician survey cognition in the context of the history, physical examination, laboratory, and other information to synthesize cognitive and clinical information into a diagnostic assessment. For busy clinicians, the demands on their time may discourage them from performing mental status testing; however, an efficient mental status examination can be as short as a few minutes; minutes that can be as important, if not more so, than an equal amount of time spent on another aspect of the examination. Unlike other aspects of the neurological or physical examination, clinicians can complete a thorough mental status examination via videoconferencing with the projection of stimuli and the use of screenshots or other methods to record patient performance.

Skill in mental status testing is not limited to any particular clinician. Neurologists, psychiatrists, psychologists, family physicians, internists, geriatricians, nurses, occupational therapists, rehabilitation specialists, speech and language pathologists, social workers, and many others can profitably learn the skill of mental status testing. All can refer to this book when questions arise about screening for memory disturbances, language disorders, visuospatial changes, problem-solving difficulties, and other brain-behavior disturbances. This handbook is a source of information and guidance on how to assess cognitive and related behavioral functions with brief screening tests, mental status scales, or neurocognitive tasks. This book can also clarify confusing procedural features of mental status testing, recommend mental status scales, and help the clinician in deciding when to refer for neuropsychological testing.

This handbook is organized into several sections. The first four chapters lay the groundwork for performing and understanding mental status evaluations, from brief examinations to the use of mental status scales and the application of a more extensive neurobehavioral status examination (NBSE). For those who wish to go directly to the examination, Chapter 5 provides an overview of testing and summarizes the examination. Subsequent chapters (6–14) amplify on specific and detailed aspects of the domains of the examination. Chapters 15 and 16 discuss mental status scales and inventories; Chapter 17 introduces neuropsychological testing; and Chapter 18 is devoted to tele-neurobehavior and computerized cognitive testing. The handbook concludes with two useful appendices summarizing the mental status tasks and amplifying on select mental status scales.

This book is not only a reflection of my 40 years of experience evaluating patients for brain-behavior disorders, but it also builds on immense contributions from my two exceptional mentors, D. Frank Benson and

Jeffrey L. Cummings, as well as the many fellows who trained in our UCLA/VAGLA program. This handbook could not have been possible without Frank Benson, who brought the clinical neurobehavioral examination to us from Boston, and Jeff Cummings, who created the original version of the workbook and encouraged my completion of this handbook. During my training, I had the great pleasure of watching both Frank and Jeff perform masterful mental status assessments of neurological patients, disclosing signs of brain dysfunction hidden to all others. Finally, I must acknowledge the many neurobehavior fellows who contributed to refining and modifying the NBSE over the last 25 years. We particularly esteem the memory of one of those former fellows, Daniel I. Kaufer, who remained a passionate advocate and contributor to the establishment of the NBSE.

Contents

FUNDAMENTALS OF MENTAL STATUS TESTING

Chapter 1

Introduction

Mental status testing, or the evaluation of cognition in the clinic and at the bedside, is among the most useful examination techniques in a clinician's tool bag. It is an art as well as a skill that can be extremely rewarding and valuable in the care of patients. Consideration of a patient's cognition is pertinent to many if not most clinical encounters. This is because cognitive dysfunction is a sensitive barometer of brain dysfunction, and brain dysfunction is sensitive to medical and physiological disturbances beyond neurological disease. In fact, mental status testing is applicable to many disorders and is an important tool for a range of clinicians and health care providers, and not just those specialized in neurologic or psychiatric diseases. Knowing how to recognize and evaluate early and subtle changes in cognition can lead to earlier diagnosis and better management of patients with drug effects or other toxic-metabolic disturbances, major organ dysfunction, inflammatory or endocrine disorders, as well as neurological disease or psychiatric disorders. Primary care providers and specialists alike can learn to assess cognition in clinical encounters, whether in-person or via telemedicine, in a process that can take as little as a few minutes, but that can be as informative, if not more so, as other aspects of the examination.

Despite the great value of mental status testing, significant barriers exist for many clinicians in acquiring these skills. Physicians and other health care providers may not understand the cognitive consequences of brain dysfunction. Some view cognition as too complex, incomprehensible, or enigmatic. These beliefs begin in professional schools, which may not devote sufficient time to teaching, or at least exposing, students to cognitive and related behavioral changes. "Neurophobia," or the intimidating effect of applied neuroscience with its neuroanatomy and neurologic examination,

extends to cognition and brain-behavior localization. Consequently, knowledge of mental status abnormalities, and confidence in its assessment, may be deficient well into postgraduate training and beyond. Another barrier to acquiring mental status testing skills is the attitude that cognitive assessment is not the role of most clinicians, either because it is too difficult, prohibitively time consuming, or simply not in their domain. Some clinicians see the assessment of mental status as solely the province of neurologists, psychiatrists, or neuropsychologists. This book aims to counter these misconceptions and show how mental status testing skills can be easily acquired, efficiently applied, and relevant to any clinician who cares for patients.

An initial step to gaining proficiency in mental status testing is understanding the concepts of mental status and cognitive domains. There is a narrow and a broad usage of the term "mental status." This handbook uses the narrow concept of mental status evaluation, which refers to methods and techniques of cognitive assessment in the clinic and at the bedside. Nevertheless, this handbook acknowledges the broader use of "mental status" evaluation to include the psychiatric interview and the neuropsychological examination, complementary and valuable areas of examination in their own right. Cognition, or the mental processes involved in perceiving, storing, understanding, and applying information, is composed of domains such as attention, language, memory, perception, and executive abilities, among others discussed further in this and subsequent chapters (Box 1.1). The term "neurocognition," incorporated into the DSM-5 (American Psychiatric Association. *Diagnostic and Statistical Manual of Mental Disorders*. 5th ed. Arlington, VA: American Psychiatric Association; 2013) for dementia (major) and mild cognitive impairment (minor), refers to cognition linked to cortical networks and neural pathways and directly affected from brain mechanisms or disease.

BOX 1.1 MAJOR NEUROCOGNITIVE DOMAINS UNDERLYING THE MENTAL STATUS EXAMINATION (MSX)

Fundamental Aspects of MSX

1. General Behavioral Observations
2. Arousal
3. Orientation
4. Psychomotor Speed and Activity
5. Attention and Mental Control

Instrumental Aspects of MSX

6. Spoken Language and Speech
7. Written Language and Reading
8. Memory and Semantic Knowledge
9. Constructional, Perceptual, and Spatial Abilities
10. Praxis and Other Motor Movements
11. Calculations and Related Functions
12. Executive Operations
13. Executive Attributes
14. Neurological Behaviors

BOX 1.2 LEVELS OF MENTAL STATUS EXAMINATION (MSX)

1. Brief MSX Screen (≤5 minutes); screens limited major cognitive domains, usually attention, language, memory, and perception (constructions).
2. MSX Scales and Inventories (≥5, >5–15, and >15 minutes); examples include the Mini-Mental State Examination and the Montreal Cognitive Assessment among many others.
3. Targeted MSX; indicated for specific clinical conditions, such as delirium.
4. Neurobehavioral Status Examination; essentially the extended MSX in neurology and neuropsychiatry, including detailed assessment of all cognitive domains.

Another initial step is knowing that there are different levels of mental status examination (MSX), depending on the context and clinical needs. Levels may be divided into four broad categories, which include a brief MSX screen; mental status scales and inventories; targeted MSX; and the extended MSX, often referred to as the "neurobehavioral status examination" (NBSE) (Box 1.2). Brief screening quickly assesses a few cognitive domains, such as attention, language, and memory, in a few minutes when urgency and expediency are indicated. Mental status scales and inventories, such as the Mini-Mental State Examination or the Montreal Cognitive Assessment (see Chapters 15 and 16), are another level of screening with semiquantitative cutoffs for detecting cognitive impairment. Targeted MSX may include isolated elements of the NBSE, or dedicated scales focused on localized neurologic dysfunction or the assessment of specific disorders, such as delirium. Finally, there is the extended MSX or NBSE. These include tasks and tests that probe cognitive domains and that include a broad range of techniques for assessing aphasia, agnosia, apraxia, perceptual deficits, frontal-executive dysfunction, and other "neurobehavioral" symptoms and signs. The NBSE may include a battery with or without a mental status scale, or they may be applied individually. Chapter 2 elaborates on how to choose between these four MSX options.

This handbook begins with general principles of mental status testing, common clinical cognitive syndromes, and essential behavioral neuroanatomy followed by chapters on cognitive assessment. The initial chapters, and the overview of MSX in Chapter 5, allow clinicians of different backgrounds to become familiar and comfortable with MSX, from brief MSX screening through to a NBSE. Chapters 6 to 13 and Appendix A are a resource for cognitive evaluation of individual cognitive domains in the NBSE, and Chapter 14, although not traditional cognition, introduces the identification of related neurologic behavioral disorders. This handbook further discusses different mental status scales and inventories (Chapters 15 and 16, Appendix B) and presents information on neuropsychological testing and computerized cognitive tests (Chapters 17 and 18). Finally, the last chapter of this handbook explains how to administer via telemedicine the mental status tests, tasks, and scales presented in this book. "Tele-neurobehavior" is the subfield of telemedicine that uses telephone, videoconferencing, or other telecommunications to evaluate neurocognition in patients who are at a different site than the examiner. The importance of "tele-neurobehavior," particularly by telephone or videoconferencing, while steadily increasing in recent years, accelerated dramatically with the need for social distancing and isolation due to the COVID-19 pandemic.

As a further introduction to mental status testing, it may be useful to put this field into a brief historical context, discuss the role of psychiatric assessment and neuropsychological testing, and conclude with an outline of the NBSE. Readers who wish to get into the examination right away may go directly to Chapter 5.

Brief History

Before developing into mental status principles and practice, it is instructive to understand the rich tradition of mental status testing. Mental status evaluation dates back to Imhotep in Ancient Egypt, Hippocrates in Classical Greece, and early Chinese dynasties, all of whom described the use of observation and inquiry for medical assessment and mental diseases. The Chinese, as far back as 2200 B.C.E., began to use what we might consider today as mental status testing in assessing candidates for fitness for public office. However, major progress in mental status evaluation did not occur until the revolutionary advances of the 19th century, spurred by the essential concept that behavior and cognition are localized in the brain.

Investigators were also stimulated by the scientific climate of that time to make measurements of human characteristics. An early proponent of brain-behavior localization and management was the brain anatomist, Franz Joseph Gall (1758–1828), who by the beginning of the 19th century had developed the pseudoscience of phrenology. According to Gall, specific elevations in the cranium reflected enlargements of brain regions responsible for a mental ability (Figs. 1.1 and 1.2). Although now discredited, phrenology helped fuel the work of Paul Broca (1824–1880), Carl Wernicke (1848–1905), and others in localizing language deficits

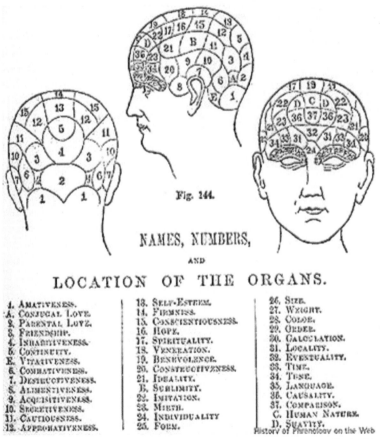

Fig. 144.

NAMES, NUMBERS,

AND

LOCATION OF THE ORGANS.

1. Amativeness.
A. Conjugal Love.
2. Parental Love.
3. Friendship.
4. Inhabitiveness.
5. Continuity.
E. Vitativeness.
6. Combativeness.
7. Destructiveness.
8. Alimentiveness.
9. Acquisitiveness.
10. Secretiveness.
11. Cautiousness.
12. Approbativeness.

13. Self-Esteem.
14. Firmness.
15. Conscientiousness.
16. Hope.
17. Spirituality.
18. Veneration.
19. Benevolence.
20. Constructiveness.
21. Ideality.
B. Sublimity.
22. Imitation.
23. Mirth.
24. Individuality.
25. Form.

26. Size.
27. Weight.
28. Color.
29. Order.
30. Calculation.
31. Locality.
32. Eventuality.
33. Time.
34. Tune.
35. Language.
36. Causality.
37. Comparison.
C. Human Nature.
D. Suavity.

History of Phrenology on the Web.

Fig. 1.1 Regions of phrenology. (Diagram from W. Mattieu Williams, *A Vindication of Phrenology*. London, 1894. Obtained through Van Wyhe, John. "The History of Phrenology on the Web." http://www.historyofphrenology.org.uk/texts/2002van_wyhe.htm.)

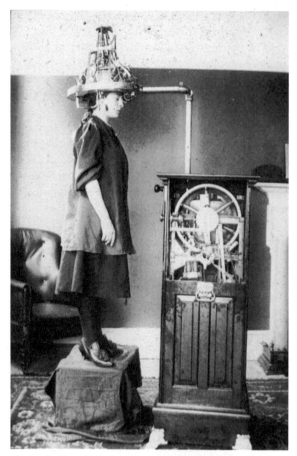

Fig. 1.2 Antique phrenology measurement instrument, 1905. (Photo Copyright © MuseumofQuackery.com http://www.museumofquackery.com/devices/psycogrf.htm.)

directly to regions of brain. In Paris, Jean-Martin Charcot (1825–1893) established clinical neurology, including descriptions of focal cognitive or behavioral deficits from brain lesions, an endeavor that involved Joseph Jules Dejerine (1849–1917), Pierre Marie (1853–1940), Sigmund Freud (1856–1939), and others. In Germany, William Wundt (1832–1920) introduced the scientific assessment of human behavior, and, by the end of the century, Sir Francis Galton (1822–1911) had laid the foundation for the assessment of cognitive abilities through tests of sensory discrimination, as well as the use of rating scales and questionnaires.

As we moved into the 20th century, both of the essential concepts for MSX, the localization of brain-behavior functions and the ability to measure cognitive abilities, began to coalesce into mental status assessment as we know it today. Psychometrics gained wide acceptance with James McKeen Cattell's (1860–1944) paper entitled "Mental Tests and Measurements" and the introduction of intelligence testing by Alfred Binet (1857–1911). The study of injured soldiers by Walther Poppelreuter (1886–1939) in World War I and by Alexander Luria (1902–1977) in World War II solidified the localizationist concepts that are the basis of the MSX. These influences were further crystallized in the postwar years as clinicians began routinely doing mental status testing in the clinic and at the bedside, applying the computer model of cognition as a flow of information processing in the "black-box" of the brain.

Psychiatry and Neuropsychology

The psychiatric interview and neuropsychological testing are related techniques for the assessment of mental status abnormalities, and their similarities and differences with the cognitively oriented MSX in this handbook needs clarification (Table 1.1). Similar to the MSX, psychiatric interviews and neuropsychological testing elicit behavioral information from patients that can be related to brain structure and function. However, the psychiatric interview primarily assesses for "productive" syndromes, such as delusions, hallucinations, and depression, rather than cognitive deficits from a normal baseline. The psychiatric interview tends to be descriptive, historical, and qualitative, but it should never be underestimated for it too is an extremely valuable tool that requires much skill. In addition, the psychiatric examination includes quantitative assessments in the form of brief, corroborative scales or inventories, and most psychiatrists usually include cognitive mental status testing in their examinations.

Compared to mental status tests, neuropsychological tests are standardized instruments with strong psychometric properties such as validity and reliability, and they have normative values. These tests are usually administered as neuropsychological batteries that are comprehensive, although requiring hours to administer and score. Neuropsychological assessment is a powerful gold standard for determining cognitive abilities, and generally serves as the standard for many mental status tests. Neuropsychology stresses

TABLE 1.1   Mental Status Examination Compared to Psychiatric Interview and Neuropsychological Testing

	Mental Status Examination	Psychiatric Interview	Neuropsychological Tests
Strengths	Short, practical Flexible tasks	Detects positive symptoms	Normative values Standardized administration Strong psychometrics
Weaknesses	Not standardized Often lacks norms	Qualitative Often not standardized	Lengthy Generally not focused
Principal Method	Neurobehavioral Clinic and bedside tests and tasks	Descriptive, quantitative, behavioral history and interview	Standardized, qualitative tests with norms
Principal Goals	Etiologic Diagnosis and neuropathology	Brain-behavior interpretation of individual	Functional cognitive assessment
Behavior Focus	Deficit ("signature") Syndromes	Productive ("positive") symptoms	Cognitive deficits and mechanisms
Parent Discipline	Neurology	Psychiatry	Psychology
Historical Basis	Development of neuroscience Clinical correlation of neuropathology	Need to care for mentally ill Need to explain mental illness	Experimental ablation studies Psychological measurement
Theoretical Basis	Syndromes are used direct neuroanatomic localization	Brain-behavior explanatory models for mental illness	Experimental and measurement models of cognition

Adapted with permission from Mendez MF, Van Gorp W, Cummings JL. Neuropsychiatry, neuropsychology, and behavioral neurology: a critical comparison. *Neuropsychiatr Neuropsychol Beh Neurol.* 1995;8:297-302.

the determination of intellectual strengths and weaknesses, individual differences, and the potential for rehabilitation, whereas the MSX emphasizes the diagnostic value of "signature" clinical syndromes, such as aphasias, amnesias, or agnosias. Compared to mental status testing, neuropsychological testing requires a controlled setting with extended testing time, special stimulus materials, delayed scoring, and lacks flexibility of administration (e.g., in test setting, test time, and variation in test application). These limit the extensive use of neuropsychological testing in the clinic or the bedside, although they remain extremely useful for specific indications. Ultimately, MSX and neuropsychological assessment are highly complementary approaches in the evaluation of patients with brainbehavior disorders. Moreover, mental status testing benefits greatly from informal validation of findings by a comparable neuropsychological test.

Conclusions

The MSX evaluates for abnormalities in neurocognition. A cognitive history precedes actual mental status testing (Fig. 1.3). Clinicians obtain an impression of the patient's mental status from descriptions and specific examples of his or her behavior and activities as provided by family members, as well as the patient. Then the clinician choses the levels of actual testing, either the brief MSX screening, mental status scales and inventories, targeted MSX, or a NBSE. The examiner often chooses elements of the NBSE as a "targeted MSX" rather than performing an extensive examination. The MSX is usually incorporated as part of a clinical evaluation involving physical examination and laboratory tests. If indicated, there may be further optional referral for neuropsychological testing in specific situations. Neuropsychological testing may be useful when clinicians suspect mild deficits

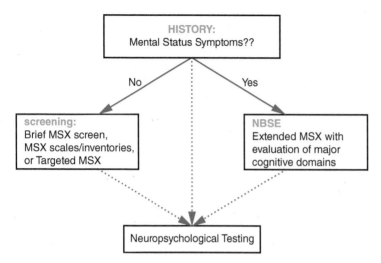

Fig. 1.3 Flow of mental status examination (MSX). *NBSE*, neurobehavioral status examination.

or when they desire an extensive, in-depth, and precise evaluation of mental functions beyond what they themselves can do in the clinic or at the bedside (see Chapter 2).

Mental status testing is an important and useful tool for most clinicians. This skill is attainable with a few basic principles and practice and can greatly contribute to patient care. Clinicians who gain proficiency in MSX are able to diagnose a wider range of disturbances and diseases that manifest with disturbed cognition. MSX is based on localization of cognition to brain areas and the ability to accurately examine these cognitive domains. Many of the coming chapters are devoted to the examination of memory, language, visuospatial skills, executive functions, and other areas of cognition.

Chapter 2

Principles of Mental Status Testing

This chapter aims to provide the foundation for mental status testing. The first step is to establish the goal or purpose for assessing cognition. This guides the decision on what level of examination is needed and whether to refer for neuropsychological testing. Second, when performing the mental status examination (MSX), there are a number of principles or key factors to consider in giving tests to patients and, afterward, in interpreting the results. Finally, there is the consideration for how to report or discuss the results with patients and families.

Goals and Levels

Mental status testing aims for the practical evaluation for cognitive problems along a medical model. The overriding goal is to screen for cognitive deficits in the clinic or at the bedside with readily available stimulus materials. Within this goal, a rapid MSX can occur with brief screening of key cognitive domains when time and circumstances are limited, such as on an inpatient service. With somewhat more time, mental status scales and inventories allow for a semiquantitative assessment of general cognition. Alternatively, the screening may use targeted tests or scales for special situations, such as delirium (see Chapter 3). For all three of these approaches, brief MSX screening, mental status scales or inventories, and targeted MSX, clinicians must be able to recognize abnormalities requiring further testing. A more extensive and comprehensive neurobehavioral status examination (NBSE) is part of a subspecialty clinical assessment for neurocognitive disorders and is a major focus of this book. NBSE is indicated when time is not an issue and the clinician can devote time to a thorough assessment of the different cognitive domains. Finally, referral for neuropsychological testing should be a consideration under certain situations, to be described later.

Brief MSX Screen (see Chapter 5)

The initial aspects of the brief assessment are observation, interaction, and orientation. The briefest assessment involves pausing to observe the patient's general behavior, such as state of alertness and wakefulness, interaction with others, and coherence of verbal output and physical movements. Clinicians often overlook the importance of just observing patients, yet this can be a very informative "MSX." If possible, engage the patient in conversation and note the quality and quantity of the interaction, including use of language and any clues to memory for recent events. Orientation, which involves asking patients to state the current date and place, is not an actual "cognitive domain," but it is a sensitive measure of either attentional or memory impairment. In the absence of a watch or other obvious display of the time, the patient's knowledge of the exact time of day can be a further extension of the assessment for temporal orientation.

Beyond observation, interaction, and orientation, clinicians can perform a brief MSX screen in approximately 5 minutes. Most clinicians can quickly examine one or two representative tasks in critical mental status areas, including awareness (arousal and attention), language (naming by confrontation), declarative episodic memory (delayed recall of a few words), and perception (three-dimensional visuospatial construction) (Table 2.1).

TABLE 2.1	Elements of the Brief Mental Status Examination Screen and Examples of Testing
Awareness	Arousal or alertness
Orientation	Orientation for time and place
Attention	Basic and complex attention
Language	Naming to confrontation and category word list
Memory	3–5 minute recall of three unrelated words
Perception	Ability to copy three-dimensional shapes

Mental Status Scales and Inventories (see Chapters 15 and 16)

When 5 to 15 minutes are available, short instruments containing a number of heterogeneous items are useful in evaluating memory plus other cognitive domains and deriving a general cognitive score. Usually, there are guidelines for administration and cutoff scores for impaired cognition. These cutoff scores may have age- and education-dependent adjustments. These instruments are useful for screening for referral for more extensive evaluation; they are less informative for assessing specific brain-behavior impairments or localization.

There are many cognitive and behavioral rating scales. Although the choice of rating scale may vary with the specific goals of the evaluation, the clinician should gain familiarity with a limited number of widely used scales, such as the Mini-Mental State Examination (MMSE) (5–10 minutes) or the Montreal Cognitive Assessment (MoCA) (10–15 minutes). Some scales are shorter and more quickly administered (e.g., the Mini-Cog or the Six-Item Screen) and others are longer and more extensive (e.g., Addenbrooke Cognitive Examination). Scales have different levels of difficulty, for example, the MMSE is easier than the MoCA, and there are differential floor and ceiling effects, for example, the MMSE shows more variance in more impaired ranges, and the MoCA shows more variance at higher levels of functioning.

Targeted MSX (see Chapters 3 and 16)

The usual mental status scales and tests may not help in differentiating specific conditions, and the clinician may want to target tests and scales to the affected cognitive domains. A major example is delirium. Here, the examiner is more concerned with an acute or subacute encephalopathy; hence the mental status focus is more on attentional systems, or even arousal. The examiner may want to use targeted scales such as the Confusion Assessment Method, the Delirium Rating Scale-Revised-98, or the Memorial Delirium Assessment Scale.

Targeted MSX is often applied to patients with specific neurologic, psychiatric, or medical illnesses. One example is HIV infection, in which there are several dedicated mental status scales sensitive to psychomotor slowing and other potential cognitive effects of HIV-associated neurocognitive disorder, for example, the International HIV Dementia Scale. Additionally, elements of the NBSE can used in isolation to target specific cognitive dysfunction or localization, such as from strokes, tumors, and other focal neurologic lesions.

The NBSE (see Chapters 6–14)

Other tasks are part of a more extended MSX, often referred to as the Neurobehavioral Status Examination (NBSE), which may take up to several hours, depending on how much is included. An extended MSX is necessary when patients have memory difficulty, language impairment, perceptual or spatial difficulty, or other instrumental problems requiring a more detailed assessment in the clinic or at the bedside. This evaluation can comprehensively examine the major cognitive domains, or parts of it can be administered in isolation as a targeted MSX (Table 2.2).

The NBSE is organized around the major cognitive domains. The "fundamental domains" include arousal, selective attention, and psychomotor activity and speed. Fundamental functions are also reflected in multidomain processes, such as orientation (place and time) and mental control. Fundamental functions are required for optimal performance of the "instrumental domains" of language, memory and semantics, perception, praxis, calculation, and executive operations and attributes. In addition, although not cognitive, the NBSE considers neuropsychiatric disturbances in socioemotional functions and the presence of disturbances in mood, affect, and thought content.

TABLE 2.2 Elements of the Neurobehavioral Status Examination and Examples of Testing

General Behavior	Appearance, attitude, personality, affect, mood
Arousal	Response to verbal and physical stimulation
Orientation	Orientation to time and place
Psychomotor Speed	Physical activity and movements
Attention	Digit span, months backward, continuous performance
Language: Verbal	Fluency, repetition, naming, comprehension
Language: Read, Write	Reading sample, writing to command
Memory	Word list learning with recognition
Perception and Spatial	Two and three-dimensional copies, search/cancellation tasks
Praxis	Limb ideomotor mime and imitation
Calculations	Simple mathematics
Executive Operations	Antisaccades, alternate tapping, GoNoGo, Luria hand sequence
Executive Attributes	Awareness of illness, proverb interpretation
Neurological Behaviors	Motivation, social, aggression, perceptive

Referral for Neuropsychological Testing (see Chapter 17)

Clinicians can request neuropsychological testing when an extensive and in-depth evaluation is desired. Neuropsychological testing is not the focus of this handbook, but in certain situations it is the gold standard for cognitive evaluation. This testing requires greater time, effort, and expense than does MSX at a clinic visit or at the bedside and is not practical for screening assessments. However, in nonurgent clinical situations in which there is time and resources for referral, neuropsychological testing can be invaluable for specific indications. Among those situations are the following:

1. To evaluate for mild deficits not detected on screening. This is particularly indicated for comparing with age and education normative data. MSX tests, including mental status scales and inventories, may not be sensitive enough to detect mild impairments, particularly among patients with higher intellectual backgrounds. In this situation, neuropsychological testing may show abnormalities for the patient's age and education.
2. To differentiate primary psychiatric conditions from dementia. For example, distinguishing the effects of a mood disorder on memory and cognition is often quite difficult and can be greatly aided by a neuropsychological assessment.
3. To determine the degree and extent of impairment. This may be important when designing a rehabilitation program for a patient, or there is a need for precise information on how the patient functions in each cognitive domain.
4. To determine detailed cognitive assessment for legal determinations, such as capacity and competence. Capacity describes decision-making ability, for example, whether to leave the hospital or accept a medical treatment. Competence, in contrast, is a legal term that refers to an individual's legal right to make these decisions. Clinicians are primarily concerned with capacity, which depends on cognition. Capacity is expressed in understanding the nature of the situation (e.g., their medical illness), the ability to express a choice, an appreciation of the alternatives and consequences, and an ability to reason rationally to reach a decision. The results of precise neuropsychological testing is better than MSX screening for providing the cognitive profile that underlies the elements of capacity.

TABLE 2.3 **Principles of Mental Status Testing**	
Administration	Interpretation
Organization of Testing	Limited Psychometrics
Testing Familiarity	Pathognomonic Sign
Patient Variables	Battery Pattern Recognition
Psychological State	Hierarchical Domains
Physical State	Process Interpretation
Test Alone if Possible	Item Difficulty and Discriminability
Context of Testing	Context Effects
Length and Speed of MSX	MSX as Part of Medical Evaluation
Encourage Responses	Assess Validity
Evaluate Responses	Examiner Biases

MSX, Mental status examination.

Principles of MSX

Mental status testing requires much skill in assessment, interpretation, and reporting. What follows are some basic principles in these areas (Table 2.3).

Principles of Assessment

1. **Organization of Testing.** The examiner begins with the choice of testing material. Generally, this involves pen with black ink or sharpened pencils without erasers, blank unlined paper, and a firm writing surface. It is best to have tests or scales that are clearly in the public domain. Choice of MSX tests or scales also depend on the patient's severity of impairment; if too severe, they may not be able to complete or perform the tests. The order of administration is additionally important. This includes the order of memory or language or attention tests in relation to each other, but also when MSX is performed in relation to the rest of the clinical examination. With mental status scales there may not be a choice of test order, but with the NBSE, it is often best to start with fundamental functions such as attention and proceed to instrumental functions such as memory and language. A further consideration is introducing the memory items relatively early, as they require returning later for delayed recall. MSX is often performed after the history and interview and before the physical examination, while the patient is still sitting.

2. **Testing Familiarity.** Assess whether the patient has taken the tests before. Many mental status tests may be subject to practice or repetition effects. Patients who have been recently or frequently tested may require alternate forms of the test. Some patients may anticipate tests and practice them such as rehearsing the day before the clinic visit or MSX. Conversely, if patients have not had occasion to be testing for a long time, for example, asking someone to copy a cube when they may not have drawn in decades, they may be given a practice trial or even shown how to initiate the task.

3. **Patient Variables.** The examiner is cautioned about specific confounders in mental status testing such as age, education, language proficiency, and intellectual background. There may be differences based on regional origin, type and extent of education, and whether they are being tested in their native language. The examiner must also determine whether there are visual, auditory, or manual impairments and adjust the testing accordingly.

4. **Psychological State.** Much of the variability in mental status testing is owing to the patient's psychological state at the time of testing. The patient may be anxious, apprehensive about testing, depressed, or otherwise indisposed to give their best performance. Often, patients feel

embarrassed or threatened by cognitive tests, which they interpret as probing their intellect, challenging their mental competency, or otherwise remind them of school examinations. The examiner must prepare the patient for the MSX by conveying the purpose for testing and putting them at ease. The examiner must also explain the nature of the tests, how the results will be used, minimize their sense of cognitive vulnerability, and discuss the confidentially of the results.

5. **Physical State.** It is obvious that patients' receptivity and performance can vary depending on their physical state at the time of the MSX. They may be quite fatigued, hungry, needing to go to the bathroom, or experiencing pain, discomfort, or the effects of a medication. Often, patients have been suffering from disturbed sleep, which can greatly alter their performance on these tests. The examiner should consider if this is the optimal time for testing or whether the MSX should be best postponed to another time.

6. **Test Alone if Possible.** Patients may not feel comfortable being tested in the presence of family or others, and this should be determined before testing. Ask the patient whether they prefer being testing alone. Explain that embarrassment from the presence of family or others may change their performance. Also note that many family members have difficulty inhibiting the tendency to jump in and answer for their loved one, rather than see them fail.

7. **Context of Testing.** Testing is preferable in a quiet room without distractions, preferably with a predetermined block of uninterrupted time. Distractions and interruptions affect the patient's performance. Optimal testing is done sitting across a table from a sitting patient and attending to them, or with a videocamera solely focused and centered on them. Sometimes it is preferable to wait to administer the tests when a quiet place is available. Also consider how the time of day of testing and the relationship to routines or other environmental factors affect the ability to do an MSX.

8. **Length and Speed of MSX.** Allot sufficient time for testing so that it is not rushed. Pause and give patients time to absorb information and to formulate their answers. Very slow patients may take time to render a response; busy clinicians who rush through the items may incorrectly grade them as impaired. In the end, practical reasons may dictate focusing the MSX on the areas of greatest concern before the patient fatigues or becomes uncooperative. Finally, consider breaking up the testing into multiple sessions; this if often a good solution.

9. **Encourage Responses.** The absence of a response is not equal to an abnormal response. It does not necessarily mean that they cannot do the task. There are many reasons why someone would not give an answer, ranging from confusion about the task to boredom, lack of cooperation, disdain for testing, depression, apathy, and many other factors. This requires patience on the part of the examiner, who must gently encourage the patient to give a response even when they give an "I don't know" answer. Positive feedback should be done to keep the patient on-track and complete testing without facilitating their answers with hints or cues. It is also best not to overtly respond to their performance, or to indicate that you consider their responses right or wrong, but rather just to continue to encourage the patients to do their best.

10. **Evaluate Responses.** During testing, note the state of the patient and how he/she relates to performance. Are they trying their best or are they getting fatigued, hungry, anxious, or experiencing pain or discomfort? If they feel uncomfortable with the result of a task or feel that they did poorly because of distractions or other reasons, offer to repeat the task. If the patient becomes emotional, agitated, or aggressive, it may be time to discontinue the testing. Alternatively, some patients give expedient answers just to placate the examiner and quickly complete the MSX. Finally, when testing patients, clinicians must also be aware of how their own responses affect patients. The examiner should keep in mind their own

emotional reaction to the patient and strive for an emotional demeanor that conveys empathy and consideration.

Principles of Interpretation

1. **Limited Psychometrics.** MSX in the clinic or at the bedside has undergone limited psychometric assessment. Few mental status tasks have been subject to the rigorous validity, reliability, standardization, and other issues that are involved in neuropsychological test development. Except for mental status scales and inventories, many lack established validity and reliability testing or normative and disease-specific data. In fact, interpretation has often relied on extrapolation from related neuropsychological norms. A major consideration in the psychometrics of MSX are their floor and ceiling effects. Tests may have floor effects in that severely impaired patients are unable to pass a "floor" of maximum impairment. There may be ceiling effects in that mildly impaired patients are unable to pass a "ceiling" of maximum normality. These considerations are important in assessing the validity of a mental status task or scale in individual patients.

2. **Pathognomonic Sign.** The approach to MSX relies on the concept of a diagnostically abnormal cutoff score. This is the traditional screening procedure in medicine and is less informative about the analog range of individual cognitive abilities. A related question is, how many items do you need to get wrong to be "abnormal?" Clinicians generally sample one item, which can be normal or abnormal, or a number of samples such that "abnormal" may be equated with two or more out of four or two or more out of six incorrect responses.

3. **Battery Pattern Recognition.** Most individual mental status tests are each influenced by multiple cognitive domains. For example, alterations in digit span can reflect changes in attention, language, or numerical ability. Consequently, an abnormality in a domain is most evident from a pattern of abnormalities across several tests, which are affected by that cognitive domain. For example, if it is attention that is affecting the digit span, then other tests influenced

by attention are also affected. A thorough MSX tests a cognitive domain with two or more tasks affected by that domain. In general, the pattern of abnormality is more reliable than that of an individual MSX test.

4. **Hierarchical Domains.** The MSX is hierarchical. In particular, impaired fundamental functions impede performance on instrumental functions. For example, abnormalities in attention will preclude accurate memory testing. This extends to syndromes, such as delirium, which affects arousal and attention, and hence the ability to distinguish underlying deficits in instrumental functions, such as memory or executive abilities. In addition, language deficits will also make it harder to test memory and executive attributes. Language is the "medium" for most MSX testing, and language impairment can preclude an accurate evaluation of other cognitive domains.

5. **Process Interpretation.** The way that a patient undertakes and performs the mental status tasks can be as informative as the actual "score" or determination of normal versus abnormal. This is the "process" approach to interpretation and requires observing and noting how the patient goes about completing a task, such as memorizing items on a memory test or copying a drawing on a perceptual test. Record or write the results just as you observe them, including not just the derived score but also their strategy in doing the tasks and the types of errors that they make during testing.

6. **Item Difficulty and Discriminability.** The examiner should give some consideration to whether individual items are appropriate to an individual patient or a particular situation. The examiner may need to take the patient's background into consideration when employing particular items. For example, on orientation questions, someone living far away may not know the county or even the exact city or suburb. If the patient has been very ill, they may have lost track of time and have temporal disorientation. Likewise, patients with limited education may not have the vocabulary for some of the items on the confrontational naming tasks, and others may use alternative regional or dialectical names.

7. **Context Effects.** As previously noted, the environment and circumstances of testing can significantly impact on the results of the MSX. Variables such as the nature of the clinic and hospital setting, with the distractions and interruptions involved, can cause differences in test performance. The other contextual factors considered in administration of an MSX, such as fatigue, anxiety, sleep disturbances, and other physiological variables, should also be considered as contextual effects in the interpretation of the results.

8. **MSX as Part of Medical Evaluation.** MSX is essentially a medical procedure and cannot be interpreted in isolation from the history, interview, and a neurological and physical examination. For example, the general physical examination may elicit signs of systemic illness that affect the MSX, and the neurological examination of cranial nerves, gait and coordination, motor and tone, reflexes, and sensation may be highly informative in clarifying a neurological origin for cognitive deficits. Similarly, when evaluating an elderly person, the MSX must be considered in light of changes seen with normal aging, both cognitive and neurological, for example, slowed cognitive speed, altered memory retrieval, presbyopia and presbyacusis, gait changes, and slowed motor movements. In addition, the clinician should integrate the MSX results with the results from neuroimaging, neurophysiological tests, and other laboratory values.

9. **Assess Validity.** Once testing is complete, it is important to consider whether the results are valid, that is, do they reflect the "truth" of the patient's mental status abilities? The examiner can briefly comment on his or her interpretation of the face validity of the testing, or whether there were concerns for motivation, possible secondary gain, or other factors that would mitigate the validity of the testing session.

10. **Examiner Biases.** Finally, the examiner must examine his or her own biases in interpreting the results. There is much subjectivity in interpreting the results of the MSX, and the examiner must honestly consider whether their interpretation was influenced by his or her attitudes. For example, MSX interpretation errors result from confirmation or expectancy bias, when the examiner sees the results that he or she expected to see; this may result from anchoring bias on a prior finding or conclusion or a framing or representative bias on how the patient presents. Three additional biases are availability bias due to a recent exposure to similar findings; attribution or affective bias from the intrusion of one's own feelings (either attributing negative intentions or feeling favorably disposed to the patient); and commission errors due to impatience and excessive haste on the part of the examiner in the MSX and interpretation.

Principles of Reporting

Reporting the results of the MSX to patients and families requires thinking about your delivery and the framing of the discussion. Reflect on your words and approach beforehand remembering that unspoken conversation may be at least as important as what is said. First, to discuss the results effectively, you need to understand their assumptions and fears. You may need to ask them how they think the patient did on these tests and what they think it means. Second, explain the limitations of testing, that is, their screening nature and the possible need to direct attention toward the specific mental abnormalities that require a more extended MSX. Third, explain your conclusions, medical terms, and any diagnosis in a simple, down-to-earth way that most people can understand. Fourth, place your discussion in the context of their preserved abilities and mental functions. Leave pauses so that they can absorb what you are saying and give them time to ask questions. Finally, ask for feedback. Ask them to repeat back to you what was said and explain what they understood. Cognitive terms and words like "dementia" or "Alzheimer disease" are understood differently by patients and families, often with misconceptions and dread. You need to plan to go over the same things again. Any bad news may induce temporary mental paralysis and they may not hear anything further. End with hopeful information and reassurance, wherever it can honestly be given.

Chapter 3

Common Clinical Disorders Affecting Mental Status Testing

It is helpful to understand how the extended mental status evaluation is altered by the commonest mental status conditions seen in the clinical setting. These can be grouped into delirium, dementia, and depression. Focal cognitive disorders are listed in the subsequent chapter on the neuroanatomy of behavior.

Delirium

Delirium is the most common brain-behavior disorder and the most frequent behavioral manifestation of medical disorders or physiological disruptions. It is an acute change in mental status with prominent changes in attention. There is a disturbance in level of awareness and a fluctuating ability to focus, sustain, and shift attention. These difficult additionally impair instrumental cognitive abilities. There is a spectrum of delirium from mild inattention and distraction to a lethargic and poorly responsive state.

Clinicians may fail to diagnose delirium because they fail to recognize and test for this syndrome. The elderly can have a "quiet" or subtle presentation of delirium that may go undetected. Yet, delirium occurs in 10% to 30% of medically ill patients, a clear majority of hospitalized elderly patients, and 80% or more of patients in the intensive care unit. The consequences of delirium include prolonged hospitalizations, increased mortality, high rates of discharge to institutions, severe impact on caregivers and spouses, and more than $4 billion of annual Medicare expenditures in the United States. Of particular importance is distinguishing delirium from dementia, the other common disorder of cognitive functioning. Delirium is acute in onset (usually hours to a few days), whereas dementia is insidious in onset and progressive. Delirium is an acute neurobehavioral decompensation with fluctuating attention, regardless of whether the patient has underlying cognitive deficits or dementia. In fact, the presence of underlying dementia is a major risk factor for delirium.

There are 10 essential characteristics of delirium (Box 3.1):

1. **Acute Onset With Fluctuating Course.** Delirium develops over hours or days but sometimes over a week or more. The course progresses to daily fluctuations of attention, arousal, and other symptoms, sometimes interposed with lucid or near normal intervals. Clinicians need to examine these patients at several points in time to get an understanding of the extent and depth of fluctuations.

2. **Attentional Deficits.** A disturbance of attention is the defining symptom of delirium. Attention is the ability to focus mental activity on a targeted external or internal stimulus to the exclusion of others. Patients with delirium cannot consistently focus, sustain, or shift their attention to relevant aspects or events, and environmental or internal stimuli, no matter how minor, can easily distract them from the topic at hand.

BOX 3.1 CLINICAL CHARACTERISTICS OF DELIRIUM

Acute onset of mental status change with fluctuating course
Attentional deficits
Confusion or disorganized thinking
Disturbed arousal
Disturbed perception
Disturbed sleep-wake cycle
Altered psychomotor activity
Disorientation and memory impairment
Other cognitive deficits
Behavioral and emotional abnormalities

Modified from Mendez MF, Yerstein O. Delirium. In: Daroff RB, Jankovic MD, Mazziotta JC, Pomeroy SL, eds. *Bradley's Neurology in Clinical Practice.* 7th ed. New York, Elsevier;2020:23-33.

3. **Confusion or Disorganized Thinking.** Patients with delirium cannot maintain a clear and coherent stream of thought. They are unable to perform organized, goal-directed behavior, and their speech reflects this disorganization. Their verbal output is poorly connected, often going from topic to topic in a tangential, circumlocutory, or totally unrelated manner.

4. **Disturbed Arousal.** Most patients have alterations in their arousal, or their readiness to react or "alert" to stimuli. This is distinct from attention and the ability to focus mental activity. Arousal refers to the ability to respond or alert; disturbances or arousal range from lethargy to stupor and coma. Most patients with delirium tend to have lethargy and decreased arousal, but some patients with delirium have increased arousal, such as those with delirium tremens. Some patients may have fluctuations that range from hypoarousal to hyperarousal.

5. **Disturbed Perception.** A dramatic feature of delirium, when present, are altered perceptions, particularly hallucinations in the visual sphere. These hallucinations are frequently animate, variable, and in color, and they may or may not be frightening to the patient. Other perceptual disturbances include illusions (distorted perceptions or sensations) and misperceptions or misinterpretations. Ultimately, the most common perceptual disturbances are missed perceptions, or failure to appreciate things that are going on around them.

6. **Disturbed Sleep-Wake Cycle.** Patients with delirium have disturbances of the normal diurnal or circadian rhythm and experience disruption of their day-night cycle. This most commonly manifests as excessive daytime drowsiness or sleeping, and sometimes wakefulness and alertness at night. There may be "sundowning," or agitation and restlessness occurring during the night.

7. **Altered Psychomotor Activity.** Delirium can be hypoactive, hyperactive, or mixed in their psychomotor activity. The most common are hypoactive with psychomotor retardation and often accompanying lethargy and decreased arousal. The less common hyperactive subtype often has accompanying agitation, perceptual disturbances, and overactivity of the autonomic nervous system.

8. **Disorientation and Memory Impairment.** Disorientation is one of the most common findings in delirium. Disorientation is not specific for delirium, however, and it occurs in dementia and amnesia as well. Among patients with delirium, recent memory is disrupted in large part by the decreased registration caused by attentional problems. In delirium, reduplicative paramnesia, a specific memory-related disorder, results from decreased integration of recent observations with past memories. Persons or places are "replaced" in this condition. For example, they tend to relocate the hospital closer to their homes.

9. **Other Cognitive Deficits.** Patients with delirium have cognitive deficits in writing and in visuospatial abilities. Writing disturbance result in poorly formed letters and words and a tendency to disturbed spatial orientation or direction of written sentences or phrases. These patients also manifest difficulties with visuospatial constructions, such as drawings, and with complex visual processing, such as visual object recognition and environmental orientation.

10. **Behavioral and Emotional Abnormalities.** Patients with delirium may have delusions, or false beliefs, that are poorly systematized and paranoid with a persecutory content. Other patients with delirium exhibit marked emotional lability or may become agitated, depressed, or quite apathetic.

Characteristics on MSX

The examiner begins with the neurobehavioral history and behavioral observations. A history of a fairly abrupt change in mental status is usually the most salient aspect of presentation. Behavioral observations then focus on overt signs of disturbed attention, fluctuations, and altered arousal. Delirium is evident in observed ease of distractibility and inability to stay on track or with the interview without having to be constantly brought back. The patient may have overt evidence of altered arousal, particularly lethargy or a tendency to fall asleep during the interview, necessitating stimulation to maintain alertness. They may be hypoactive and psychomotor slowed, or there may be hyperactivity. If conversation is elicited, the examiner listens for the organization and coherence of their verbal output. Finally, the examination should evaluate for behavior disturbances, including agitation and irritability, signs of perceptual alterations such as responding to hallucinations, and changes in emotional lability and mood.

The examiner then proceeds to evaluate attention with specific testing. The most common are assessments of orientation and recitation tasks. Orientation for time and place can be disturbed from attention deficits, as in delirium, or from memory impairment, as in dementia. Ask the patient for time, date including year, and place, including city. Patients should be within 4 hours of time and a few days of the date and know the city if not the exact place that they are at. The most common recitation task is repetition of digits forward, delivered one per second in a steady voice beginning with four digits and gradually increasing (or decreasing) the number of digits as needed (see Chapter 7). The patient must repeat the entire sequence immediately after presentation. The examiner gives them two trials at each level, with a normal performance of at least five (preferably six) digits forward. Similar recitation tasks are letters forward and reversal tasks such as digits backward, spelling backward (e.g., the word "world"), or counting backward (by 3 from 20 or by 7 from 100). These tasks are harder than forward recitation and involve other aspects of mental control, particularly working memory, a frontal executive ability. Other attentional tests are continuous performance tasks, such as the "A vigilance test," in which the patient must indicate whenever the letter "A" appears among 20 random letters presented one per second, or in a string of written letters. There should be no errors of omission or commission.

Considering that attention is required for instrumental cognitive functions, attentional deficits may preclude completion of tests in other cognitive domains. Nevertheless, the examiner should screen language, memory, visuospatial abilities, and executive functions. A language examination should listen for evidence of aphasia and obtain a written sample from the patient. The written sample can reveal linguistic disturbances, or the graphomotor alterations described for delirium. A simple memory test for these patients is to ask them to remember the examiner's name or three words for 5 minutes, and simple visuospatial screening involves having them copy a simple construction, such as cube. The examiner may screen for executive dysfunction with simple alternating hand movements between one hand fisted and the other open palm down on the table.

The usual mental status scales may differentiate delirium from other cognitive disturbances, and there are a number of targeted delirium scales that can augment the mental status examination (MSX) (see Mariz J, Castanho TC, Teixeira J, Sousa N, Cerreia Santos N. Delirium diagnostic and screening instruments in the emergency department: an up-to-date systematic review. *Geriatrics.* 2006;1(3):22). The Confusion Assessment Method (CAM) is a widely used instrument for screening for and diagnosing delirium, which requires an acute (hours to days) and fluctuating course and difficulty focusing plus either disorganized, irrelevant thinking for an alteration in arousal. There are a number of variants or modifications of the original CAM. The Delirium Rating Scale-Revised-98, a revision of the earlier Delirium Rating Scale, is a 16-item scale with 13 severity items and three diagnostic items that reliably distinguish delirium from dementia, depression, and schizophrenia. Other scales have unique aspects. For example, the Delirium Triage Screen assesses level of consciousness and attention in less than 1 minute; the Richmond Agitation-Sedation Scale has a 10-level scale that assesses level of arousal; and the Neelon and Champagne Confusion Scale combines both behavioral and physiologic signs of delirium. The diagnosis of delirium may be facilitated by the use of these instruments; however, the best assessment remains a careful MSX focusing on abnormal attention and other specific areas disturbed in delirium, as described earlier.

The physical examination may show evidence of systemic or medical illness, meningismus, signs of increased intracranial pressure, or focal neurologic abnormalities. Delirium is associated with three nonspecific movement abnormalities: an action or sustention tremor of high frequency, asterixis, or brief lapses in tonic posture, especially at the wrist; multifocal myoclonus or shock-like jerks; choreiform movements; dysarthria; and gait instability. There may be agitation or psychomotor retardation, apathy, waxy flexibility, catatonia, carphologia ("lint-picking" behavior), and autonomic hyperactivity.

Dementia

Dementia is an age-related disorder that is growing in importance in proportion to the increasing age of our population. Dementia is an acquired impairment in multiple areas of intellectual function not due to delirium and includes a compromise in memory, language, and other cognitive functions. These cognitive impairments are generally severe enough to interfere with quality of life, social adjustment, and elder independence. Alzheimer disease (AD) is the most common cause of dementia. AD affects at least 6% of people over age 65 years and, in some studies, nearly half of those over age 85 years. More than 5.5 million Americans have AD, and the numbers may reach 14 million by the year 2050 in proportion to the aging population. Furthermore, AD costs approximately 90 billion health care dollars per year and is one of the greatest causes for the loss of independence in the elderly.

After memory loss, language impairment is the second most common disability among patients with AD. The pattern of language changes in AD constitutes a specific loss of linguistic competencies involving semantic aspects rather than syntactic or phonologic abilities. The first abnormality is word-finding difficulty with a decreased ability to generate lists of words in a given category. Perception and spatial abilities are additionally impaired early in the usual course of the disease. With disease progression, there is eventual prominent involvement of executive operations and attributes, as well as a more global impairment in all cognitive domains. The application of the National Institute on Aging-Alzheimer Association criteria facilitates making the diagnosis of AD and are summarized in Box 3.2.

BOX 3.2 NATIONAL INSTITUTE ON AGING-ALZHEIMER ASSOCIATION CRITERIA FOR PROBABLE ALZHEIMER DISEASE

Criteria for all-cause dementia: core clinical criteria. Dementia diagnosed when there are cognitive or behavioral (neuropsychiatric) symptoms that:
1. Interfere with the ability to function at work or at usual activities; and
2. represent a decline from previous levels of functioning and performing; and
3. are not explained by delirium or major psychiatric disorder;
4. cognitive impairment is detected and diagnosed through a combination of history-taking and an objective cognitive assessment;
5. the cognitive or behavioral impairment involves a minimum of two domains.

Probable Alzheimer disease dementia: in addition to Dementia criteria, the following are other clinical criteria specifically for Alzheimer's disease:
1. Insidious onset over months to years;
2. clear-cut history of worsening of cognition by report or observation; and
3. the initial and most prominent (predominant) cognitive deficits are:
   A. amnestic presentation.
   B. nonamnestic:
      i. language presentation;
      ii. visuospatial presentation;
      iii. executive dysfunction;
      iv. other (i.e., ideomotor apraxia)
4. Other dementias or neurologic disease has been ruled-out.
5. The term "Major Neurocognitive Disorder," often used in lieu of dementia, is actually broader than the traditional definition of dementia as it requires a substantial decline in only one cognitive domain.

From McKhann GM, Knopman DS, Chertkow H, et al. The diagnosis of dementia due to Alzheimer's disease: recommendation from the National Institute on Aging-Alzheimer's Association workgroups on diagnostic guidelines for Alzheimer's disease. *Alzheimers Dement.* 2011;7(3):263-269.

Characteristics on MSX

AD often begins with a long preclinical period, often 3 to 6 years in duration, during which episodic memory deficits occur without other symptoms of dementia. The first symptom of AD is usually progressive difficulty with "recent" memory or the ability to encode information and store it for later recall. AD patients have decreased delayed recall on word-list learning with a decreased primacy effect. They also have early decreased paired associate and logical paragraph learning. They are unable to use cues or production priming to improve memory and may have an accelerated rate of forgetting. Early on, the retrieval of old remote memories is relatively preserved, but this too becomes compromised as the disease advances, with the development of a temporal gradient of progressively better recall for the most remote information. In addition, there is relative preservation of procedural memory or the learning of motor tasks until the late stages of the illness, and confabulation is usually not present until several years after onset of the illness.

In AD, initial word-finding difficulty progresses to poor naming (anomia) and impaired comprehension. At onset, memory deficits usually overshadow the language problems, but some patients with AD present with early aphasia. Early in the course, there may be an inability to retrieve words with circumlocution and poor word-list generation, particularly for words in a given semantic category. As the disease progresses, difficulty naming becomes apparent and spontaneous speech becomes increasingly empty. Semantic aspects, grammatical complexity, and prepositional content undergo progressive deterioration with relative sparing of basic syntactic and phonologic aspects of language. Verbal paraphasias (whole-word substitutions) occur and become progressively less related to the target word as the disease advances. With further progression, impaired comprehension of speech and writing with relatively spared verbal repetition and reading aloud suggest a transcortical sensory aphasia. At this stage, the listener may be unable to follow a coherent line of thought in the verbal output and this may be complicated by inappropriate intrusions from earlier conversations or testing and by literal paraphasias and neologisms.

Speech, the mechanical aspect of language production, remains normal throughout most of the course of AD. In late phases of the illness, however, reiterative speech disturbances can appear. There may be echolalia, the tendency to repeat the words of others; palilalia, the tendency to repeat their own words; and logoclonia, repetition of the final syllable of a word. Terminally, vocalization is reduced to the production of repetitive sounds unrecognizable as language, or even to complete mutism.

Visuospatial impairment is a third early manifestation of AD. It is evident as an inability of patients to make drawings and other constructions or to orient themselves in their surroundings. Basic visual functions are spared, but there are early decreases in visual attention and visual search, contrast frequency sensitivity, and global pattern recognition. Simple drawing tests reveal an inability to copy elementary figures or three-dimensional representations accurately. Disturbances in clock drawing are particularly sensitive to disruption in AD. Patients with environmental disorientation get lost easily in unfamiliar surroundings, lose their way while driving, and eventually become disoriented in their own homes. Left hemispatial neglect may occur, along with decreased right occipitoparietal metabolism and blood flow. As the disease progresses, patients may develop visual agnosia, or the inability to recognize objects despite adequate visual input. Some patients have specific visual agnosic difficulties, such as prosopagnosia, or the failure to recognize familiar faces. Advanced patients with impaired self-recognition may develop the "mirror sign" in which patients misidentify their own images when they encounter a mirror. In addition, some patients with AD develop complex auditory disorders, sensory aprosodia, or an interhemispheric disconnection syndrome.

Apraxia is rarely an early component of the illness but occurs in 70% to 80% of patients in middle stages of the disease. Apraxia is the inability to perform learned motor acts in the absence of impaired primary motor and sensory function. Several mechanisms for apraxia occur in moderate to severe AD. First, patients manifest ideomotor apraxia with spatial and temporal errors in execution of a motor act or with the use of a body part as a substitute for an object (such as using the index finger to pantomime brushing the teeth). Second, patients have ideational apraxia with difficulty in sequencing events of a complex motor plan, such as filling and lighting a pipe. Third, patients have conceptual apraxia with difficulty choosing the correct motor acts due to content or tool-selection errors. Finally, patients with AD may have dissociation apraxia with disconnection of language from the motor system.

Subtle executive impairments occur early in AD. Frontal-executive disturbances include impairments in insight, planning, goal-oriented behavior, abstractions, judgment, and reasoning. The earliest manifestations are decreased awareness of their deficits and impaired performance on executive tests, such as Trailmaking B. The lack of concern for their deficits may mask and delay their presentation for a dementia evaluation. The initiation of activity decreases, and patients appear less motivated or engaged. Other abilities mediated by the frontal lobes are impaired in AD including working memory, sustained and divided attention, disengagement of attention, set changing, response inhibition, and motor programming.

Personality and social behavior are not markedly changed during the early phases of AD. These preserved behaviors allow patients to continue functioning socially and often lead others to underestimate or excuse the patient's cognitive disabilities. Thus it is not uncommon to discover that individuals with severe memory impairment, empty speech, impaired calculation abilities, and impaired abstraction continue in their employment, and their dementia becomes manifest only when some novel or demanding situation arises.

As the disease progresses, however, a range of behavioral symptoms can emerge. The most common is indifference and apathy, but patients with AD are prone to agitation, anxiety, irritability, aggression, poor impulse control, disinhibition, and wandering. An initial loss of spontaneity may be followed by a prolonged period of restless hyperactivity with purposeless pacing and carphologia (purposeless handling and picking). These behaviors may occur from underlying frustration or may be an early sign of physical discomfort. With progression to the later stages of the illness, disinhibited, agitated, and self-centered behaviors become more apparent. In late stages, about one-quarter of patients with AD manifest significant aggression, most commonly verbal in nature, but hitting, pushing, and shoving also occur. In addition to agitation and aggressive acts, wandering and pacing are significant management problems in these patients. Additional neuropsychiatric symptoms include depression and delusions and hallucinations. Patients with AD also experience disturbances of sleep, appetite, and sexual behavior.

Depression

Severe depression, particularly in the elderly, can be associated with prominent cognitive dysfunction. Even in younger, otherwise cognitively normal individuals, severe depression can result in cognitive dysfunction. About half of elderly individuals who present with both major depression and reversible or irreversible cognitive impairment develop irreversible cognitive deficits within 5 years. Moreover, depressed patients with reversible cognitive deficits have a 4 to 5 times greater risk of developing an irreversible dementia within 3 years, compared with those without cognitive deficits. These findings suggest that severe depression in the elderly may unmask or disclose early, preclinical dementing disorders. Significant depression affects about one-third of patients with dementia.

Patients with depression with cognitive impairment tend to have more intense psychiatric symptoms, cognitive complaints, and "I don't know" answers than patients with depression without dementia (Table 3.1). These patients suffer from more intensive hopelessness, helplessness, guilt, self-deprecatory feelings, and anxiety than cognitively unimpaired elderly patients with depression, and they are more likely to demonstrate delusions. In addition to neurovegetative disturbances, such as loss of appetite and sleep disturbances, patients with depression-associated dementia have prominent cognitive complaints, especially difficulty concentrating and poor recent memory. Patients with depression are often acutely aware of their memory problems, and complaints may be out of proportion to the actual degree of impairment. In addition, patients may give many "I don't know" responses or fail to make or complete a response on mental status testing. These "I don't know" responses may indicate a tendency to report only answers of which they are sure. In sum, distinguishing features of depression versus dementia include evolution over weeks or less and possible precipitant factors, awareness and memory complaints, vegetative signs, normal or inconsistent orientation, normal speech and language, memory improvement on recognition (retrieval deficit), lack of rapid forgetting and intact incidental memory,

TABLE 3.1 Characteristics of Depression-Associated Cognitive Impairment		
History	**Mental Status Changes**	**Neurologic Examination**
Age >60 years	Mini-Mental State Examination >21	No focal deficits
Subacute onset	Hamilton Depression Scale >21	Masked facies
Discrete course	Variably disturbed effortful cognition	Stooped posture
Past history mood disorder	Psychomotor slowed	Slow, hypophonic speech
Family history mood disorder	Attentional deficits; ease of confusion	Bradykinesia
Prominent depressive symptoms	Memory impairments	EEG: first REM rebound
Emphasizes cognitive deficits	Abnormal delayed recall	Normal P300 evoked response
Aware of cognitive deficits	Better recognition (retrieval deficit)	MRI/CT: enlarged lateral ventricles
"I don't know" answers	Poor organization for encoding	MRI: frequent white matter lesions
Antidepressants improve	Retain "primary" effect	PET: prefrontal hypometabolism
	More comparable recent-remote	Abnormal dexamethasone
	Better recall of unpleasant events	Suppression test
	Decreased verbal (letter) fluency	
	Adequate confrontational naming	
	Omit detail on constructions	
	Executive deficits: abstraction, set maintenance, perseveration, flexibility time perception, initiation	
	Verbal and performance IQs are more comparable	

CT, Computed tomography; *EEG*, electroencephalogram; *MRI*, magnetic resonance imaging; *PET*, positron emission tomography; *REM*, rapid eye movement.

absent agnosia or apraxia or marked perception/spatial disturbances (incomplete and careless), and an overall attention and motivation deficit.

Characteristics on MSX

This "depression-associated dementia" is worse for measures that depend on effort, speed, and attention. All cognitive tasks that are effortful are impaired including amount of behavioral initiation and verbal responses and the spontaneous elaboration of information or detail. Some patients have cognitive deficits primarily from failure of effort secondary to their depression. Others have a more profound depression with slowed processing speed, including start phenomena and decision times. This psychomotor retardation may impair performance on timed tests, such as the Digit Symbol Test. Attentional deficits lead to

poor concentration, disorientation, impaired analysis of detail, and increased irrelevant thoughts. Throughout testing, errors of omission are more evident than are errors of commission, and there may be substantial variations in performance from test to test.

Depression can impair performance on memory tests in subjects of all ages, especially in the elderly. Learning new information, recent memory, and free recall suffer the most in depression. There is poor effortful memory that improves with recognition tasks and with repetition priming. On learning curves, patients with depression learn fewer words than nondepressed persons, but they may retain the normal primacy and recency benefits. Memory dysfunction in depression usually improves with recognition tasks and indicate a predominant retrieval deficit. This suggests poor encoding strategies form decreased effort or attention. When retrieving remote memories, patients with depression may have difficulty and may more easily retrieve unpleasant experiences, the so-called negative contents response bias in depression. All these memory deficits are at least partially related to inattention and distractibility, leading to poor organization and encoding of stimulus materials. If patients with depression are provided structure and organization, their memory deficits become less apparent.

There are a number of other cognitive changes associated with depression. Although they do not have cortical-type aphasias, there are impairments in verbal fluency or word-list generation and in syntactic complexity. Naming is impaired but not to the same degree as verbal fluency. On visuospatial tasks, patients with depression omit details on tests of copying and construction. Patients with depression have

multiple deficits in executive functions, such as ability to give abstract interpretation of proverbs, maintain set, manifest cognitive flexibility, perform dual tasks, and perceive time. Furthermore, abnormalities in initiation and perseveration are associated with relapse and recurrence of geriatric depression.

On neurologic examination, there is overt slowing and lack of spontaneity. Facial movement is diminished, and gross motor slowing with increased muscle tension is present. Speech is slowed and hypophonic, and speech pause time (the silent interval between phonations during automatic speech) is elongated.

The differential diagnosis of the three common brain-behavior disorders discussed in this chapter can be difficult. We include a summary of features that are helpful in distinguishing between them (Table 3.2).

TABLE 3.2	**Differential Diagnosis of Delirium, Dementia, and Depression**[a]		
Clinical	**Delirium**	**Dementias**	**Depression**
Course	Acute onset; hours, days, or more	Insidious onset[b]; months or years; progressive	Insidious onset, at least 2 weeks, often months
Attention	Markedly impaired attention and arousal	Normal early; impairment later	Mild impairment
Fluctuation	Prominent in attention arousal; disturbed day-night cycle	Prominent fluctuations absent; lesser disturbances in day-night cycle	Absent
Perception	Misperceptions; hallucinations, usually visual, fleeting; paramnesia	Perceptual abnormalities much less prominent[c]; paramnesia	May have mood-congruent hallucinations
Speech and language	Abnormal clarity, speed, and coherence; disjointed and dysarthric; misnaming; characteristic dysgraphia	Early anomia; empty speech; abnormal comprehension	Decreased amount of speech
Other cognition	Disorientation to time, place; recent memory and visuospatial abnormalities	Disorientation to time, place; multiple other higher cognitive deficits	Mental slowing; indecisiveness; memory retrieval difficulty
Behavior	Lethargy or delirium; nonsystematized delusions; emotional lability	Disinterested; disengaged; disinhibited; delusions and other psychiatric symptoms	Depressed mood; anhedonia; lack of energy; sleep and appetite disturbances
Electroencephalogram	Diffuse slowing; low-voltage fast activity; specific patterns	Normal early; mild slowing later	Normal

[a]The characteristics listed are the relative and usual ones and are not exclusive.
[b]Patients with vascular dementia may have an abrupt decline in cognition.
[c]Patients with dementia with diffuse cortical Lewy bodies often have a fluctuating mental status and hallucinations.
Modified from Mendez MF, Yerstein O. Delirium. In: Daroff RB, Jankovic MD, Mazziotta JC, Pomeroy SL, eds. *Bradley's Neurology in Clinical Practice*. 7th ed. New York, Elsevier;2020:23-33.

Chapter 4

Essential Behavioral Neuroanatomy

The interpretation of the mental status examination depends on an understanding of behavioral neuroanatomy. As in the rest of neurology, the examination leads to localization, followed by a differential diagnosis of disease processes. This chapter gives the essentials necessary for localization of mental status abnormalities in the brain. It includes the different cortical lobes and the limbic structures that line the medial aspect of the cerebral hemispheres and contribute to memory and emotions. It covers the essentials only, as it would require the entire book for a complete and exhaustive review of behavioral neuroanatomy.

This chapter has three parts. The first part discusses general brain-behavior principles. They involve hemispheric specialization and cerebral dominance, disconnection phenomena, and the "anomalous dominance pattern." The second part discusses the regional localization of specific behaviors in the brain. This section assumes a "localizationist" view that testable neurocognitive domains are located in different brain regions or centers. The last part of this chapter challenges this localizationist view and introduces neural networks and circuits. It emphasizes that, although we use a modular centers approach for localization of neurocognitive disorders, the reality is that they arise from changes in complex and distributed, interconnected circuits.

General Brain-Behavior Principles

The brain is composed of two cerebral hemispheres (telencephalon) along with subcortical white matter and basal ganglia, corresponding thalamic and hypothalamic nuclei (diencephalon), the brain stem, and the cerebellum. The six-layered neocortex is a convoluted structure, organized into gyri and sulci, which spans four major lobes: frontal, temporal, parietal, and occipital. The brain contains approximately 86 billion neurons, with 100 trillion synapses, resulting in numerous and complex networks. Histological areas of the brain are composed of "Brodmann areas" (BA) (Fig. 4.1), which aid in localizing brain-behavior functions.

A basic principle of brain organization of importance to the mental status examination is the presence of hemispheric specialization and the related concept of cerebral dominance. The strongest evidence of differences between the two brains comes from the occurrence of distinct disorders from focal lesions in the left and right hemispheres (Table 4.1). Further evidence for hemispheric specialization comes from studies on "split-brain" patients. To prevent seizure generalization, some patients have undergone a surgical transection of the corpus callosum, the main interhemispheric fiber bundle, with resultant inability to transfer information between the two hemispheres. The split hemispheres may manifest different emotional states along with interhemispheric cognitive differences evident on specialized testing of each side separately (Fig. 4.2). With the left hand they may not be able to name (tactile anomia), perform learned motor movements (ideomotor apraxia), or write without linguistic errors (agraphia), whereas with their right hand they may not be able to copy or perform visuospatial tasks (dyscopia, left hemineglect).

Hemispheric specialization implies that there is cerebral dominance for cognitive functions in one hemisphere versus the other. Most of this focuses on language dominance, although the most common overt phenotypic expression is hand preference. The early work of Paul Broca, Karl Wernicke, and others demonstrated language in the left hemisphere localized in two hubs: the Broca area (BA 44, 45) for language production in the left inferior frontal region, and the Wernicke area (BA 22) for

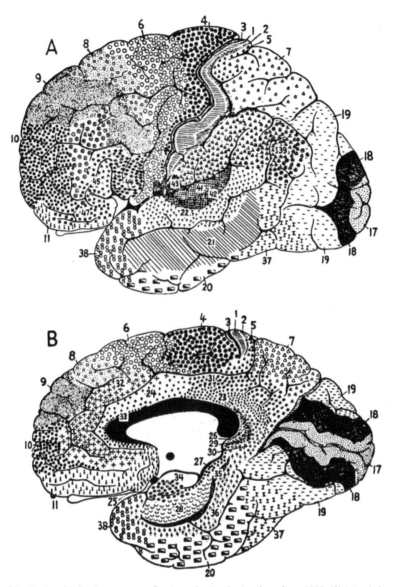

Fig. 4.1 Neuroanatomy of the brain with Brodmann areas: Brodmann's classic drawings from 1909. **(A)** Lateral view. **(B)** Medial view. (Photo number L0061107. Vergleichende Lokalisationslehre der Grosshirnrinde in ihren Prinzipien dargestellt auf Grund des Zellenbaues/[K. Brodmann] Leipzig: Barth, 1909. Wellcome Library, London).

language comprehension in the left superior temporal gyrus. Broca further suggested an association between the dominant hand and the dominant hemisphere for language, and the majority of right-handed persons are left-hemisphere dominant for language. In contrast to the left hemisphere, the right hemisphere has a dominant role for global visuospatial processing.

It may also have a "dominant" role in emotion, for example, determining the emotional prosodic aspects of communication and the emotional state of a speaker from tone of voice (Table 4.1); however, the valence theory of emotion suggests that negative emotional tendencies arise from the right hemisphere and more positive emotional tendencies from the left.

TABLE 4.1 Signature Left and Right Hemisphere Deficits
Left Hemisphere Abnormalities
Aphasias
Alexia and agraphia
Ideomotor apraxia
Acalculia and Gerstmann syndrome
Loss of detail in drawings/constructions
Somatotopagnosia or autotopagnosia
Associative visual agnosia
Color anomia or color agnosia
Right Hemisphere Abnormalities
Visuospatial difficulties
Abnormal visuospatial constructions with decreased overall pattern
Environmental disorientation or topographagnosia
Dressing apraxia
Left hemispatial neglect
Anosognosia
Aprosodia and amusia
Face discrimination difficulties

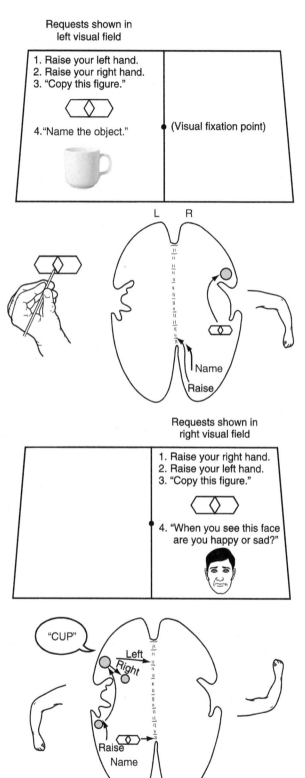

Fig. 4.2 A commissurotomy typically leaves patients with the split-brain syndrome, i.e. disconnected left and right hemisphere (labeled "L" and "R"). Each of their hemispheres can be tested individually by showing commands and figures or objects in the contralateral visual field. Top, written commands (raise left or right hand; copy figure) and request to name a cup are shown in isolated left visual field before the patient can move his/her eyes, hence they are only received by the right hemisphere. Since connections to the ipsilateral motor area are intact, the patient can raise the left hand and use it to copy the figure. However, since the right hemisphere is unable to transmit information through the corpus callosum to the dominant left cerebral hemisphere, which governs language function, they are unable to produce the name for "cup". Bottom, the left hemisphere perceives written commands and figures or objects which are projected to the isolated right visual field before the patient can move his/her eyes, hence they are only received by the left hemisphere. Patients can raise the right hand but has difficulty raising the left hand and processing the visual figure sufficiently to make a good copy. In contrast, because the language areas are usually in the left hemisphere, they are able to say the name of the object. (Modified from Kaufman DM, Geyer HL, Milsten MJ. Aphasia and Anosognosia. In: Kaufman, Myland (Eds) Kaufman's Clinical Neurology for Psychiatrists. 8th Ed. Elsevier; 2016).

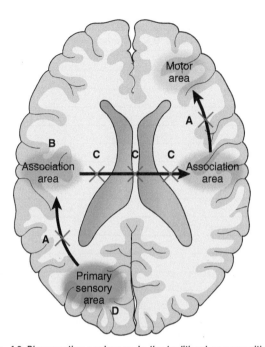

Fig. 4.3 Disconnection syndromes. In the traditional neurocognitive center model, distinct disconnection syndromes occur from disease or lesions that damage their interconnecting pathways. In this illustration, association fibers (A) can be damaged within the hemispheres, disconnecting primary sensory areas (D) form association areas (B) or association areas from motor areas. Disconnection syndromes can also result from disconnection of commissural fibers (C) between the hemispheres, such as part of the corpus callosum.

As seen from hemispheric specialization and split-brain studies, there can be disconnection between hemispheres and between different neurocognitive centers within each hemisphere (Fig. 4.3). Norman Geschwind described how disconnection of cortical centers, such as the Broca area and Wernicke area, could produce language syndromes that were distinct from those due to lesions in the Broca area or Wernicke area. The phenomena of disconnection syndromes led to an entirely different understanding of the origin of mental status deficits or neurocognitive disorders, for example, alexia without agraphia (reading difficulty without writing impairment) from disconnection of visual input to the left hemisphere language areas. The concept of localized disorders from disease in neurocognitive centers or their disconnection has continued to be useful for mental status testing, despite our current understanding that the brain is composed of widely distributed, but interconnected, neural networks, discussed in the final section of this chapter.

One further general principle is that of the "anomalous dominance pattern." As described by Geschwind and others, this term indicates an alternative brain organization among left-handers that challenges the neat description of hemispheric specialization. Most right-handed individuals show anatomic differences between hemispheres, such as a larger left planum temporale (located on the surface of superior temporal gyrus) for Wernicke area, consistent with hemispheric specialization. In contrast, most left-handed individuals, rather than an inverse hemispheric dominance, have an "anomalous" pattern characterized by less hemispheric specialization. This manifests as decreased exclusive or predominant localization of traditional left or right hemisphere functions and a greater likelihood of bilateral representation compared with the majority of right-handers. One of the first things that mental status examiners determine is the patient's handedness, as this is pertinent to the localization value of many lesions.

Brain-Behavior Localization (see Table 4.2)

FRONTAL LOBES

The frontal lobes are much of what defines being human. We have the largest frontal/total brain quotient of the animal kingdom, making up more than one-third of the entire cortex. Lying anterior to the central sulcus, the frontal lobes consist of motor cortex and prefrontal cortex. The motor cortex includes not only primary motor cortex but also the premotor area for initiation and planning movements, the supplementary motor area for complex movements involving sequencing and coordination, and the frontal eye fields for overseeing saccadic eye movements. The much larger, prefrontal cortex is the seat of the highest cognitive functions and the main target of this discussion. The prefrontal cortex consist of at least six major behavioral divisions divided into two major groups: the lateral "executive-cognitive" group for goal-oriented behavior, and the medial "frontolimbic" group for socioemotional behavior.

(Text continues on p. 31)

TABLE 4.2   Brain Localization of Cognitive and Behavioral Disturbances

The following lists are not exhaustive, and localization is approximate for many items. B = bilateral; L = left; R = right.

Frontal Lobes

Abstraction impairment on idioms and proverbs (B, L>R)

Amusia and aprosodia, expressive (R)

Apathy, abulia, and akinetic mutism (B)

Aphasia, non-fluent or Broca (L)

Aphemia or isolated verbal language expression difficulty (L)

Attentional disengagement (R)

Complex problem-solving difficulty (L>R)

Compulsive or repetitive behaviors (B?)

Delusions or impaired reality testing (especially with temporal limbic involvement) (R)

Depression (L)

Design fluency impairment (L)

Disconnection ideomotor apraxia (L)

Disinhibition (B)

Dysexecutive syndrome (B)

Emotional lability (R>L)

Empathy impairment (R>L)

Environmental dependency, echolalia, echopraxia, imitation/utilization behavior (B)

Feedback responsiveness impairment (B)

Frontal lobe personality change (R)

Insight impaired and loss of personal and social awareness (R>L)

Jocular affect, euphoria (B, R>L)

Judgment impairment (B)

Manic-like affect (R)

Motor programming difficulty (B, L>R?)

Perseveration, intrusions, stimulus-bound (B, R>L?)

Phonagnosia, or inability to identify voices (R)

Psychomotor slowed, poor initiation (B)

Response inhibition impairment (B)

Set changing difficulty (L>R)

Social dysregulation (R>L)

Social judgment, tact, and social responsibility impairments (R>L)

Theory of mind impairment (R>L)

Verbal fluency or word-list generation impairment (L)

Working memory impairment (B)

Temporal Lobes (Lateral Neocortical and Mesial Limbic)

Amnesia, particularly declarative, episodic memory loss (B)

Amusia, receptive difficulty in music appreciation (B, R>L)

Aphasia, fluent, Wernicke (L)
Aprosodia, receptive difficulty in the melody and intonation of language (R)
Auditory agnosia (B, R>L)
Auditory perception disturbances (B, R>L)
Biological motion, difficulty in detection (B, R>L)
Conduction aphasia (L)
Contralateral superior quadrantanopia (L or R)
Cortical deafness (B)
Emotional empathy impairment (R)
Emotional learning or conditioning impairment (B)
Emotional reaction impairment (B)
Expert visual system disturbance (B, R>L)
Kluver-Bucy (placid, hypermetamorphosis, hyperoral, hypersexual, visual agnosia) (B)
Landmark agnosia (R)
Prosopagnosia, or impaired recognition of familiar faces (B, R>L)
Pure word deafness (B or L)
Rhythm agnosia (L)
Semantic anomia (L)
Semantic knowledge difficulty (B)
Sense of perceptual familiarity altered (R)
Social concepts impaired (R)
Surface agraphia (L)
Temporal lobe personality changes (B, R or L)
Theory of mind impairment (R>L)
Topographagnosia, or environmental disorientation from landmark agnosia (B, R>L)
Visual hallucinations, formed (R)
Visual word form alexia (L)
Word-selection anomia (L)
Parietal Lobes
Acalculia, or abnormal calculation (L>R)
Agency attribution impairment (R)
Agraphia, or writing disturbance (L)
Akinetopsia, or abnormal movement detection (R)
Alexia, or reading disturbance (L)
Alexithymia, or inability to recognize one's feelings (R)
Anarithmetia, or loss of basic mathematical processes (L)
Anosodiaphoria, or loss of concern for illness (R)
Anosognosia, or loss of awareness or denial of illness (R)
Aphasia, transcortical sensory (L)

(Continued)

TABLE 4.2   Brain Localization of Cognitive and Behavioral Disturbances   *(Cont'd)*
Asomatognosia, or the loss of awareness of parts of one's body (R)
Attentional disengagement and disorientation (B, R>L)
Balint syndrome, or simultanagnosia, optic ataxia, oculomotor apraxia (B)
Body identity disorders or distortions (R)
Constructions with impaired basic form (R)
Constructions with impaired detail (L)
Contralateral inferior quadrantanopia (L and R)
Depersonalization or derealization (R)
Depth perception impairment (global stereopsis, monocular depth cues) (R)
Digit agnosia or difficulty knowing fingers or toes, and right-left confusion (L)
Dressing apraxia (R)
Egocentric spatial disorientation (R)
Environmental disorientation from topographic memory impairment (R)
Facial discrimination impairment (R)
Gerstmann syndrome (acalculia, agraphia, right-left confusion, digit agnosia) (L)
Gestalt grouping perceptual impairment (R)
Ideomotor apraxia (L)
Idiokinetic apraxia (L>R))
Neglect, hemispatial, contralateral sensory or body, or conceptual (R)
Oculomotor apraxia (B, R>L)
Optic ataxia (B, R>LR)
Planotopokinesia, or impaired map reading (R)
Spatial acalculia (R)
Spatial agnosia including visual search difficulty (R)
Visual line orientation impairment (R)
Occipital Lobes
Alexia without agraphia (L)
Apperceptive visual agnosia (B)
Associative visual agnosia (L)
Body form and body action agnosia (B)
Color agnosia, color anomia, and color aphasia (L)
Cortical blindness (B)
Figure-ground disturbance (B, R>L)
Hemiachromatopsia (L or R)
Homonymous hemianopsia (L or R)
Stereopsis disturbances (B)
Visual hallucinations, unformed (B)
Visual illusions (R>L)
Visual synthesis disturbance (B, R>L)

The executive-cognitive prefrontal group enables goal-orientation by allowing deliberation between stimulus and immediate response, thus permitting a weighing of options, choices, and the potential outcomes of responses. The largest executive-cognitive division, the dorsolateral prefrontal cortex, has the greatest role in the strategic planning of goals. It receives input from the mediodorsal thalamic nucleus and interconnects with parietal and temporal association areas. It facilitates goal-orienting behavior through executive operations, such as working memory and complex attention (mental control), task setting and shifting, and task maintenance. These executive operations are evident in alternate or motor programming tasks, and they influence reasoning, decision-making, and judgment abilities. The adjacent executive-cognitive division, the ventrolateral prefrontal cortex, further enables goal-oriented behavior by reconciling stimuli and responses with the stored representations of past similar experiences. This division contains the Broca area on the left, which participates in language production (fluency) and syntax (rules for combining words into clauses or phrases); the corresponding area on the right participates in intonation and prosody.

The "frontolimbic" group is engaged in integrating emotion and social behavior. Disease here can significantly impair social propriety and interactions. This region interconnects with emotionally important areas, such as the insulae, the amygdalae, and other limbic regions. Frontolimbic divisions include the ventromedial, orbitofrontal, and dorsomedial prefrontal cortices, and output occurs through the anterior cingulate cortex. The ventromedial cortex links emotional meaning to scenarios ("affective valuation"), facilitates emotion by reconstituting somatic states when exposed to certain experiences, and contributes to the experience of empathy. On the right side, the ventromedial cortex is particularly involved in valencing social scenarios and experiences, in understanding the feelings of others, in "theory of mind" (appreciating that others have thoughts, feelings, and beliefs), and, generally, as part of the social brain (dedicated social-interpersonal neural systems). The theory of mind circuit also includes the temporal pole, temporoparietal junction, posteromedial (precuneus, posterior cingulate) cortex, and

posterior superior temporal sulcus; the related social brain includes the temporal pole, orbitofrontal cortex, subgenual anterior cingulate cortex, anterior insula, posterior superior temporal sulcus, and temporoparietal junction. The orbitofrontal cortex runs into the ventromedial region and contributes to learning from reward and punishment. The orbitofrontal cortex is additionally involved in controlling or inhibiting rapid, "in-the-moment" responses to stimuli. The dorsomedial prefrontal cortex, which often includes the frontal pole, considers more long-term outcomes and the potential feedback from different courses of action. It is crucial for reflecting on delayed or "what-if" scenarios and for considering the "self" or self-aware perspectives. Finally, it is worth considering the anterior cingulate cortex, a part of the limbic system, and its relationship to frontolimbic areas. The anterior cingulate is a "motor" limbic area that motivates action for choosing the best available response. The dorsal anterior cingulate cortex (more properly the anterior midcingulate cortex) is engaged in set change detection in influencing response choices, whereas the subgenual and pregenual portions are more involved in emotional assessment.

Although useful for brain-behavior localization, the functions of the different divisions of the prefrontal cortex are not entirely distinct or discrete. There is much overlap, and many clinical disturbances, such as environmental dependency (drawn to external stimuli) and abstracting ability, are products of more than one division. They are, nevertheless, a guide to localization in the prefrontal cortex.

TEMPORAL LOBE NEOCORTEX

The temporal neocortex, along the dorsolateral side of the lobe, is associated with auditory processing and language. The primary auditory area is the transverse gyrus of Heschl (BA 41) located on the surface of the superior temporal gyrus. It has a tonotopic map that corresponds to the distribution of frequency-responsive cells in the ear. Auditory input to Heschl gyrus is through the medial geniculate body and output is through ventral and dorsal auditory streams. The ventral stream, which travels anteriorly in the temporal lobe, is a "what" stream or a semantic circuit for sound identification and for speech and word meaning. The dorsal stream, which curves around the posterior end of the Sylvian fissure, is a "where" stream or phonological circuit involved in sound localization and in communication with the Broca area. The comprehension of phonemes or decoding of speech sounds occurs in the Wernicke area (BA 22) located in the left planum temporale. The corresponding region on the right participates in the analysis of tones and music. In addition, the posterior superior temporal sulcus is involved in the detection of biological motion.

The temporal pole (BA 38) integrates information about words, objects, or persons to derive its significance or meaning (semantics). It is a convergence zone that combines sensory or perceived features into multimodal semantic knowledge that transcends any individual feature or modality. The left temporal pole is associated with verbal semantic memory, and the right temporal pole with other perceptual input, particularly if emotionally or socially relevant. The temporal pole is part of the circuitry for theory of mind and the social brain and contributes to social semantic knowledge.

Several other regions of the temporal neocortex are noteworthy for their neurocognitive significance. The temporoparietal junction is involved in body-related processing for self-awareness, and agency (attribution as the source of actions), and distinguishing self from others. As part of the circuitry for theory of mind, the area is critical for perspective-taking. The fusiform face area (BA 37), which is located in the posterior fusiform gyrus of the inferior temporal cortex, processes the configural aspects of faces. This area becomes activated not only when viewing faces but also when viewing familiar classes of visual stimuli that involve "expert" within-class discrimination, for example, cows for dairy farmers, plants for botanists, automobiles for car specialists, and other similar distinctions.

INSULA

The insula, embedded in the Sylvian fissures under the opercular lips of temporal and frontal lobes, receives input from somatosensory cortex and sensory relay nuclei of the thalamus and has strong connections to amygdala. The anterior insula is important for emotional awareness and contributes to emotional empathy or affect sharing. It is particularly involved with monitoring signals generated in the body and in "interoceptive awareness" of internal body states and sensations. The posterior insula is a sensory association area for somatic sensations. It passes on the information to the anterior insula, where the emotion component of experience reaches awareness.

PARIETAL LOBES

Much of the parietal lobe is for tracking the external world from the viewpoint of a body-centered (egocentric) map. The parietal lobe processes somatosensory signals for spatial attention and localization, all in relation to the person's body. The parietal lobe includes superior and inferior parietal lobules separated by the intraparietal sulcus and the precuneus located on the medial side of the lobe.

Superior parietal lobule. The superior parietal lobule disengages and shifts attention to a new target and facilitates visually guided reaching as part of the dorsal attention system. It is essentially the terminus of the dorsal "where" visual stream, and provides information about the location, direction, and velocity of a visual target. Together with the frontal lobes, it programs a plan to intercept a visual target using attentional shifts, saccadic eye movements, and head, arm, or body movements.

In addition, the superior parietal lobule contains maps of the body and its surrounding peripersonal egocentric space. This region has access to a personal somatotopic map in the nearby postcentral gyrus. Lesions in this lobule on the right contribute to disturbances of eye and hand movements to visual stimuli (optic ataxia and oculomotor apraxia) and to body identity disorders or distortions including derealization and depersonalization.

Precuneus. The precuneus is actually the medial aspect of the superior parietal lobule and a major component of the posteromedial cortex (including posterior cingulate cortex) and the default mode network. It is one of the most metabolically active regions of the brain. When people are not engaged in goal-directed tasks, the precuneus is continuously processing information about the surrounding world. It particularly gathers and integrates past information regarding the self and the external spatial world, participating in the retrieval of autobiographical memory. With the posterior cingulate (posteromedial cortex), the precuneus is involved in self-related tasks, conscious self-awareness, and theory of mind interpretations. In addition, the precuneus is engaged in mind-wandering and visuospatial imagery.

Intraparietal sulcus. The intraparietal sulcus works with the superior parietal lobule in visual saccades, reaching, and spatial navigation. The lateral part of the sulcus assess the salience of a visual stimulus then programs covert attentional shifts to the stimulus, followed by visual saccades to look directly on the stimulus. The medial and adjacent intraparietal areas contribute to visually guided reaching movements of the upper limb and incorporates them in a body-centered perspective. The posterior intraparietal sulcus contributes binocular and monocular depth cues. Part of the horizontal segment of the intraparietal sulcus on the left contains a center for the digital processing of quantities and the use of syntactic rules and symbols for calculation. Patients with primary acalculia ("anarithmetia") from lesions in this parietal area usually have "neighborhood" cognitive difficulties in localization on their personal body maps.

Inferior parietal lobule. This critical association area has two parts: the supramarginal gyrus (BA 40), and the angular gyrus (BA 39). Together, they constitute an integration zone for different sensations. The inferior parietal lobule monitors sensory signals representing movements of both the self and others. The supramarginal gyrus on the left specifically encodes learned motor sequences and stores these "praxicons" as spatiotemporal movement formulas associated with the meaning of the actions (action semantics). The praxicons connect to the left frontal motor areas for translation and implementation of these programs. Lesions of the supramarginal gyrus and its connections can result in ideomotor apraxia, or difficulty performing learned motor movements. The angular gyrus on the left integrates information from language areas with visual symbols and motor programs for reading and writing. Lesions in the angular gyrus can disrupt reading, writing, and contribute to Gerstmann syndrome (acalculia, agraphia, digit agnosia, and right-left confusion).

OCCIPITAL LOBES

The occipital lobe processes vision. A lesion of the occipital striate cortex (BA 17) will produce an area of blindness (scotoma) in the contralateral visual field,

and disease involving both left and right visual cortices can result in cortical blindness. Cells of the primary visual cortex respond to visual lines and their orientation, detect edges, and interpret contours and boundaries of visual objects. Two cortical visual streams, the ventral stream and the dorsal stream, arise from the primary visual cortex. The ventral or "what" stream to the temporal lobe represents foveal vision and processes color and object recognition. The ventral stream includes the extrastriate body area, sensitive to human bodies or non-face body parts, and the occipital face area, sensitive to facial features but not to facial identity. It projects to the previously discussed fusiform face area for configural face processing in the temporal fusiform gyrus. In contrast, the dorsal "where" stream represents peripheral vision and processes location, spatial relationships, and visual motion. Lesions involving the dorsal stream can result in neglect of the contralateral visual hemifield. Finally, a part of the dorsal stream participates in the perception of visual motion.

LIMBIC SYSTEM

Broca originally defined the limbic (limbus, or border, of the hemispheres) lobe as the parahippocampal and cingulate cortex, but Papez' original medial limbic circuit included much more. Papez' circuit incorporated the hippocampus, fornix, and mammillary bodies, mammillothalamic tract, anterior thalamic nuclei, cingulate gyrus, entorhinal cortex, and hippocampus. Paul McClean and others expanded the limbic system even further, to include the amygdala, septal nuclei, and portions of hypothalamus, habenula, raphe nuclei, ventral tegmental nucleus, nucleus accumbens, basal nucleus (of Meynert), and posterior orbitofrontal cortex.

Hippocampal formation. The hippocampus and septal nuclei make up a subsystem of the greater limbic system. The hippocampal formation is associated with explicit or declarative memory, either episodic (context, time, and place dependent) or semantic facts, but not implicit memory, such as procedural learning. The hippocampal formation forms a portion of the medial wall of the temporal horn of the lateral ventricle. It consists of the hippocampus proper along with the dentate gyrus and the subiculum. The main input to the hippocampus is through the entorhinal cortex and

TABLE 4.3   Neuroanatomy of Declarative Memory From Hippocampal Formation
Hippocampal Formation
• Associated with storage and encoding of information
• Gives time-spatial context
• Involved in associative learning
• Dentate gyrus, discriminates between very similar contexts (projects to CA3)
• CA3 (cornu ammonis 3), completes memory from partial or incomplete patterns
• CA3, tags and temporarily stores information
• CA3, consolidates memory via continued autoassociation
• CA1 (cornu ammonis 1), compares match between CA3 and entorhinal inputs
• CA1, engaged in novelty detection (to subiculum)
• CA1, vivid autobiographical memory
Entorhinal cortex (BA 28) (entry to hippocampus, especially via dentate gyrus)
• Convergence of all sensory regions prior to hippocampus
• Associated with retrieval of stored information
• Integrative role in consolidation and retrograde amnesia
• Contains grid spatial neurons that provide a spatial coordination system
Parahippocampal Cortex (~BA 34+)
• Supports egocentric scene perception
• General associative and contextual knowledge, spatial and nonspatial
• Parahippocampal place area and landmark identification
• Involved in novel activity along with hippocampus
Perirhinal Cortex (BA 35, 36) (also frontal)
• Relative memory familiarity (lesions affect recognition)
• Early pattern completion, distinguishes known from unknown
• Preliminary filter to hippocampus; selects information to pass on to entorhinal cortex
• Recency memory effect and facilitates fast autoretrieval

the dentate gyrus, but it also receives input from the hypothalamus, the septal nuclei, and the amygdala. The cortex transitions from six layers to three as the entorhinal area enters the hippocampal formation. Output is largely through the subiculum to the fornix, which connects with the septal complex and the mammillary bodies-anterior thalamic nucleus-cingulate gyrus. The hippocampus proper has three fields, CA1, CA2, and CA3, which have distinct roles in the memory process before long-term storage in neocortical areas (Table 4.3). The overlying parahippocampal cortex functions in support of scene perception and contains the parahippocampal place area, which responds to contextual objects and landmarks. The adjoining perirhinal cortex additionally responds with memory familiarity. Finally, the nuclei that make up the septal complex (lateral, medial, nucleus accumbens) are situated below the corpus callosum and just in front of the anterior commissure. The nucleus accumbens in particular is a major reward center of the brain.

Amygdala. The amygdala is a nuclear complex located inside the temporal lobe. The basolateral nuclei of the amygdala receive sensory input, which is primarily projected to the centromedial nucleus, which, in turn, project to other behaviorally relevant areas of the brain. The amygdala attaches an affective or emotional dimension to sensory input and initiates autonomic and endocrine responses through connections with the hypothalamus and brainstem. The prefrontal cortex is of particular importance in the appreciation of emotions generated in the amygdala. The amygdala also informs the hippocampus of the emotional significance of the signals. There is emotional conditioning such that the next time a person experiences the same pattern, the learned emotional response is more quickly elicited.

Cingulate cortex. The cingulate cortex lies deep within the longitudinal cerebral fissure and sits over the corpus callosum, along with its output tract, the cingulum. The anterior cingulate gyrus includes pregenual and subgenual sections; the midcingulate includes anterior and posterior sections; and the posterior cingulate includes the posterior cingulate gyrus and retrosplenial cingulate cortex. The subgenual anterior cingulate cortex, which lies inferior to the genu (knee) of the corpus callosum, determines the autonomic expressions of emotion, whereas the pregenual section participates in the storage and retrieval of emotional memories. The anterior midcingulate is involved in error detection and conflict monitoring, signaling the most preferred option. It also participates in cognitive aspects of empathy. The posterior cingulate sections receive input from the posterior parietal cortex and from the hippocampal formation and are involved in visuospatial orientation and in retrieval of autobiographical memories.

SUBCORTICAL STRUCTURES

A number of subcortical structures are important considerations in mental status assessment. The thalamus is primarily a sensory relay center with access to the cortex; however, thalamic lesions can result in anomia and aphasia from left thalamic lesions, and hemispatial neglect from right thalamic lesions. Disorders of the cerebellum include cerebellar cognitive-affective syndrome with disturbances in executive function, language, visuospatial processing, and personality due to damage to lobules VI-IX and their connections to prefrontal cortex. Brain stem disorders can affect arousal and sleep. The upper brain stem contains the ascending reticular activating system, which functions for arousal and activation of the cerebral cortex. Attention depends on the brain stem as well, particularly for the mechanism for actual movement of attention. Disorders of sleep and breakthrough hallucinations can result from problems in the brain stem, especially the serotonergic dorsal raphe nucleus but also the norepinephrine-producing locus coeruleus. Finally, the habenula is a central node in the antireward network as it tonically inhibits dopamine neurons in the substantia nigra, ventral tegmental area, and the nucleus accumbens (reward).

Basal ganglia. There are two divisions of the basal ganglia. The dorsal division is primarily motor and cognitive, and the ventral division, which is associated with paralimbic cortical areas, is involved in emotional operations. The dorsal division (globus pallidus, caudate nuclei, putamen) includes frontal-subcortical tracts and direct and indirect pathways whose imbalance can lead to compulsive or repetitive behavior. Psychomotor speed is a function of the dorsal basal ganglia, the substantia nigra, and their white matter connections from frontal lobe regions. The ventral division (ventral or limbic striatum) includes structures of the basal forebrain, such as the ventral pallidum, olfactory tubercle, bed nucleus of stria terminalis, and nucleus basalis of Meynert. It includes central parts of the reward system, such as the nucleus accumbens and the dopaminergic structures of the midbrain (substantia nigra and ventral tegmental area). There is a motivation-action-reward loop that involves the ventral division and the prefrontal cortex. Finally, the claustrum, a thin structure between the insula and putamen, is a poorly understood basal ganglia postulated to have a role in consciousness.

Hypothalamus. The hypothalamus is the region of the brain that is most important for psychophysiological behaviors such as feeding, drinking, sex, and aggression. It is the primary center for the control of endocrine and autonomic function. The preoptic area (medial and lateral preoptic nucleus) makes up the anterior portion of the hypothalamus. In addition to a lateral zone, a medial zone contains the majority of the hypothalamic nuclei, and a thin periventricular zone abuts the third ventricle. "Releasing hormones" from the hypothalamus indirectly control the anterior pituitary. In contrast, the posterior pituitary receives direct innervation from hypothalamic neurons that release the neurotransmitters vasopressin and oxytocin. Oxytocin functions for uterine contraction and milk production in women and results in an increase in nonsexual social interaction.

Different regions of the hypothalamus control sexual behavior, eating and dietary behavior, and aggression. Neurons in the preoptic area and nearby anterior hypothalamus contains testosterone, estrogen, and prolactin receptors. Stimulation of these areas initiates sexual behavior, especially in response to visual input, whereas lesions of the preoptic area reduce copulatory behavior. In male monkeys, activity in the medial preoptic area increases during sexual arousal but decreases during the sexual act, possibly from inhibition from other areas of the brain. Temporal-amygdalar damage, for example, can lead to a release of sexual arousal from the preoptic area. The ventromedial nucleus is a "satiety center," which regulates food consummation through receptors responsive to leptin, the satiety hormone generated by adipose tissue. Lesions here can cause hyperphagia (excessive eating) and obesity. The ventromedial nucleus interconnects with a "hunger center" in the lateral hypothalamic zone. Similar to the release of sexual arousal, changes in eating behavior may be more commonly associated with right frontal and temporal lobe damage rather than with hypothalamic lesions. Finally, the medial hypothalamus and periaqueductal gray of the midbrain (connected to amygdala and prefrontal cortex) control the expression of aggression. Stimulation of the dorsomedial nucleus in animals produces aggressive behavior, and exposure to threat activates the ventromedial nucleus in support of aggressive behavior.

Neural Networks and Circuits

In the last few decades, many imaging techniques have expanded our understanding of behavioral localization in the brain and moved us beyond the lesion model of cognitive centers and their disconnection. The brain has interconnected and distributed networks or circuits that mediate brain-behavior functions. Cognitive tasks occur, not in individual brain centers working in isolation, but in networks consisting of several discrete functionally interconnected brain regions.

The realization of distributed neural networks has challenged the basic assumptions of the classical lesion model that we use in mental status assessment. For example, today we know that it takes more than the Broca area or Wernicke area for Broca aphasia or Wernicke aphasia, respectively. To have a complete Broca aphasia syndrome, there must be damage extending beyond the traditional Broca area (BA 44, 45) to involve its underlying white matter tracts and the adjacent anterior insula. Likewise, isolated destruction of the Wernicke area (BA 22) does not necessarily result in decreased auditory comprehension, which may require damage extending to involve the underlying white matter and adjacent areas, such as the inferior parietal region.

Understanding of structural and functional tracts in the brain is essential for brain-behavior localization. Diffusion tensor imaging has been valuable in clarifying the clinical importance of large white matter tracts in addition to the corpus callosum. Clinicians can consider lesions involving association tracts (intrahemispheric) such as arcuate fasciculus, superior and inferior fronto-occipital fasciculi, superior and inferior longitudinal fasciculi, uncinate fasciculus, and cingulum. For example, lesions of the uncinate fasciculus impair memory-guided decision-making and severing of the anterior cingulum is a psychosurgical treatment for intractable depression or obsessive-compulsive disorder. Resting-state functional magnetic resonance imaging has also disclosed large-scale, statistically interconnected brain networks. Clinicians can consider lesions involving the default mode, salience, fronto-parietal central executive (control), dorsal and ventral attention, lateral visual, and other networks (Fig. 4.4). For example, disturbance of the internally oriented default mode network characterizes Alzheimer disease, whereas disturbance of the externally oriented salience network characterizes behavioral variant frontotemporal dementia.

A further consideration is the use of neurocomputational algorithms to form a comprehensive map, or connectome, of brain-behavior disorders. These techniques depend on the assumption of simultaneous activation at multiple levels with consequent top-down, as well as bottom-up, effects. To generate a connectome of the connectivity architecture of the brain, one first defines computational nodes and then measures the structural or functional connectivity between them. These interconnected nodes undergo nearly simultaneous iterative computation of the "best fit" neuronal effects. This permits a topology with graph theory yielding short average path-length between nodes, highly connected hub regions, and strongly interconnected hub regions, or rich club networks. The resultant connectome can reveal maladaptive circuits, the presence of distant hypofunction, or signs of transneuronal degeneration. Ultimately, "localization" of brain-behavior disorders and the interpretation of the mental status examination may depend on understanding how they affect underlying networks.

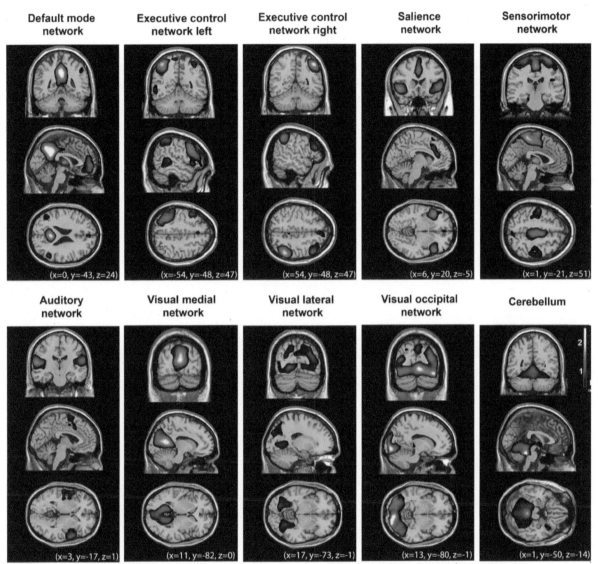

Figure 1. Cerebral networks identified with fMRI. Resting State Networks and Consciousness (2012)
Lizette Heine, Andrea Soddu, Francisco Gómez, Audrey Vanhaudenhuyse, Luaba Tshibanda, Marie Thonnard,
Vanessa Charland-Verville, Murielle Kirsch, Steven Laureys, and Athena Demertzi doi:10.3389/fpsyg.2012.00295

Fig. 4.4 Illustration of resting state functional neural networks. Cerebral networks identified with functional magnetic resonance imaging. Resting state networks and consciousness. (From Heine L, Soddu A, Gómez F, et al. Resting state networks and consciousness. Alterations of multiple resting state network connectivity in physiological, pharmacological, and pathological consciousness states. *Front Psychol.* 2012;3:295.)

Conclusions

Behavioral neuroanatomy requires an understanding of variations in hemispheric specialization, in cognitive centers and their disconnection, and on recent developments in neural networks and circuits. This understanding is still based on knowledge of where cognitive functions tend to be localized in the cortical lobes, limbic system, and subcortical structures of the brain. Subsequent chapters expand on this localization when discussing aspects of the Neurobehavioral Status Examination.

MENTAL STATUS TESTING

Chapter 5

Overview of the Mental Status Examination

The mental status examination (MSX) employs a cognitive domain approach, examining fundamental aspects, such as arousal and attention, and instrumental aspects, such as language, memory, perception, and executive abilities. The mental status examiner often starts with a more limited screening procedure, either a brief MSX, mental status scales, or a targeted MSX, which can be composed of isolated parts of the neurobehavioral status examination (NBSE). Here we will expand on the brief MSX and outline the major elements of the NBSE.

Brief MSX

For most clinical encounters, either in-person or by telemedicine, the clinician may quickly probe wide areas of the patient's cognition with a brief MSX. This has the advantage of being able to assess critical cognitive domains in 5 minutes or less; clinicians can quickly examine one or two representative tasks in awareness, orientation, attention, language, memory, and perception (Table 5.1). The subsequent NBSE sections discuss these cognitive domains in greater detail.

Step 1: Awareness. The brief MSX starts with deliberate observation of the patient's general behavior with the most prominent focus on determining their state of alertness and wakefulness. Although most patients requiring mental status testing are sufficiently aware and awake, occasionally there is evidence of disturbances of arousal, such as lethargy, drowsiness, sleepiness, stupor, and coma. In situations in which the patient lacks significant awareness, the examiner can check for arousal with verbal stimulation (loudly calling their name) or applying mild physical discomfort (sternal pressure, pinching the Achilles tendon).

TABLE 5.1 Steps in a Brief Mental Status Examination	
Awareness	Observation for awareness; if necessary, loudly call name, sternal pressure, pinch Achilles tendon.
Orientation	What is the date (day, month, year, day of week, time)? Where are we; the name of this place, city, state, floor/location?
Attention	Digit span forward (until misses two trials at a level); If necessary, subtraction by 7s from 100 (or by 3s from 20).
Language	Naming of six common items in the room or pictures/drawings; if necessary, ask for as many names of animals in a 1 minute.
Memory	Give three to four unrelated words for subsequent recall in 1 or more minutes; (during delay period, can ask for three recent or current events).
Perception	Copy a three-dimensional "Necker" cube; if necessary, add two-dimensional drawing (e.g., intersecting pentagons).

Step 2: Orientation. The examiner asks the patient to state the current date and place. Orientation in the clinical setting is a sensitive general measure of awareness, attention, and memory. In the absence of a watch or other obvious display of the time, the patient's knowledge of the exact time of day can be a further extension of the assessment for temporal orientation. For place, asking about their floor or location in the building is of additional value.

Step 3: Attention. Proficiency in attention is a prerequisite for adequate performance in instrumental abilities, such as memory and perception. The examiner most commonly screens the patient's ability to

To the patient: "I am going to read some lists of numbers to you.
After I have finished each list, please repeat them for me in the same order I read them."
Read numbers at the rate of one per second.

Correct	Incorrect	
☐	☐	3 – 7 – 2
☐	☐	4 – 9 – 5
☐	☐	5 – 1 – 4 – 9
☐	☐	9 – 2 – 7 – 4
☐	☐	8 – 3 – 5 – 2 – 9
☐	☐	6 – 1 – 7 – 3 – 8
☐	☐	2 – 8 – 5 – 1 – 6 – 4
☐	☐	9 – 1 – 7 – 5 – 8 – 2
☐	☐	4 – 6 – 1 – 5 – 8 – 2 – 7
☐	☐	2 – 8 – 5 – 7 – 1 – 9 – 4

Longest number of digits: _____

Fig. 5.1 Digit Span test.

maintain attention with a digit span. Random digits are given, one per second, starting with three (Fig. 5.1). The patient is asked to recite them back in the same order. Two trials are given at each ascending level until the patient misses both trials. His/her digit span is the level just before missing both trials. If necessary, the examiner can do other serial recitation tasks that include subtracting from 100 by 7s (or the easier version of subtracting from 20 by 3s).

Step 4: Language. Most MSX depends on understanding verbal commands and the ability to give verbal responses. Abnormal language function (aphasia) can therefore compromise subsequent aspects of the MSE. Two subtests—naming ability and word-list generation (verbal fluency)—are particularly sensitive to language disturbances and act as good screening tests. First, ask the patient to name six common items pointed out in the room or as pictures/drawing. If more language information is desired, have the patient generate the names of as many animals as he or she can in 1 minute, with the expectation of generating at least 12.

Step 5: Memory. The examiner can screen declarative episodic memory through the patient's ability to recall a list of words. One easy test in the clinical setting is with a three to four word-learning task with a 1

or more minute delay before asking for their recall. To avoid continued rehearsal, the patient must do other cognitive tasks during this recall or "interference" period, such as recalling three current events in the news and performing the perception task from Step 8. One can also save the orientation questions for this interference period.

Step 6: Perception. Visuospatial skills depend on a number of areas of the brain, which can harbor perceptual deficits without demonstrable abnormality on other MSX tests. The ability to copy a three-dimensional cube drawing is a common visuospatial perceptual screening test (Fig. 5.2). Abnormalities can involve its three-dimensional perspective, the presence of parallel faces, the number of surfaces, and the placement of internal lines. The examiner can add two-dimensional drawings if the patient is quite impaired (e.g., copying intersecting pentagons).

Although a detailed evaluation is not necessary in all patients, a more extensive assessment is indicated if the brief MSX discloses problems or if the patient complains of ongoing cognitive difficulty. In this situation, the clinician may choose additional mental status tasks from the NBSE that offer information of value for a particular patient's deficits. Although this can also be performed through formal psychometric examinations,

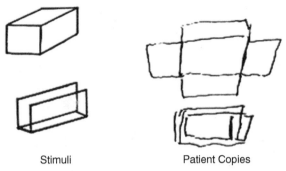

Stimuli   Patient Copies

Fig. 5.2 Examples of copies of three-dimensional drawings. (Modified from Mendez MF, Cummings JL. *Dementia: A Clinical Approach.* 3rd ed. Philadelphia, PA: Butterworth-Heinemann (Elsevier); 2003.)

the clinician can obtain excellent information from the NBSE, and in many instances, this provides information unavailable from any laboratory study.

Overview of the NBSE

The following is an outline of the NBSE, which can take a few minutes to several hours to complete, depending on how much of it is done. It is organized into 14 "domains" (Table 5.2), which are much expanded with many more tests or tasks elaborated on in Chapters 6–14. This is not the only possible organization of the NBSE, but it is one method that has proven practical in terms of the hierarchical order of testing and the ability to localize dysfunction in the brain. The examiner can use elements of the NBSE for targeted MSX or can modify them for patients with visual or auditory impairment. The examiner needs to consider the patient's education, intellectual background, and facility with English before. Finally, the examiner must perform the NBSE as part of the overall neurological examination.

TABLE 5.2 Neurobehavioral Status Examination Domains	
FUNDAMENTAL aspects of the mental status examination	
General behavioral observations	Awareness, appearance, attitude, affect
Arousal	Response to verbal and physical stimulation
Orientation	Orientation to time and place
Psychomotor speed and activity	Spontaneity, speed, and latency of verbal and motor movements and responses
Attention and mental control	Digit span backward and forward, serial 7s or 3s, other serial reversal tasks and continuous performance tasks
INSTRUMENTAL aspects of the mental status examination	
Spoken language and speech	Fluency (spontaneous and work lists), comprehension, repetition, naming
Written language and reading	Reading paragraph and regular, irregular, and nonsense words; writing to dictation and spontaneously
Memory and semantic knowledge	Word-list recall/recognition; retrieval of historical information; identifying misnamed words
Constructional, perceptual, spatial	Two- and three-dimensional copies; hemispatial neglect tasks; clock task
Praxis and other motor movements	Limb ideomotor pantomime, imitation, gesture recognition; ideokinetic fine motor tasks
Calculations and related functions	Simple mathematics, right-left orientation, digit recognition
Executive operations	Verbal and nonverbal fluency, alternate tapping set-shifting, motor programming/Luria hand sequences; Go-No-Go response inhibition
Executive attributes	Insight for illness and circumstances; abstraction of similarities, idioms, or proverbs
Neurological behavioral examination	Motivation and emotion, social behavior, psychophysiological behaviors, content (speech and language, thought, behavior), altered perceptions

1. **General Behavioral Observations.** The experienced examiner begins with a thoughtful inspection of the patient's overt behavior and interactions with others and the environment. The patient's general behavior may be the only method of assessment available in a very uncooperative, agitated, or arousal-impaired patient. Yet, careful behavioral observations in and of themselves can provide a very informative mental status assessment.

   If the patient is sufficiently awake and aware, further consideration of his/her general behavior includes attention to the patient's appearance, attitude, and affect. For example, a slovenly appearance with poor personal hygiene can reflect dementia, psychosis, depression, apathy, and other behavioral disturbances. Specific findings such as neglect of one side of the body can indicate a focal hemispheric insult. Patients may be cooperative, indifferent, disinterested in the interview, or hostile. The examiner also considers their prevailing affect, whether it reflects anger, depression, fear, or other emotion. The examination of a violent or agitated patient requires unique considerations. Always use a calm, nonthreatening tone of voice, and never examine a violent patient alone, keeping an open, unimpeded exit quickly accessible to you. Additional aspects of behavioral observations are discussed in Chapter 6.

2. **Arousal.** An adequate state of arousal is a prerequisite to other cognitive functions. Arousal is the state of awareness or responsiveness to environmental stimuli. A disturbance of arousal is usually evident on initial patient presentation. States of arousal include alertness, wakefulness, lethargy, clouding of consciousness, sleep, obtundation, stupor, and coma. Disorders of arousal arise from brain stem lesions, bihemispheric metabolic or structural disturbances, or disorders causing increased intracranial pressure.

   If a disturbance of arousal is suspected, the examiner evaluates the patient's response to verbal and, if necessary, physical stimulation. Patients with abnormal arousal may need vigorous stimulation to maintain a conversation, or even keep their eyes open. Record the nature of the stimulus necessary to evoke a response and the character of that response. Thus if the patient awakens to loudly calling his or her name but eventually drifts off, necessitating restimulation, this pattern should be recorded. If firm rubbing of the sternum or a pinch of the Achilles tendon is needed to evoke a response, both the stimulus and the degree of response should be recorded. The examination also assesses whether the patient waxes and wanes, has spontaneous movements, maintains eyes open, or visually tracks environmental stimuli.

3. **Orientation.** Further assessment of the "sensorium" includes a determination of orientation to time and place. In some patients, deficits in arousal may preclude the opportunity to pursue the MSX much further, but the examiner should still attempt to assess orientation as much as possible. The least common disorientation occurs to person, that is, the loss of personal identity, and usually indicates a psychiatric as opposed to a neurological disorder. The most common disorientation occurs to time, that is, day of the week, date, month, year, season, and time. Patients who are off 3 days on the date, 2 days on the day of the week, or 4 hours on the time of day may be significantly disoriented to time.

   The next most common disorientation occurs to place, that is, clinic or hospital, city, county, state, and specific floor or localization in a building. In addition to inquiring whether the patient knows where they are, the examiner can ask what kind of a place it is and under what circumstances they are there. The assessment of orientation can extend all the way to an evaluation of their understanding of their medical situation.

4. **Psychomotor Speed and Activity.** Psychomotor speed is often difficult to assess beyond observation of cognitive or motor activity. Decreased speed, activity, and movements can reflect psychomotor speed or a neurological or psychiatric disorder, for example, bradykinesia, decreased facial expressiveness, or overall paucity of movement. Conversely, there may be signs of increased speed or activity, such as fidgetiness and inability to sit still, hand wringing

stereotypical movements or mannerisms, and tremors or other movement disorders. Causes of decreased psychomotor speed and activity include delirium, dementia, depression, parkinsonism, frontal lobe disease, or catatonia. Causes of increased psychomotor speed and activity include delirium, agitation, anxiety, mania, psychosis, delirium, or akathisia.

The examiner should consciously note spontaneity in movements, the overall speed of movements, and the latency in initiating responses. Individual differences in psychomotor speed may occur from the patient's personality and regional or cultural background, and large variations in psychomotor speed occur from state conditions such as fatigue, anxiety, or sleep disturbance. Nevertheless, interpretation of psychomotor speed can be based on intraindividual differences, as informed by history or by comparison to prior examinations. It is sometimes useful to record the speed of counting (e.g., count as fast as you can for 10 seconds) or speed of reciting the alphabet.

5. **Attention and Mental Control.** Attention is the ability to concentrate awareness or to focus mental activity on one thing to the exclusion of others. Elements of attention include selectivity and the ability to sustain, divide, and shift attention. In addition to difficulty concentrating, patients with abnormal attention may have impersistence, distractibility, and increased vulnerability to interference. Attention requires the ascending reticular activating system in the upper brain stem, the reticular nucleus of the thalamus for modulating sensory input, prefrontal cortex for complex attention, and parietal cortex for shifting attention. Abnormal attention is the hallmark of delirium, the most common cause of behavioral disturbance among hospitalized elderly patients.

The most common clinical tests of attention are serial recitation tasks, and the most common serial recitation task is the Digit Span test (Fig. 5.1). The examiner speaks a series of digits, one per second and in a clear voice, and asks the patient to repeat the sequence. If the patient can correctly repeat three digits, the examiner presents four digits, and then five digits, until the patient incorrectly repeats a string of digits twice at the same level. A normal performance is a forward digit span of 7 ± 2, regardless of age. This task may also be performed as a nonverbal sequence span test. The examiner asks the patient to serially tap four blocks (or objects, spots, or squares) in the same sequence as presented by the examiner. The test can be done with or without verbal counting. In the reverse digit span, the patient repeats digits in reverse order, beginning with the last number. The elderly have a modest decline in the reverse digit span but can normally reverse a string of three or more digits. A more difficult serial recitation is the Serial 7s Test. The examiner asks the patient to subtract by 7s beginning with the number 100, for example, 93, 86, 79, 72, 65, et cetera. Mathematical competence is required for this task. If serial 7s is too difficult, the examiner may do the serial 3s test, that is, subtract by 3s beginning with the number 20. Other common serial reversal tasks include spelling "world" backward, reciting the months of the year in reverse order beginning with December, or reciting the days of the week backward. A different set of "attention" tasks require continuous performance or alternating sequences and are described in Chapter 7.

6. **Spoken Language.** Language is the brain's use of symbols for communication. Language is distinct from speech, which is the verbal expression of language. The spoken language examination evaluates verbal fluency, auditory comprehension, repetition, and naming. In addition, prosody, or the inflection and melodic quality of speech, is an ancillary part of the spoken language examination. The different language disorders or aphasias have different patterns of impaired language skills. In right-handed individuals, aphasias result from focal lesions in the left-hemisphere, perisylvian language zones, whereas disturbances of prosody usually occur from right-hemispheric abnormalities. Aphasia also develops as part of the cognitive deficits of Alzheimer disease or other dementias. Speech disorders, as distinct from the aphasias, are limited to the verbal expression of language, and include the dysarthrias, stuttering

and stammering, and logoclonia (repetition of the last syllables).

The language examination evaluates fluency (spontaneous and word-list generation), comprehension, repetition, and naming in a systematic fashion. The fluency examination starts with engaging the patient in conversation and listening to the patient's spontaneous discourse. Some elements of fluency are quantity (in U.S. English normal is approximately 100 ± 50 words/minute), flow (uninterrupted without word-finding pauses, hesitancy, or effort), phrase length (four or more words/phrase), absent agrammatism or telegraphic output (loss of prepositions, conjunctions, and other "functor" words), and normal prosody. During the course of conversational speech, also listen for the information content, for the presence of paraphasic errors (word or phonemic substitutions), and for dysarthric speech. These aspects of conversational discourse can distinguish between fluent and nonfluent aphasias (Table 5.3). For word fluency, also ask the patient to generate a list of as many animals as possible (or other category of items) in 1 minute. Normal subjects can list 18 ± 6 animals/minute without cueing. The patient may also generate as many words as possible that begin with the letters "F," "A," or "S" (the Controlled Oral Word Association Test in English).

Normal subjects can list $15 + 5$ words/minute for each letter. Tests of auditory comprehension include responses to simple commands, for example, "close your eyes" or "touch your nose," followed by multiple step commands, for example, "point to the floor and then point to the window." The examiner can also ask yes-or-no questions, for example, "Are you sitting down?" "Is a hammer good for cutting wood?" "Does March come before April?" "If the lion was killed by the tiger, which animal is dead?" Tests of repetition involves asking the patient to repeat "No ifs ands or buts," "The quick brown fox jumped over the lazy dog," and other sentences. Finally, tests of naming involve asking the patient to name at least six items, pictures, or drawings of common objects; for example, watch, ring, button, collar, nose, chin; plus six lower-frequency items, for example, eyelashes, eyebrows, lapel, shoe laces, sole or heel of shoe, watch band, or crystal.

7. **Written Language and Reading.** The language examination is not complete without an assessment of reading comprehension and writing. These aspects of language are important enough to deserve their own "domain" and emphasis on the MSX. The examiner may be able to localize brain disorders of reading (alexias) and of writing (agraphias) to specific areas of the brain. Examples of reading and writing syndromes are the central and peripheral alexias and disturbances of the direct (reading-by-sight) and indirect (reading-by-sound) reading pathways resulting in syndromes such as alexia with agraphia, alexia without agraphia, surface dyslexia, deep dyslexia, and others. There are comparable agraphia syndromes, as well as graphomotor disturbances (see Chapter 8).

The examiner asks the patient to read aloud and to perform various written commands comparable to the verbal commands. Reading tasks should include a paragraph for reading comprehension and a list of regular words (with expected symbol-to-sound pronunciation), irregular words, and nonsense words that can follow symbol-to-sound

TABLE 5.3 **Conversational Discourse in Fluent vs. Nonfluent Aphasias**		
	Fluent Aphasia	**Nonfluent Aphasia**
Quantity	>100 words/minute	<50 words/minute
Flow	Uninterrupted	Interrupted, hesitant, effortful
Phrase length	5.8 words/phrase	1.2 words/phrase
Agrammatism	Absent	Present, "telegraphic"
Prosody	Normal	Dysprosody
Content	Empty	High-content words
Paraphasic errors	Word, phonemic substitutions	Often absent
Speech	Normal	May sound dysarthric

rules. The examiner evaluates for errors in reading-by-sight ("regularization" or reading irregular words by sound) and in reading-by-sound ("lexicalization" or reading nonsense words as if they were real words). The examiner further requests the patient to write one sentence to dictation, complete with punctuation, and another sentence of their own composition. Errors in writing extend from the purely lexical to difficulties with graphomotor expression (see Chapter 8).

8. **Memory and Semantic Knowledge.** Memory has multiple dimensions. These include short-term memory (immediate recall), working memory (manipulation of short-term memory), recent memory (new learning), and remote memory (retrieval of old information). Short-term memory, which patients, families, and clinicians often mistake for recent memory, overlaps with complex attention and mental control and is tested with Digit Span and related tests. In dementia and memory disorders, clinician are most concerned with disturbances in recent memory (classical "amnesia") and in the retrieval of remote information. This amnesia is usually antegrade or on-going, and episodic (with temporal and spatial tags) rather than semantic (knowledge of facts). Classical amnesia implies injury to the limbic system, either both hippocampi in the temporal lobes or the midline limbic structures. Verbal amnesia may be more impaired with injury in left hemispheric limbic structures, and visual memory with lesions in right hemispheric limbic structures. Amnesia results from Alzheimer disease, head trauma, strokes and other lesions involving limbic structures, Korsakoff syndrome, epilepsy, and anoxic injury to the hippocampi. Semantic knowledge, particularly for naming, is specifically impaired in semantic dementia.

A common way to assess recent memory is a word-list learning task (Table 5.4). For the screening examination, a list of 3 or 4 words may suffice; however, for the more extended examination, a list of 8 or 10 words with multiple initial repetitions is preferable. The examiner reads the word list and asks the patient to immediately recall as many words as possible from the list. The examiner repeats this process four or five times. After an interference interval, which can range from 10 to 30 minutes, during which time the patient's attention is engaged in other tasks, the examiner tests the patient's spontaneous recall of the 8 or 10 words. Normal individuals learn most of the list after three or four repetitions and spontaneously recall two-thirds or more of the words on delayed recall. The examiner then checks recognition memory and retrieval by giving categorical and/

TABLE 5.4 **Examples of Word-List Learning Memory Test**						
Immediate Repetitions				**10-30-Minute Delayed Recall**	**Recognition**	
					Category Cue	**Multiple Choice**
	Trial 1	Trial 2	Trial 3	Trial 4		
Cabbage						
Table						
Dog						
Chevrolet						
Baseball						
Rose						
Belt						
Blue						
TOTALS:						

The "Interference Period" label appears as a vertical divider column between the Trial 4 column and the Delayed Recall column.

or multiple-choice clues for the words that are not recalled. Normal elderly patients recognize most of the 8 to 10 words. The examiner further screen visual memory by evaluating delayed recall for three or four figures previously drawn by the patient or three or four items previously hidden in the room. The examiner assesses retrieval of remote information by asking the patient about three or four past public events that have occurred during the individual's lifetime and asking them to elaborate. Finally, there may be a need to test semantic knowledge, most commonly by asking the meaning of words that the patient missed on prior confrontational naming ("What is a…?").

9. **Constructional, Perceptual, and Spatial Abilities.** Perceptual disturbances are a sensitive indicator of brain disease, particularly involving occipital cortex and parietal cortex. Specific disorders include visual agnosia (inability to visually recognize objects despite intact primary visual functions), abnormal facial discrimination, prosopagnosia (inability to recognize familiar faces), color agnosia and achromatopsia, abnormal spatial localization, simultanagnosia (inability to visually attend to more than one item or area at a time), and topographagnosia (inability to spatially orient in the environment). The easiest way to screen for complex visual disturbances is through constructional tasks such as drawings (Fig. 5.2). First, the examiner asks the patient to copy a simple two-dimensional figure, such as a triangle; a complex two-dimensional figure, such as overlapping pentagons; and a three-dimensional figure, such as a cube. These drawings may show abnormal spatial relationships, absence of detail, stimulus-boundedness (closing-in and drawing over the master copy), loss of three-dimensional perspective, or neglect of one part of the drawing. Second, hemispatial neglect may also be evident on line bisection or figure cancellation tasks. The patients must either bisect lines in half or scan for specified figures on a piece of paper centered in front of them. Third, many clinicians use the clock drawing task to screen for visuospatial difficulties. The freehand drawing of a clock is a sensitive measure of visuospatial difficulty but is also affected by attention, language comprehension, numerical knowledge, and executive abilities. The administration of the clock drawing task involves the presentation of a blank paper with the instructions to "draw the face of a clock." After the initial clock-drawing attempt, the examiner instructs the patient to indicate the time as "10 after 11" or "5 past 4." Various scoring systems distinguish normal elderly subjects from those with early dementia. These scoring systems, along with additional complex visual processing tasks, are discussed in Chapter 10.

10. **Praxis and Other Motor Movements.** Praxis is the integration and performance of learned, complex motor acts. Ideomotor apraxia is a disturbance of these motor acts despite the presence of normal elementary motor, sensory, and language functions. The inability to perform the movement reflects left parietal, left frontal, or callosal dysfunction; the substitution of a part of the body for the imagined object is a nonspecific symptom of brain dysfunction. Other forms of apraxia are conceptual apraxia with difficulty understanding what a movement correctly signifies and limb-kinetic apraxia with difficulty with fine motor movements. Other "apraxias" are often not praxis problems at all. For example, dressing "apraxia" is actually a visuospatial deficit resulting in problems orienting to a garment. The examiner asks the patient to pretend to use an object (transitive actions) and to demonstrate symbolic gestures (intransitive actions). The examiner tests both upper limbs, first the dominant limb and then the nondominant one, with commands to pantomime an action. Examples of praxis commands are "wave goodbye," "beckon someone to come," "hitchhike," "brush your teeth with a pretend toothbrush," "comb your hair with a pretend comb," and "open a door with a pretend key." If the patient fails to perform the movement on verbal command, then the examiner pantomimes the action and asks the patient to imitate it. Should the patient continue to have difficulty, ask him/her to explain what the action signifies or represents. Finally, for limb-kinetic praxis, the examiner asks the

patient to do rapid finger tapping and to pick up a coin from a table without sliding it.

11. **Calculations and Related Functions.** Loss of calculation ability can be due to primary or secondary acalculia. Primary acalculia (or "anarithmetia") is most commonly a disturbance of numerical ability that results from disease in the left parietal region affecting the horizontal intraparietal sulcus. Secondary acalculias include aphasic acalculia due to a disturbance of the comprehension of symbols and spatial acalculia due to a disturbance of the placement of numbers in a calculation.

The patient performs two or more addition problems, two or more subtraction problems, and two or more simple multiplication problems, using paper and pen. A written assessment allows for a greater process interpretation of any errors in attempting to solve the calculation problems, such as carryover and placement errors. In the presence of primary acalculia, the examiner also evaluates for other neighborhood deficits that constitute Gerstmann syndrome, including agraphia out of proportion to any reading disturbance, right-left disorientation, and digit (finger) agnosia or loss of knowledge. For right-left orientation, the examiner asks the patient to identify body parts on the left and right side of both his/her own body and the examiner's body. For digit gnosis, the examiner asks the patient to point to named fingers or to state, with occluded vision, the number of fingers between two fingers touched by the examiner.

12. **Executive Operations.** Executive functions deal with goal setting, strategic planning, follow-through, and self-monitoring of progress. In other words, they include the ability and drive to formulate long-range goals, the steps and program to meet those goals, the motivation to act on those steps, and the ability to monitor and reassess progress in attaining those goals. The prefrontal cortex and their connections through the caudate nuclei are the main source of executive functions, which are reflected in various testable "operations." Lesions of the dorsolateral frontal cortex may produce decreased verbal and design fluency, decreased set-shifting, and impaired motor

programming with perseverations or impersistence. Lesions of the orbitofrontal region may produce disinhibition and impulsivity with decreased response inhibition. Lesions of the medial frontal lobe may produce apathy, aspontaneity, and decreased verbal output. There is no sharp separation of these manifestations; most patients have mixtures of these symptoms. Ultimately, the MSX of executive functions can be insensitive, but the history provides important information on a change in personality with decreased goal-directed behavior, disinhibition, and apathy.

Executive abilities work through specific, testable operations that may corroborate the historical evidence of altered executive functions. First, there may be a decline in verbal (e.g., "F" word/minute) fluency and the number of free-form designs/minute. Second, there may be changes in the ability to change set. In the alternate tapping task, the examiner asks the patient to tap twice every time the examiner taps once and to tap once every time the examiner taps twice (Fig. 5.3). The examiner randomly presents a sequence of taps and monitors the patient for errors of omission or commission. Third, there may by difficulty in motor programming. One test of motor programming involves the Luria Three-Step Hand Sequence or Slap-Side-Fist. The examiner first demonstrates this task three times. The patient must then reproduce the sequence with the examiner for three more times followed by six times on their own. Fourth, there may be difficulty inhibiting responses. In the Go-No-Go test, the examiner asks the patient to tap once every time the examiner taps once but not to tap at all if the examiner taps twice (Fig. 5.3). Similar to the alternate tapping task, the examiner randomly presents a sequence and monitors the patient for errors of omission or commission. Finally, the patient may manifest observable stimulus-bound behavior such as the compulsion to imitate the examiner's movements or to utilize ambient objects.

13. **Executive Attributes.** Along with executive operations, there are executive "attributes" that emerge as products of executive functions. Prominent executive attributes are decision-making and judgment, which rely on the presence of

Alternating Programs

1. "Tap twice when I tap once"

2. Run three trials: 1-1-1

3. "Tap once when I tap twice"

4. Run three trials: 2-2-2

5. Perform the following series:

1-1-2-1-2-2-2-1-1-2

Go-No-Go Test

1. "Tap once when I tap once"

2. Run three trials: 1-1-1

3. "Do not tap when I tap twice"

4. Run three trials: 2-2-2

5. Perform the following series:

1-1-2-1-2-2-2-1-1-2

Fig. 5.3 Executive operations.

logic and reasoning. It is very difficult to test a patient's judgment; responses to questions such as "what would you do if you saw a fire in a theater?" may be unreliable. In everyday life, good decision-making and judgment is the presence of personally and socially appropriate goals, strategies, and procedures, and the best assessment of judgment are examples or observations of behavior from the patient's daily life. One caution is to not depend on verbal self-reports, as these patients can give a good verbal plan in contrast to their actual follow-through behavior.

Testable executive attributes include insight and the ability to abstract. Insight relates to the awareness and understanding of their illness and its consequences. On asking patients about their condition, those with executive dysfunction may have anosognosia or denial of illness and anosodiaphoria or decreased emotional appreciation of illness (disturbances that may also occur from right parietal lobe disturbances). The ability to abstract is a related feature that is disturbed in dementia,

psychosis, and other neuropsychiatric conditions. The examiner asks the patient to interpret similarities, idioms, and proverbs. Concrete interpretations indicate disturbed abstraction ability. Examples of similarities include orange-banana, lie-mistake, poem-statue, watch-ruler, and child-midget. Common idioms include the meaning of "level-headed," "narrow-minded," and "warm-hearted." Examples of proverbs include relatively familiar ones such as "People who live in glass houses shouldn't throw stones." Unfamiliar proverbs are preferable because their interpretation precludes a rote remembered interpretation.

14. **Neurological Behavioral Examination.** The examiner cannot separate the neurocognitive examination from alterations in behavior. As previously emphasized, positive "psychiatric" behaviors can be due to neurological disorders, and brain-behavior disorders can lead to apathy and emotional changes, socioemotional problems, delusions, hallucinations, and many other behavioral disturbances.

During the interview and examination, the examiner appraises the patient's motivation and emotion, alterations in social or psychophysiological behavior, and whether he or she has any special preoccupations. Emotion may be evident from the patient's affect or emotional expression. Mood disorders are manifestations of emotional disturbance. Social behavior includes responsiveness to social cues and maintaining social boundaries, and changes in social behavior may indicate acquired frontal lobe or temporal lobe disorders. Psychophysiological behavioral disturbances involve sexual behavior, dietary changes, and aggression or violence. Special preoccupations involve disorders of language or thought content, and altered perceptions, such as illusions or hallucinations.

Conclusions

This chapter presents the elements of a brief MSX and a very basic outline of the domains of an NBSE. The following chapters greatly expand on each of these different domains and the repertoire of tests available to clinicians who want to explore a neurocognitive area in greater depth.

Chapter 6

The Neurobehavioral History and Behavioral Observations

Obtaining a history and observing the patient are the first steps in a comprehensive mental status examination (MSX). Obtaining a history involves a skilled interview, a targeted cognitive history, and an evaluation of the patient's personal background. Except for telephone encounters, the examiner should be able to make important observations of the patient's behavior while conducting the interview and history taking. In addition to an excellent history, a skilled examiner can make an effective visual assessment of the patient either in-person or by videoconferencing.

The Neurobehavioral History

INTERVIEWING TECHNIQUES

The opening and introduction must focus on putting the patient at ease and establishing rapport. The examiner is establishing a relationship. To this end he or she first addresses the patient, introducing him- or herself while looking and speaking directly to the patient. Although initial small talk can help put some patients at ease, it should be minimal, and the examiner should not talk about him- or herself. The introduction requires some preparation, not only in knowing the patient's medical information but also how to pronounce the patient's name and what the expectations might be. The examiner must briefly explain the purpose and nature of the examination, his or her role, and the goals of interview. Other aspects of the opening and introduction include attending to one's own attitude and body language (i.e., conveying an empathic attitude), the environment (i.e., if in-person, sitting at the same level and about 2 feet from the patient), and the patient's verbal and nonverbal cues (i.e., cooperative or hostile toward the interview) (Box 6.1). Rapport is most facilitated if the examiner searches for the patient's

underlying emotions and areas of concern and adjusts his or her demeanor accordingly.

The interview then proceeds with open-ended questions, allowing the patient to talk freely in their responses. Open-ended questions include "Why are you seeing a doctor today?"; "Tell me your problem and how it started?"; and "What difficulty do you want to talk about?" At the beginning, the examiner listens attentively, minimizing interruptions and distractions. In fact, much of the interview involves just listening while occasionally repeating the patient's words ("echoing") and giving nonverbal encouragement to continue

---

BOX 6.1 MENTAL STATUS INTERVIEW

Opening and Introduction

Preparation (know medical record, pronunciation of patient's name)
Establishing rapport
Introducing oneself directly to patient
Interviewing patient alone if possible or appropriate
Attending to interview environment and where you are in relation to patient or videocameras
Explaining goals and your role

Open-Ended Questions and Active Listening

Determineing when to interview family/caregivers
Open-ended questioning:
  e.g.: "Tell me your problem?" or "Why are you seeing a doctor today?"
Active listening with echoing and encouragement
Facilitation of free speech from the patient
Do not rush the patient's explanation or description

Closed-Ended Questions

Specific questions clarifying the patient's responses
Clarifying particularly with examples of mental status difficulty
Assure that patient understands and avoid jargon
Summarizing problem in patient's own words
Neurobehavioral review of systems
Personal history

talking. Let this first part of the initial interview follow the patient's train of thought. Of course, the examiner may need to probe with additional open-ended questions and provide structure to help patients who have trouble ordering their thoughts or just giving a history.

Directed questions probing specific cognitive and behavioral areas follow later. These close-ended questions focus on obtaining more in-depth information. For example, if the patient reports memory loss, then the examiner asks about the type, duration, and impact of memory difficulty. The examiner should ask for clarification particularly with examples. In asking close-ended questions, it is important to assure that the patient understands the questions by not rushing, using the patient's own words, and avoiding jargon, technical terms, or long sentences. It is often helpful to assure comprehension by asking the patient to repeat back their understanding of the questions. Conversely, it is also helpful to briefly summarize what the patient said in his or her own words.

Two additional points in the interview are note-taking and the presence of family or others. First, note-taking, now often directly on the computer, need not interfere with listening to the patient. If in-person, the body is positioned in a "golden triangle" facing the patient as much as possible while maintaining intermittent eye contact. Incidentally, everyone in the room should be situated with ready access to the exit in case of an emergency. Second, determine if the patient would rather be interviewed alone, with a separate interview with the caregiver or informants. The examiner should not direct initial questions to family, caregivers, or others unless and until it is clear that the patient cannot provide history. Cognitive deficits or behavioral disorders can interfere with the patient's ability to provide history, and the examiner often needs to interview family members or friends but only if the patient agrees or cannot give history. Furthermore, patients may lack the insight into their disorder and may deny or minimize any difficulty, and the contrast between the patient's history and that of the caregiver can reveal valuable information.

COGNITIVE HISTORY

The examiner elicits a chief cognitive complaint from the patient, family, and/or caregivers. The examiner asks the patient to describe their specific behavioral difficulties, including the onset and progression. Common chief complaints are problems forgetting recently learned information, word-finding difficulty, or getting lost in familiar surroundings. As noted, it is important to get specific examples of the mental status difficulties. In addition to the chief complaint, obtain a neurobehavioral review of systems encompassing the major cognitive domains with questions on arousal and attention, language, memory, visuospatial abilities, motor movements, calculations, and "executive" or goal-directed behavior (Box 6.2). The past medical history further includes neuropsychiatric disorders and neurological conditions that could impact on behavior.

The examiner may reserve specific cognitive questions for family and caregivers that require their particular perspective. These involve the neurobehavioral

BOX 6.2 MENTAL STATUS REVIEW OF SYMPTOMS

Does the patient have any of the following?

Clouded or "foggy" thinking
Confabulation
Decreased ability to stay alert and awake
Decreased initiation of activity
Decreased retrieving old information
Delusions
Depression, mood problems, or anxiety
Dietary changes
Difficulty with calculations and manipulating numbers
Difficulty following through or completing usual activities
Disorientation to time and place
Distractibility
Ease of forgetting
Episodes of confusion
Getting lost in familiar surroundings
Hallucinations, illusions, or other perceptual phenomena
Impaired reading or writing
Impropriety in social behavior
Inability to find items in their visual environment
Inability to get around in space
Inability to speak clearly
Learning impairment for new information
Poor concentration
Poor memory for recent events
Poor performance of goal-oriented behavior
Poor performance of learned motor tasks
Repetitive behaviors or thoughts
Slowed thinking
Stereotypical or other movement disorders
Understanding of spoken words is impaired
Word-finding difficulty

review of systems but worded as informant observations. For example, for memory, the examiner can ask whether the patient has had trouble with recent memory, such as remembering daily household events, where the patient puts things, and what they were recently told. A particular area for questioning for family and caregivers is the nature of the patient's overall pervasive pattern of behavior. For example, the history provides the most important information for personality changes from frontal-executive dysfunction including decreased goal-directed behavior (initiation of productive behavior, follow-through, monitoring and correction, success and completion), disinhibition, and apathy and disengagement. Other dysexecutive symptoms and signs include deficits when there is a history of poor problem-solving and impaired judgment. Is the current pattern of behavior a change from a prior level of functioning? Compare the current pattern of behavior with premorbid functioning based on educational, occupational, economic, and marital attainment, performance, and stability.

As part of the cognitive history, the examiner gets a functional history for activities of daily living, such as dressing, personal hygiene, continence, the pattern of eating and sleeping, and instrumental activities, such as making change at a store, balancing their accounts, cooking a meal, or driving an automobile. The functional history also evaluates whether there is a decline in their usual occupational activities. The functional history extends to an assessment of who is taking care of most of the responsibilities, what the living and safety situation is, what the status of caregiving is, and whether there is other support.

PERSONAL HISTORY

Several personal characteristics may impact on mental status testing, specifically the patient's age; education; sex, ethnic, and socioeconomic background; and language proficiency. It is important to emphasize these as part of the history because they may influence the interpretation of performance on any subsequent mental status tests.

Age. The examiner must be aware of how the patient's age could impact on the neurobehavioral status examination (NBSE) and MSX. Five characteristics of behavioral evaluation in the elderly may affect the mental status assessment. First, the range of

"normality" broadens with age, and there is increased overlap between disturbed cognition and some of the changes of normal aging. This is reflected in neuropsychological tests, which have age-stratified norms. Second, cognitive changes occur at different rates for different cognitive functions as people get older. For example, there are age-associated decreases in psychomotor speed, and older people perform less efficiently on time-dependent mental tasks. Third, mental status testing may not be entirely comparable between the elderly and the young. Even after age-adjustment, there is a cohort effect due to differences in generational experiences and education with regard to taking these tests. Fourth, older patients have physical difficulties that can affect the mental status testing. Changes in vision, hearing, sleep patterns, health status, and drug effects, all of which are more common in older people, can affect cognition and behavior. Because of these age-associated changes, the interpretation of mental status tasks and rating scales in the elderly must be done with these considerations in mind.

Longitudinal and cross-sectional studies on aging have shown a decline in the speed of neuronal processing, selective attention, memory, and certain aspects of higher cognitive function (Box 6.3). The elderly have a decreased ability to concentrate and maintain attention over prolonged periods. This is consistent with increased daytime somnolence, fragmented sleep and decreased deep sleep (stage III, IV) and rapid eye movement sleep. Short-term/working memory, for example, the ability to temporarily retain a telephone number, is more difficult. New learning, although slower, is relatively spared, as are old well established memories. However, it is the retrieval of old information at the time that is needed, which is of greater concern to older people. Moreover, they can "forget" where the car keys are or what someone's name is one moment but bring it to mind later.

Education. Education is a major factor in performance on mental status tests. Very few tasks are truly independent of educational effects. This is clearly reflected on neuropsychological measures, in which tests are routinely normed for educational level with scores directly correlated with the extent and quality of formal education. Studies have demonstrated education effects on tasks ranging from the simple digit span forward to perceptual or spatial tasks, but are

BOX 6.3   SUGGESTED MENTAL STATUS FEATURES OF NORMAL AGING

1. Fundamental functions
   a. Tonic underarousal and decreased sensory processing
   b. Slowed neuronal processing and increased stimulus persistence
   c. Decreased complex, divided, and sustained attention
   d. Interference from redundant or irrelevant material
2. Memory
   a. Decreased short-term/working memory
   b. Well-preserved long-term remote memory
   c. Decreased retrieval of long-term memory when needed
3. Language
   a. Richer narrative style
   b. Decreased active naming (individual within-class names)
4. Perception and spatial abilities
   a. Decreased perception
   b. Increased spatial segmentation
5. Socioemotional and neuropsychiatric
   a. Decreased excitability and impulsivity; more cautious
   b. Disengagement and fewer risk goal-oriented behaviors
   c. Decreased flexibility and tolerance for change

generally worse for verbal tests, including language and verbal memory. In fact, poorly educated but cognitively normal persons can score lower than mildly impaired but well-educated individuals.

The mental status examiner needs to consider education on two levels. First is the extent of education. The examiner needs to determine the last grade or level completed in school and whether the patient was in special education classes. Those with eight or fewer completed years of formal education may perform one or more points lower than expected on verbal tasks, whereas those with three or fewer completed years of education may perform one or more points lower than expected on all mental status tasks. A second consideration is the quality of the education. The mental status examiner needs to consider the equivalency of the educational experience. The same extent of formal schooling can mean very different educational experiences, particularly in the United States where great discrepancies may exist between suburban and inner city schools or large urban schools compared with small rural ones.

Sex, Ethnic, and Socioeconomic Differences. There are limited data on sex differences in mental status assessment in the clinical encounter and at the bedside. Sex differences are reported, but few remain unquestioned, and the overlap in performance between men and women is the predominant finding. In general, men show more lateralization effects than women, and this is particularly the case for strongly right-handed men. Reports suggest that women may do better on tests of verbal skills, particularly speech production and word generation, whereas men may do better than women on perceptual and spatial tasks, particularly spatial orientation, and on mathematical tasks, particularly spatially based mathematics. Some studies suggest that left-handed males (and homosexual males) perform comparable to right-handed women. All of these purported group differences, however, are small and do not apply to any particular individual, who may be superior in any cognitive domain regardless of sex or sexual orientation.

The effects of race or ethnicity on mental status tests are also controversial. A major stumbling block is the confounding effects of education and socioeconomic status. These have proven difficult to disentangle on neuropsychological measures, and more so on screening mental status tests. Nevertheless, lower socioeconomic status and the lack of corresponding advantages do affect performance on these tests. For example, patients from inner city backgrounds may have decreased practice and greater unfamiliarity with tasks used to screen cognition, such as letter-based word fluency or three-dimensional drawing tasks, exemplified by cube drawing. In addition, different socioeconomic backgrounds may emphasize different abilities that are evident on mental status screening, such as manual skills over intellectual attainment.

Language Proficiency. Performance on mental status testing is very dependent on language proficiency. There is great variability in language facility among individuals of different educational, occupational, and cultural backgrounds. In many countries, mental status examiners may need to evaluate bilingual patients. Broadly defined, bilingualism is the use of two or more languages in everyday life; however, there is a large range of language competency based on "balance," simultaneous versus sequential language acquisition, and the age of acquisition and proficiency of the second language. The truly balanced bilingual, who is equally fluent in two languages, is rare. Most bilinguals have a dominant base language and a less dominant second language, and this variation in bilingualism is a factor in mental status testing. Sequential bilinguals often learned their languages in two different environments and may have separate modular lexicons, and relatively simultaneous bilinguals learned their languages in the context of frequent code switching and fluent interchange, resulting in a single interconnected system with easier switching. With aging and disease, there is a tendency to retreat to the first language, with increased cross-language interference and code switching from the deactivated language. Moreover, bilinguals may use specific languages for different purposes, in different social functions, and with different people. Consequently, their performance on mental status testing can depend on whether the linguistic environment matches the preferred language, the language used by the examiner, or the social situation.

Behavioral Observations (In-Person or Videoconferencing)

Nonverbal and verbal cues are informative as to the patient's cognitive and emotional state. Initial general behavioral observations are an important part of the NBSE. The minute that the examiner sees the patient for the first time, he or she automatically starts to make behavioral observations. Information is evident in the patient's interactions with the examiner, staff, family, and the medical environment. Even when a patient is mute, incoherent, or refusing to answer questions, the clinician can obtain a wealth of information through careful observation. Behavioral observations include the following eight areas (Box 6.4).

Alertness and Attention. First observe whether the patient is fully awake, alert, and responding to the

BOX 6.4 LIST OF BEHAVIORAL OBSERVATION AREAS

1. Alertness and attention
2. Appearance and personal hygiene
3. Psychomotor speed and movements
4. Speech and communication
5. Eye and facial behavior
6. Contextual propriety and disinhibition
7. Social interactions and personality
8. Attitude and affect

environment (see Chapter 7). General behavior may range from falling asleep during the interview to agitation and combativeness. On initial interaction with the patient, it may be evident that there is a dulling of cognitive processes and a general impairment of sharpness or focus. Attention is further evidenced in the patient's ease of distractibility; his or her attention may wander so much that it must be constantly brought back to the subject at hand. Behavioral observations can be indicative of a delirium, encephalopathy, or fluctuating alertness as is seen in dementia with Lewy bodies.

Appearance and Personal Hygiene. The examiner takes note of the patient's general appearance and grooming. Observe for hygiene (cleanliness, body odor, shaven, grooming), dress (cleanliness, dirty, neat, ragged, seasonally appropriate), and anything salient (rings, earrings, makeup). A slovenly, disheveled appearance with poor personal hygiene can reflect self-neglect from dementia, delirium, psychosis, depression, apathy, and many other disorders. Patients with dementia often fail to match their clothes or dress in multiple layers. Specific findings such as neglect of one side of the body can indicate a focal hemispheric insult.

Psychomotor Speed and Movements. Psychomotor speed is an informative cognitive function (see Chapter 7). Other than the latency and speed of response, the patient's physical activity can reflect psychomotor retardation or generalized slowing of body movements. Patients may manifest rigidity, bradykinesia, apathy, waxy flexibility, or catatonic posturing. Conversely, the examiner describes any hyperactivity such as agitation, restlessness, fidgetiness and wringing of hands, pacing, and any aimless, purposeless activity, such as carphologia ("lint-picking" behavior).

The examiner observes for the presence of any active movement disorders starting with abnormalities of gait and posture. Gait disorders and difficulty manipulating a hallway or walking into a room may inform on the presence of neurological deficits and visuospatial functioning. Other movements include choreoathetosis, tics, tremors, twitches, compulsive behaviors, gestures, mannerisms, and semipurposeful stereotypies. Stereotypical movements are repetitive, coordinated movements that resemble purposeful acts but have no clear purpose. In addition, observe for perseverative or repetitive behaviors or environmentally dependent behaviors, such as utilization and imitation behaviors or echopraxia. In delirium, for example, there can be action or sustention tremors of high frequency (8–10 Hz); asterixis or brief lapses in tonic posture, especially at the wrist; multifocal myoclonus or shock-like jerks from diverse sites; choreiform movements; dysarthria; and gait instability.

Speech and Communication. Changes in the quantity, flow, rate, rhythm, volume, and tone of speech can indicate neurological disease. The examiner evaluates how much verbal behavior is initiated by the patient. If the patient does communicate, then the examiner determines whether there is a dissociation between what the patient says and what he or she will do. This could be the main manifestation of frontal abulia or a dysexecutive state. Note the coherence or intelligibility of speech. Incoherent speech may be caused by poor articulation, dysarthria, or apraxia of speech (see Chapter 8). Finally, evaluate speech content for cognitive and behavioral dysfunction. Slow and loosely connected thinking and speech may be present, with irrelevancies, perseverations, repetitions, and intrusions. Frontal lobe dysfunction can manifest as speech that is circumstantial, tangential, or conveys a special preoccupation.

Eye and Face Behavior. The examiner specifically evaluates the patient's eye contact or any avoidance of gaze, the length of gaze, the sense of staring, and how easily gaze is "locked" on another visual stimulus. This is challenging via videoconferencing but can be done by having the patient focus on the camera in lieu of the examiner's face. Often patient's with Balint syndrome are evident when they struggle to visually locate someone or something that may be directly in front of them. In addition, the examiner evaluates facial expression for the classic emotions of fear, surprise, disgust, anger, happiness, and sadness. Facial expression may reveal decreased expressivity and a fixed smile suggestive of a frontal lobe syndrome. It may help for the examiner to consider the activity of the corrugator supercilii and zygomaticus major facial muscles. The corrugator lies at the medial end of the eyebrows and draws the eyebrows downward in a frown. The zygomaticus lies on the corner of the mouth and draws the mouth angle up and outward in a smile.

Contextual Propriety and Disinhibition. Behavior is context dependent; hence it is informative to assess whether the patient's behavior is inappropriate to the situation at hand. This includes emotional detachment or loss of insight into their condition or the circumstances of their clinical contact or hospitalization. It also includes out-of-context laughter or crying, which may suggest pseudobulbar affect. There may be intrusive verbal and nonverbal behaviors, such as personal commentary or intrusion into others' personal space. For example, the manifestation of private behaviors in public would be inappropriate, as would be excessive familiarity with strangers.

Social Interactions and Personality. During the interview, the examiner appraises the patient's personality and social interactions. This is an important part of assessing brain function. Personality refers to habitual patterns of behavior and is composed of character traits or dispositions to behave in a particular manner. Personality assessment may reveal frontal lobe or temporal lobe personality changes. The assessment starts by observing the patient's interaction with others and continues by assessing the "greeting ritual," that is, did the patient make eye contact, smile, lean forward, and shake hands or otherwise greet the examiner. The examiner goes on to observe how the patient interacts during the interview and the rest of the examination. One major clue is whether the patient is "in the conversation." The patient may be emotionally detached or cognitively distant or speaking about totally unrelated items or events.

Attitude and Affect. Patients may be uncooperative, indifferent or apathetic, disinterested in the interview, or they may be suspicious, defensive, and hostile. Regardless of the patient's attitude, the examiner always uses a calm, nonthreatening tone of voice. The examination of a violent or agitated patient can be particularly difficult. In an in-person setting, do not examine these patients alone, leave the room door open, and sit so that one can exit the room unimpeded if necessary.

Affect refers to the expression of emotion, and mood refers to the patient's emotional state (see Chapter 14). Specifically, affect is the examiner's observation of the patient's expressed emotional state based on the patient's facial expressions, behavior, and interactions. Characteristics of affect include type, range, intensity, lability, congruence, and appropriateness. Affect has emotional range from broad to restricted, intensity from blunted and flattened to heightened, and stability from unmoved to labile. When affect is constricted, both the range and intensity of expression are reduced. In blunted affect, emotional expression is further reduced. To diagnose flat affect, virtually no signs of affective expression should be present; the patient's voice should be monotonous, and the face should be immobile. In addition to neurological disorders, changes in affect can, of course, indicate primary psychiatric disorders such as depression, anxiety, euphoria, and mania. The examiner notes the appropriateness to content as affect may or may not be congruent with mood or with the situation and context.

Clinical Implications

A significant issue in mental status testing is clarification of the patient's or family's "memory" complaint. This term is often used widely to refer to most cognitive difficulties, such as attentional difficulty, word-finding problems, visuospatial disorientation, calculation problems, and executive function disturbances. The examiner must clarify this at onset by asking for their examples of "memory difficulty." These examples could quickly clarify that the neurobehavioral complaint really involves finding or comprehending words or the ability to initiate and follow-through on tasks, that is, executive dysfunction. If the examples are insufficient, the examiner can pursue further examples or questions for greater clarification. Moreover, if the patient or family continue to describe "short-term memory" difficulty, they may be referring to a problem anywhere along the memory stream (see Chapter 9). Some examples of their memory problems are forgetting what they went to get at the store or not remembering the last lines on a page. These examples tend to be attentional difficulty with poor registration, and subsequent mental status testing could point to physiological or related disturbances, such as sleep disorders, medication effects, or medical illnesses. At other times, the examples are clearly those of long-term "recent" memory such as inability to learn new information, particularly what just happened in the last few hours or days. These examples are more consistent with declarative episodic memory as one might see in patients with memory impairment from hippocampal disease. In summary, clarification of the cognitive history is an essential part of the mental status evaluation.

One of the most salient disorders of emotional expression is pseudobulbar affect. In this disorder, the mental status examiner observes the patient to cry, laugh, or manifest an intermixed laugh-cry without much provocation. The crying and laughing can be prominent and frequent; however, careful behavioral observations may reveal only a mild tendency to crying or laughing, not always evident to patients or even families. These patients have pseudobulbar palsy with overt changes in affect triggered by trivial stimuli. In pseudobulbar palsy, the patient's laughs, cries, or laugh-cries are incongruent with the intensity of their mood and their contextual situation. Other features of pseudobulbar palsy may include dysarthria, dysphagia, bifacial weakness, increased mandibular reflex, preserved or increased palatal reflexes, and weak tongue movements. Pseudobulbar affect is secondary to bilateral interruption of supranuclear innervation of bulbar motor nuclei of the lower face and brainstem centers. Bilateral strokes, multiple sclerosis, amyotrophic lateral sclerosis, progressive supranuclear palsy, and severe brain trauma are the most common causes of this syndrome.

Conclusions

This chapter illustrates how the mental status evaluation is aided by interview techniques, cognitive history, personal history, and behavioral observations. Some conditions, such as frontal lobe personality changes, may be predominantly evident on history and behavioral observations, irrespective of the MSX. Nevertheless, the neurobehavioral history and behavioral observations are necessary for setting the stage for mental status tests and for targeting specific areas of the NBSE.

Chapter 7

Arousal, Attention, and Other Fundamental Functions

Fundamental functions, or disturbances of the "sensorium," are a prerequisite to instrumental functions. They include arousal, basic attention, "mental control," and psychomotor speed. The multimodal aspect of orientation to time and place, although dependent on memory, is also affected by attentional deficits, and is therefore discussed here. Alterations in fundamental functions decrease efficiency of cortical functioning, and hence affect the validity of the assessment of instrumental functions such as memory, language, or executive functions.

Fundamental Functions and Orientation

AROUSAL

Arousal is a psychophysiological readiness to react or respond to stimuli. Most patients requiring mental status examination do not need to be examined for arousal; however, some patients fluctuate in level of alertness and awareness. Basic arousal is present if there is nonspecific, nonreflex responsiveness to any verbal or physical stimuli. Arousal results from activation of the cerebral cortex and is centered in the ascending reticular activating system (ARAS) in the upper brain stem (primarily midbrain) with projections to the intralaminar and centromedian thalamic nuclei, the autonomic and endocrine systems in the dorsal hypothalamus, and, ultimately, the neocortex. Neurologists often divide disorders of arousal into those that affect the brain stem, with associated brain stem neurological findings, and those that more diffusely affect the neocortex. Primary states of arousal include alertness or wakefulness, lethargy or somnolence, sleep and hypnosis, obtundation, stupor or semicoma, and coma (Table 7.1). In addition, there are related coma-like states that include the vegetative state, the minimally conscious state, akinetic mutism, coma vigil, and locked-in syndrome.

The primary arousal states vary in responsiveness to environmental stimuli. Patients with lethargy or somnolence tend to drift off if not stimulated, and those with obtundation require vigorous or greater than normal verbal or physical stimulation to arouse. Patients with stupor or semicoma are limited to responses to noxious or painful stimuli by groaning or withdrawal to pain, and those with coma are totally unresponsive except for reflex action, including decorticate or decerebrate posturing, depending on whether the dysfunction is above or below the red nucleus in the midbrain, respectively. The definition of coma additionally specifies the absence of normal sleep-wake cycles documented on electroencephalography. These categories of disturbed arousal are not discrete, and there is a continuum of arousal from alertness to deep coma. In contrast, coma-like states, such as vegetative state and minimally conscious state, have some apparent responsivity, with eye openings and sleep-wake cycles.

ATTENTION

"Everyone knows what attention is. It is the taking possession by the mind, in clear and vivid form, of one out of what seem several simultaneously possible objects or trains of thought. Focalization, concentration, of consciousness are of its essence. It implies withdrawal from some things to deal effectively with others and is a condition, which has a real opposite in the confused, dazed, scatterbrained state, which in French is called distraction, and Zerstreutheit in German."

William James, The Principles of Psychology, Vol. 1, Chapter XI. Attention. 1890, pg 404.

Basic attention is selective attention. As explained by William James, attention is the ability to focus and concentrate arousal and mental activity on a targeted external or internal stimulus to the exclusion

TABLE 7.1   States of Arousal

	Stimulation for Arousal	Verbal Response	Eye Response	Motor Response	Physiology
Alert	Normal	Coherent response	Eyes open and fixate/track/contact	Moves and orients body	Normal wakefulness, normal EEG
Sleep, lethargy, somnolence	Voice or physical-mild	Coherent response	Eyes open and fixate/track/contact	Moves and orients body	Slow wave or sleep EEG
Obtundation	Loud voice or physical-strong	Incoherent (± mumbled)	Eyes open and fixate/track/± contact	Moves ± orients body	Slow wave EEG
Stupor or semicoma	Physical- pain or noxious	None (may groan)	None (eyes may flicker)	Withdrawal only; aimless movement	Slow wave EEG
Coma	None	None	None	Reflex ± decorticate or decerebrate	Slow wave EEG
Coma-Like States					
Vegetative or apallic state (unaware of self, environment)	None	None	Eyes open; random eye movements; do not fixate/track/contact	± None	Sleep-wake cycle, diffuse cortical damage; preserved brain stem, hypothalamic function
Minimally conscious sate	Inconsistent responses	None ± yes/no or intelligible speech	Eyes open ± fixate/track/contact	None ± purposeful movements/may follow simple commands	Sleep-wake cycle, diffuse cortical damage; partial preservation of conscious awareness
Apathetic akinetic mute (look lethargic or somnolent)	Inconsistent responses (± orient to sound)	None spontaneously; minimal responses ± short, soft/whispered	May have eyes open and fixate/track/± contact (± vertical gaze palsy)	Minimal but definite movements	Lesion in midbrain, subthalamus, or frontal-ACG interrupts ARAS
Coma vigil (look awake day and night)	Inconsistent responses (± septal rage)	None spontaneously; minimal responses ± short, soft/whispered	Eyes open and fixate/track/± contact	Minimal but definite movements	Lesion in septal region, anterior hypothalamus, frontal-ACG or bilateral OFC
Decreased Motivation States					
Apathy	Normal	Minimal responses ± short, soft/whispered	Eyes open and fixate/track/contact	Minimal but definite movements	Variable, may be normal
Abulia (difficult to distinguish from apathy, but more severe and normal mood)	Normal	Minimal responses ± short, soft/whispered	Eyes open and fixate/track/±contact	Minimal but definite movements	Variable, may be normal

(Continued)

TABLE 7.1	States of Arousal (*Cont'd*)				
	Stimulation for Arousal	**Verbal Response**	**Eye Response**	**Motor Response**	**Physiology**
Catatonia	Normal	Minimal responses ± short, soft/ whispered	Eyes open ± fixate/track/ contact	Minimal but definite movements; postures, catalepsy	Variable, may be normal
Conditions Mistaken for Coma					
Locked-in syndrome	Normal	None	Eyes open ± fixate/track/ contact; blink movements (may communicate by blinking)	Reflex ± decorticate or decerebrate	Variable, may be normal
Brain death	None	None	None	None	No cortical or brain stem functions/reflexes (e.g., gag or corneal) and positive apnea test

ACG, anterior cingulate gyrus; *ARAS,* ascending reticular activating system; *EEG,* electroencephalogram; *OFC,* orbitofrontal cortex.

of others, that is, to avoid being distracted by extraneous stimuli. Like arousal, attention works by enhancing neocortical processing and is a prerequisite for effective instrumental cognitive abilities. Attention is more of a distributed system than arousal, and many areas of the brain can disrupt attention. Attention depends on the brain stem, both arousal from the ARAS and the mechanism for actual movement of attention; the reticular nucleus of the thalamus for modulating and "gating" the sensory input so that selectivity emerges; the parietal cortex for ipsilateral disengaging and contralateral shifting attention and its spatial distribution (particularly right parietal); and the prefrontal cortex for the mental control or complex aspects of shifting, maintaining, and dividing attention (Fig. 7.1). Given the distributed system mediating attention, this cognitive

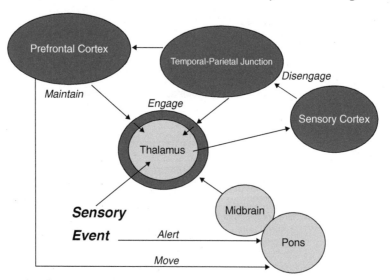

Fig. 7.1 Attentional pathways. The diagram illustrates the processes of attention including engagement, disengagement, maintenance, interaction with alerting, and the ability to move the attentional "spotlight."

process is quite vulnerable to metabolic disruptions. Patients with abnormal attention have difficulty concentrating and experience impersistence, ease of distraction, and increased vulnerability to interference. Abnormal attention is the hallmark of delirium (see Chapter 3), the most common cause of behavioral disturbance among hospitalized elderly patients.

MENTAL CONTROL

Mental control is the management of attention. It is a heterogeneous concept that includes complex attention and short-term or working memory. Complex attention involves the ability to maintain attention, divide attention between two or more stimuli, shift attention between stimuli, vigilance or readiness to shift attention, and spatial attention. These complex attentional activities interact with working memory, an aspect of executive functions (see Chapter 13). Maintaining or sustaining attention is altered in most clinic or bedside tests of attention. Divided attention, however, can be quite difficult to test independent of executive functions. The ability to shift attention involves mechanisms for engaging, disengaging, and actual movement of the attentional spotlight. Vigilance has an optimal level; for example, hypervigilance leads to easy distraction to irrelevant stimuli, as is the case in delirium tremens. Spatial disorders of attention, such as hemispatial neglect and Balint syndrome, are discussed in Chapter 10.

PSYCHOMOTOR SPEED

Speed of processing and latency of response onset are cognitive abilities that can be very sensitive to aging, white matter disease, frontal lobe disorders, and other conditions. "Psychomotor" speed combines or conflates, two general neurological processes, basic cognitive speed and basic motor speed. The former is a mental decision-making process, and the latter is basic motor reaction time or speed of movement. Psychomotor speed is particularly a function of the basal ganglia (striatum, globus pallidus, subthalamic nucleus, substantia nigra) and their white matter connections from frontal lobe regions (dorsolateral, orbitofrontal, anterior cingulate, supplementary motor area). These frontal cortical areas promote action through input to the striatum (caudate nuclei and putamen), which, in turn, directly inhibits the globus pallidus (and,

less directly, the subthalamic nucleus), thus releasing the thalamus and other structures for action selection and motor execution. Some neurological and neuropsychiatric disorders result in increased speed, but most slow basic mental decision times, both response choice and response selection, even beyond basic motor reaction time. Slowed psychomotor speed and delayed latency of response initiation are common in delirium, frontal conditions, advanced dementia, and, of course, parkinsonian disorders; whereas increase speed may occur in hyperkinetic delirium and agitated, anxious, or manic patients.

ORIENTATION

As discussed in Chapter 5, orientation is a very sensitive, although nonspecific, measure of an altered mental status. Orientation to time and place is a multimodal characteristic and not a specific property of the brain. Orientation to time is usually the most sensitive, followed by orientation to place. Many people are frequently mildly disoriented in time and place, off a day or so on the date or confused about the building location or floor, which may vary depending on the context or time of day. Pathological disorientation for time and place occur from disturbances of attention such as delirium, from memory disorders such as dementia, and from other cognitive deficits in language, semantics, perception, or executive abilities. In contrast to disorientation to time and place, disorientation for person or personal identity is not usually a manifestation of cognitive impairment and likely reflects a primary psychiatric disorder, such as a dissociative state.

Testing of Fundamental Functions and Orientation

AROUSAL

A disturbance of arousal is usually evident on initial patient presentation. Is the patient alert or dull, wide awake or drowsy? If the patient is not alert, can he or she be aroused to full awareness or will arousal produce only partial awakening? If the patient is aroused, can attention be sustained or does the patient drift back into sleep? Can the patient keep his or her eyes open, or do they remain shut; are the eyes fixed or do they follow movements?

If a disturbance of arousal is suspected, the examiner evaluates four aspects of the arousal examination. First, the examination assesses whether the patient is awake and responding to the environment. Alternatively, he or she may need stimulation for arousal. For verbal stimulation, clinicians loudly call the patient's name while tapping them. If physical stimulation is necessary, clinicians apply sternal pressure or pinch the Achilles tendon. A description of the extent of stimulation necessary for responsiveness is a gauge of the level of wakefulness and provides useful data for later comparison. Second, the examiner notes the type of responsiveness to stimulation. Evaluate whether the patient maintains eyes open and visually fixates, tracks stimuli, or attains eye contact. Note the presence of any verbal responses, reactive movements to stimulation, reflex actions, or posturing. The examiner can semiquantify the eye, verbal, and motor responses with various scales, such as the Glasgow Coma Scale (Table 7.2). This assessment for arousal must take place in the context of a thorough neurological examination that particularly focuses on the presence of brain stem signs, such as pupillary size, symmetry, and reactivity; extraocular movements including oculocephalic reflexes ("Doll's Eyes Maneuver"), respiratory pattern, and long tract findings or upper motor neuron signs.

BASIC ATTENTION AND MENTAL CONTROL

If responsive, first ask the patient whether he or she feels "foggy" and cloudy or sharp and clear in thinking. Assess their conversation with an appraisal of how "interviewable" they are. Further assess by asking them to count the number of raised fingers on your hand. Verbal incoherence may provide a solid indication of disrupted attention, as patients with disturbed attention tend to ramble, lose the train of their conversation, and fail to maintain coherence in thought. The examiner may rate the patient's overall ability to stay with the interview on a subjective rating scale of 0 (highly distractable) to 5 (fully attentive). In addition, observe the patient's overall behavior for hypoactivity, hyperactivity, or movement abnormalities, such as myoclonus or tremors.

Basic attention is difficult to assess directly and is usually evaluated through complex attentional tasks that involve other abilities, particularly sustained attention and vigilance tasks, both requiring short-term/working memory. Any one bedside test of attention has limited sensitivity and specificity because they are affected by effort and other cognitive domains. It is therefore best to administer three or four different types of attentional tasks and mentally "factor analyze" the common denominator of attention from the tasks (Fig. 7.2).

Serial Recitation Tasks. Bedside tests of attention include serial recitation tasks, continuous performance tasks, alternate response tasks, and spatial attention

TABLE 7.2	Glasgow Coma Scale					
	1	**2**	**3**	**4**	**5**	**6**
Eye	Does not open eyes	Opens eyes in response to painful stimuli	Opens eyes in response to voice	Opens eyes spontaneously	N/A	N/A
Verbal	Makes no sounds	Incomprehensible sounds	Utters inappropriate words	Confused, disoriented	Oriented, converses normally	N/A
Motor	Makes no movements	Extension to painful stimuli (decerebrate)	Abnormal flexion to painful stimuli (decorticate)	Flexion/ Withdrawal to painful stimuli	Localizes painful stimuli	Obeys commands

The scale is composed of three tests: eye, verbal, and motor responses. The three values separately as well as their sum are considered. The lowest possible Glasgow Coma Scale score (the sum) is 3 (deep coma or death), whereas the highest is 15 (fully awake person).
Coma: No eye opening, no ability to follow commands, no verbalizations (3-8).
N/A, Not applicable.
From Teasdale G, Jennett B. Assessment of coma and impaired consciousness. A practical scale. *Lancet*. 1974;2:81-84.

1. Digit span:

Tell the patient, "I am going to read a list of numbers. Listen carefully and when I am finished, repeat the same numbers after me." Present the digits in a normal tone of voice at a rate of one digit per second.

Forward task: Repeat in same order; Reverse task: repeat in backwards order

	(3)	(4)	(5)	(6)	(7)	(8)
F____	249	8527	29683	571946	8159362	39815147
R____	174	5297	63851	294738	4192751	

2. Verbal "A" Test:

Tell the patient, "I am going to read you a long series of letters. Whenever you hear the letter A, indicate by tapping the desk." Read the following letter list in a normal tone at a rate of one letter per second.

LTPEAOAICTDALAAANIABFS
AMRZEOADPAKLAUCITOEAB
AAZYFMUSAHEAVAARAT

Omission Errors: _____
Commission Errors: _____

3. Months of the year in reverse-

Dec, Nov, Oct, Sept, Aug, July, Jun, May, Apr, Mar, Feb, Jan

4. Subtraction backwards from 20 by 3's –

20...17...14...11...8...5...2...

Fig. 7.2 Attention and mental control battery. The examiner administers more than one task that share the property of testing attention. A normal performance is expected on three or more of these tasks.

tasks (Box 7.1). Alternate response tasks are also measures of executive operations and are discussed in Chapter 13, and spatial attention tasks are discussed with visuospatial abilities in Chapter 10. The most common serial recitation task is the Digit Span Test in which the examiner presents a series of digits, one per second in a clear voice, and the patient is asked to repeat the entire sequence immediately after presentation (see Chapter 5). The examiner explains, "I am going to repeat a series of numbers. Please immediately repeat the same numbers after I give them to you." Perceptual clumping is avoided by the use of random digits and a regular rhythm of presentation. If the patient can correctly repeat three digits, the examiner presents four digits, and then five digits, and so forth at increasing series. If the patient incorrectly repeats a string of digits, then another string of digits at the same series level is repeated. The examiner stops when the patient incorrectly repeats two strings of digits at the same series level. A normal performance is correct recitation of seven (±2) digits, and a patient attaining fewer than five digits may have a significant attentional problem. This task may be performed as a nonverbal sequence span test using visual stimuli. The

BOX 7.1 CLINICAL ATTENTION TASKS

General

1. Ask the patient if he or she feels "foggy" and cloudy versus sharp and clear in thinking
2. Assess overall behavior including presence of myoclonus or tremors
3. Assess conversation, interviewability, and verbal incoherence
4. Note distractibility on scale of 1–5

Serial Recitation Tasks

1. Digit Span Test
2. Nonverbal Sequence Span Test
3. Backward Digit Span
4. Serial 7s and Serial 3s Tests
5. "World" backward
6. Months (or weekdays) backward
7. Auditory Letter Span
8. Serially Order Digits
9. Modified Clinical N-Back Test
10. Paced Auditory Serial Addition Test

Continuous Performance Tasks

1. Repetitive Tapping Task
2. "A" Cross-Out Test
3. Figure Cancellation Test
4. Trailmaking Test, Part A
5. Computerized Timed Tasks

Alternate Response Tasks, Overlap With Executive Functions; see Chapter 13

1. Alternate Tapping Task
2. Go-No-Go Test
3. Anti-Saccades Task
4. Trailmaking Test, Part B
5. Digit Symbol and Symbol Digit Substitutions Tasks

Spatial Attention Tasks, Overlap With Visuospatial Functions; see Chapter 10

1. Hemispatial and Neglect Testing
2. Balint syndrome, optic ataxia, and oculomotor apraxia

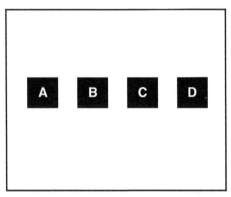

Fig. 7.3 Nonverbal sequence span test. The examiner instructs the patient to repeat a tapping sequence beginning with a sequence of three or four and escalating until patient misses two at a single level. There may or may not be accompanying verbal commands or responses (e.g., "A-D-C-A", etc.).

examiner asks the patient to serially tap four squares or blocks in the same sequence as tapped by the examiner (Fig. 7.3). The test can be done with or without verbal input from the examiner or verbal responses from the patient.

The serial recitation tasks also include reversal tasks in which the patient recites digits in reverse order, the spelling of a word such as *world* backward, or the results of subtracting by ones, threes, or sevens from a predetermined number. In the backward digit span, the patient repeats digits, beginning with the last number and in reverse order to the first number. The instructions and methodology are the same as for the forward digit span with the examiner continuing until the patient incorrectly repeats two strings of digits backward at the same series level. A normal performance is correct backward recitation of five (±2) digits, and a patient failing at three or fewer digits may have a significant attentional problem. A more difficult serial recitation is the serial 7s test. The examiner asks the patient to subtract by 7 beginning with the number 100, for example, 93, 86, 79, 72, 65, et cetera. The number of errors are the number of incorrect subtractions; if the patient makes an incorrect subtraction at one level, the examiner corrects the patient and instructs the patient to continue subtracting from the corrected number. Alternatively, the subsequent "correct" subtractions are determined from the incorrect number, that is, if the patient subtracts 7 from 100 as 94, then the subsequent correct subtraction is 87 and not 86. Clearly, mathematical competence is required for this task, but an alert patient should be able to get three or more subtractions in a row. If serial 7s is too difficult, the examiner may do the serial 3s test, that is, subtract by 3s beginning with the number 20. Another common serial reversal task is spelling a word, such as "world," backward. In contrast to the serial subtraction tasks, the word backward tasks are best scored by "error of place," that is, a correct performance would require a "d" in the first place, an "l" in the second, and so on. For example, the score for a response of "d-r-l-o-w" is 3 as the "r" and "l" are absent or in the wrong place, and the score for a response of "d-o-w" is 1. Additional reversal tasks include the months of the year in reverse order beginning with December and reciting the days of the week backward. The item is missed if it is absent or if it is in the wrong sequence.

The examiner can escalate the level of difficulty of these serial recitation tasks with three techniques. First, the examiner can use an auditory letter span rather than a digit span. The auditory letter span can be forward or backward. Repeating back a series of random letters is harder for most people than is repeating back a series of digits. Second, the examiner can ask the patient to serially order digits by asking the patient to reorder a forward digit span in an ascending order from smallest to largest. For example, if given the series "2-1-3," the correct answer would be "1-2-3." Most people can serially order four or more digits. Third, the examiner can do a modified clinical version of the "N-back" in which the examiner recites a long series of digits and, when the examiner stops, the patient must say the next to last digit in the sequence ("N-1"). The value of this test is that it can be easily escalated in difficulty to N-2, N-3, and so on. Most people have difficulty beyond this level. Finally, there is a bedside version of the difficult Paced Auditory Serial Addition Test (PASAT). The PASAT requires the addition of the last numbers in a sequence, and it can be administered as cumulative addition (adding the last number to the prior sum) or simply adding the last two, three, or more numbers. This test is rarely done at the bedside as it is quite challenging for most people.

Continuous Performance Tasks. These tasks are useful for sustained attention or vigilance. Continuous performance tasks include a simple motor repetitive tapping task in which the patient must keep tapping an index finger on a table until the examiner instructs the patient to stop. Another continuous performance task is the "A" Cross-Out Test, in which the patient must indicate the letter "A" among random letters. In the "A test," the examiner recites a list of 30 or more letters, one per second, and instructs the patient to tap on a table only when they hear the letter "A." An abnormal performance includes any errors of omission in which the patient fails to tap for an "A," or errors of commission in which the patient taps for a letter other than "A." This test can also be done visually by asking the patient to cross out the letter "A" in a written paragraph or on a piece of paper with random letters scattered on the page (Fig. 7.4). Alternatively, the patient can cross out every instance of a particular letter in a magazine or newspaper paragraph. More than a single omission in 60 seconds suggests a disturbance in sustained attention. Harder versions of this continuous performance measure involve indicating a target letter whenever it appears in a specific sequence, for example, "A" only when followed by "B" or crossing out whole words that have a certain letter.

Other related continuous performance tests overlap with other cognitive functions. Visual search tasks, which overlap with visuospatial processing, may be administered timed or untimed and involve searching for a letter, figure, or drawing on a piece of paper (Fig. 7.5). Alternatively, the examiner may simply recreate a similar visual search cancellation task on a piece of paper by randomly placing target letters or figures among nontarget ones on a piece of paper and asking the patient to mark the targets. There should

BEIFHEHFEGICHEICBDACHFBEDACDAFCIHCFEBAFEACFCHBDCFGHE
CAHEFACDCFEHEFCADEHAEIEGDEGHBCAGCIEHCIEFHICDBCGFDEBA
EBCAFCBEHFAEFEGCHGDEHBAEGDACHEBAEDGCDAFGBIFEADCBEACG

CDGAACHEFBCAFEABFCEDEFCGACBEDCFAHEHEFGICHBIEBCAHCDEFB
ACBCGBIEHACAFCICABEGFVEFAEABGCGFACDBEBCHFEADHCAIEFEG
EDHBCADGEADFEBEIGAGGEDACECEDCABAEFBCHDACGVEHCDFEHAIE

Fig. 7.4 "A" cross-out test. The examiner asks the patient to cross-out every letter "A" in the sample. The examiner determines errors or omission and commission.

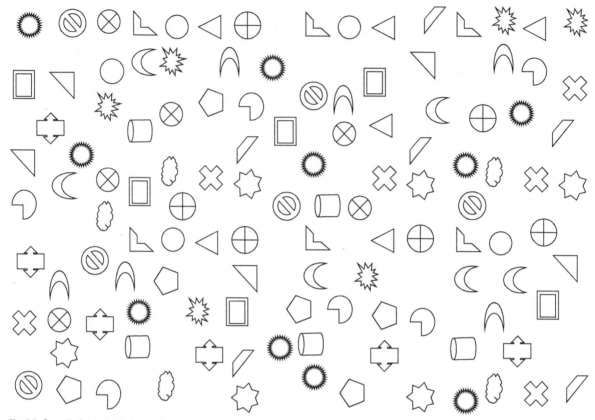

Fig. 7.5 Cancellation task. The instructions are to circle all the figures ⬤ that appear on the form. Score 10/124.

be at least 60 stimuli and 10% targets, and the patient should be able to locate all of them. Another important timed visual search test, which also overlaps with executive functions, is the Trailmaking A Test (Fig. 7.6). The patient must draw a line connecting 25 randomly arrayed numbered circles in ascending numerical order (1-2-3, etc.). After a practice sample, the examiner tells the patient to go as fast as possible without lifting the pencil or pen, points out errors as they occur so that the patient can correct them, and times the overall performance. On the standard timed version, which also reflects psychomotor speed, an average completion time is less than 30 seconds and an impaired completion time is greater than approximately 78 seconds. The examiner can give a version of the Trailmaking A Test in an untimed version to assess strictly for errors (as is done in the Montreal Cognitive Assessment). Although computerized versions of these tests are not routine in clinic or at the bedside, computerized versions easily provide scored results and measures of psychomotor speed (Chapter 18). Finally, another group of mental control tasks, the alternating sequence tasks, greatly overlap with executive operations and the assessment of response inhibition. These tasks are introduced in Chapter 5 and further discussed in Chapter 13.

PSYCHOMOTOR SPEED

Psychomotor speed is one of the most important cognitive functions but surprisingly infrequently assessed. This cognitive function varies greatly from individual differences and the patient's state on testing. The use of timed tasks, preferably computerized, would be the best measures, but many things can be done at the bedside or in clinic. The observation of overall speed of movements and latency of responsiveness are

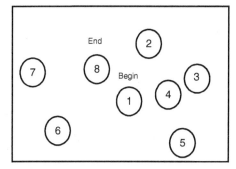

PRACTICE CONNECTING THE NUMBERS: Draw a line from 1 on up

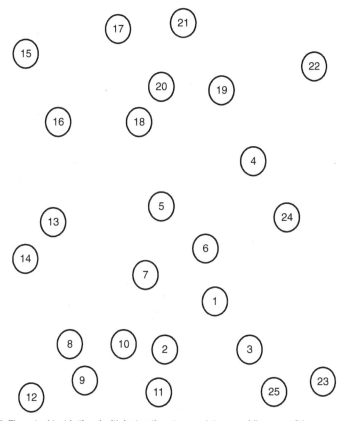

Fig. 7.6 Trailmaking A. The actual test is timed with instructions to complete as rapidly as possible.

obvious first steps in assessing psychomotor speed. Other than direct observation, changes in psychomotor speed are reflected in the patient's overall physical activity and movements. Abrupt or rapid movements, fidgetiness, or brisk gestures and pressure of speech all reflect increased psychomotor speed, and bradykinesia, delayed thoughts or speech, and slowed verbal output

all reflect decreased psychomotor speed. Two easy bedside tests are having the patient count from one as fast as possible and recording the number reached in 10 seconds, or asking the patient to recite the alphabet, or write it in uppercase letters, as fast as possible. The written alphabet should take the patient 30 seconds or less to accomplish. Another timed test is to have the patient draw lines between a series of three to five dots as rapidly as possible. Patients may also grasp a measuring pole at the bottom, let it go, and then grasp it as fast as possible before it falls. The distance between the original and final grasp reflects reaction time. Routine finger tapping is also indicative of psychomotor speed and should be tested with both the left and right index finger for approximately 10 seconds each. A modification of this requires the patient to perform a repetitive movement with the opposite hand, such as supination and pronation, while having them finger tap with the other hand. As noted, the Trailmaking A is a timed test that can give a more precise measure of psychomotor speed. Ultimately, computerized tests can yield the most precise measures of psychomotor speed, both decision times and motor reaction times (see Chapter 18).

ORIENTATION

On assessing orientation, the examiner should be prepared to prevent patients from quickly referring to their watch or to a wall calendar or from turning and asking caregivers or family for the answers. Patients may be temporally disoriented to day of the week, date, month, year, season, and current time. Ask the patient to tell you what time it is at the present moment. Normal subjects are orientated to within four hours of the time, three days of the date, and two days of the week, but they should know the month and year. Patients should not be disoriented to place, but they may be off on the floor or ward if they are hospitalized or the city/location if they were taken there without their full awareness. They should know the state and their city or residence. In addition to time and place, the examiner probes for orientation to their current situation and the reason for the clinic or hospital contact.

Clinical Implications

Disturbed states of arousal, from lethargy to coma, have varied causes ranging from structural neurological lesions to toxic-metabolic disturbances. Depressed arousal suggests a disturbance involving either the brain stem or the neocortex of both hemispheres. Disorders of arousal from brain stem dysfunction usually have a neurological cause, such as strokes, tumors, or other focal lesions of the brain stem, or from pressure on the brain stem from supratentorial mass lesions and increased intracranial pressure, herniation syndromes, or cerebral edema. In contrast, disorders of arousal from bihemispheric cortical dysfunction often have a toxic-metabolic cause, such as drug overdose, hypoxia, alcohol abuse, major organ insufficiency, sepsis, and many others.

Coma-like states result from contained damage to the brain, either both cortices or the upper brain stem and mesial frontal regions. A vegetative state is a coma-like state from bihemispheric cortical damage, most commonly due to anoxic encephalopathy, with the retention of brain stem function, most notably sleep-wake cycles. It is critical to distinguish vegetative state, which may be "persistent" after 4 weeks and "permanent" after 6 months, from the minimal conscious state in which the patient retains some residual, albeit inconsistent, responsiveness to stimulation indicating partial preservation of conscious awareness. A major distinguishing feature between vegetative state and minimal consciousness is the presence of purposeful eye movements, such as visual fixation and pursuit, evident at some point in time among patients with the minimally conscious state. They are essentially wakeful states with minimal spontaneous or reactive speech and movement and an indifference to pain, thirst, and hunger. Akinetic mute and coma vigil states are related disorders of arousal from midbrain-diencephalic and medial frontal lesions, respectively. Both have retained eye fixation and pursuit and rare but definite verbal and motor responses or spontaneous behaviors. They differ in that coma vigil patients tend to maintain their eyes open, giving an appearance of a continuously alert state. The "apathetic" akinetic mute state follows lesions that interrupt the ARAS but not the corticospinal or corticobulbar tracts, and the more alert appearing coma vigil state may be associated with similar septal-frontal lobe lesions. Finally, locked-in syndrome is a unique disorder of brain stem paralysis (usually dorsal pontine lesions) that may be confused with decreased states of arousal. Patients who have locked-in syndrome, who are unable to speak or move due to motor paralysis, can communicate through eye blinks and, when preserved, eye movements.

Other psychomotor disorders, such as apathy, abulia, and catatonia, suggests disturbances or arousal but are actually disturbances of motivation, hence they are briefly discussed here and in Chapter 14. In addition to psychiatric conditions such as depression, clinicians must consider neurological etiologies in these disorders because they may be symptoms of dementia, particularly if frontally predominant. Apathy is prominently decreased emotional reactivity and interests, which results in decreased initiation and maintenance of overt behavior. In contrast, abulia is a primary absence of "initiative" and involves profoundly decreased motor initiation of purposeful and spontaneous speech and movements without a primary decreased emotional reactivity. Clinically, it is difficult to distinguish abulia from apathy, but when distinguished, abulia usually indicates bifrontal disease with absent productive behavior. Catatonia are inhibitory or excitatory psychogenic motor behaviors, which may include mutism, posturing, waxy flexibility (catalepsy), and stereotypical movements. Inhibitory catatonic symptoms include unresponsiveness to verbal and physical stimuli, mutism, the assumption of an inappropriate or bizarre posture for a long period of time, and catalepsy or the maintenance of a body position into which they are placed.

Many neurological disorders affect psychomotor speed, particularly those involving the basal ganglia or the frontal-subcortical white matter tracts. Some of these disorders produce parkinsonism with bradyphrenia and bradykinesia. Others produce frontal apathetic or abulic states with associated increased latency of responsiveness or slowed thought and action. A common error in mental status evaluations is to misinterpret all psychomotor retardation as depression when, in fact, it is one of these conditions. Additional considerations include medical conditions such as hypothyroidism and the effects of sedative or tranquilizing medications.

Finally, and perhaps most important from a clinical point of view, the most common disorders affecting fundamental functions affect attention and lead to delirium (discussed in Chapter 3). The polysynaptic and distributed neuroanatomy for attention is not only vulnerable to many toxic-metabolic disturbances, but also to psychological disturbances, physiological changes such as poor sleep or fatigue, or the effects of medications. Patients may experience a range of attentional difficulty, from mild problems concentrating, mild forgetfulness, inefficient retrieval of information when needed, all the way to the full delirium syndrome. In addition to delirium, there are other specific disturbances of attention including hemispatial neglect (see Chapter 10) and attention deficit hyperactivity disorder. This later condition is more of a disturbance of the executive control of attention rather than of basic attention itself.

Conclusions

Fundamental functions are necessary to higher cognition. Although arousal may not be comprised in most patients requiring mental status evaluation, it is important to consider in patients who may be fluctuating in alertness, such as patients with delirium, encephalopathies, or dementia with Lewy bodies. Attention and mental control are processes that mediate memory, language, and other abilities and are easily disturbed from medical conditions, physiological changes, or medications. A completely accurate assessment of memory, for example, is not possible if the patient is inattentive. Once the mental status examiner has concluded that fundamental functions are sufficiently intact, the examiner is ready to undertake an evaluation of instrumental cognition.

Chapter 8

Language and Speech

Language is the usual "medium" for communication during mental status assessment. Like fundamental functions, the examiner must assess language early as disturbances can affect the rest of the examination. The first consideration is that language and speech are not the same. Language is the brain's use of symbols for communication, and speech is the verbal motor expression of language. By this definition, language includes all symbolic communication whether spoken or written, sign language or Braille, or codes such as Morse Code or musical notation, and others. Speech, in contrast, is restricted to the verbal modality.

To assess language, the examiner must divide language functions into their components. The most basic division is by spoken or written modality, hence this chapter is organized into Part 1 Spoken Language and Speech and Part 2 Written Language and Reading. Within these divisions, language testing includes encoding outgoing sequences of symbols (fluency, repetition, naming) and decoding incoming symbols (comprehension). Additional important aspects of the language examination focus on the association of language symbols with their meanings (semantics), prosody or the intonation of verbal output, the occurrence of paraphasic or word errors, and the evaluation of motor speech.

The neural network subserving language function is a large system involving distributed regions and circuits. Despite their neuroanatomic impression, the classical modular centers and their disconnections remain useful for clinically characterizing language disorders if they are conceived as "hubs" of distributed neural networks. The classical model, known as the Wernicke-Lichtheim-Geschwind Model, focuses language functions around the perisylvian region of the left hemisphere (Fig. 8.1). This model is anchored anteriorly in the Broca area in the inferior frontal region for production (fluency) and syntax (rules for combining words into clauses or phrases), and posteriorly in

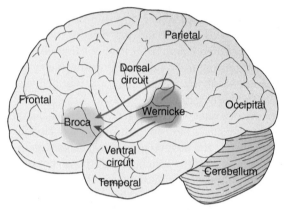

Fig. 8.1 The left perisylvian language circuit.

the Wernicke area in the superior temporal cortex for comprehension of phonemes (units of sound of a language) and facilitation of their semantic connections. Connections between the two travel along a dorsal, word sound or phonological circuit and along a ventral, word meaning or semantic circuit.

Part 1. Spoken Language and Speech

Aphasia (or "dysphasia") is the loss or impairment of language caused by brain damage. With aphasia, there is a loss of ability to produce and/or understand written and/or spoken language. The aphasic syndromes are predominantly fluent versus nonfluent, which is a better dichotomy than "expressive" versus "receptive," as all language impairments have an expressive component. The examiner further characterizes the aphasic syndromes in terms of the ability to comprehend, repeat, and name. These four characteristics—fluency, comprehension, repetition, naming—are the key to an aphasia examination, particularly for spoken language. Moreover, all those with aphasia have, to varying degrees, disturbances of reading and writing. In fact, disturbances in writing, in particular, is one way to assure the presence of an aphasia, rather than a primary speech problem.

Before describing the examinations there are some special issues to consider. First are differences depending on the hemispheric "dominance" of the individual. Left-hemisphere language dominance is present in strongly right-handed people, or approximately 90% of individuals. Those with left-handedness or a family history of left-handedness have less hemispheric specialization for language with more bilateral representation in the brain, particularly for more posterior language functions. Because of their greater bilaterality of language, compared with strong lateralized right-handers, left-handers who are language-impaired are less likely to fit into typical aphasia syndromes and more likely to have an initial aphasia with a better recovery. The incidence of true right-hemisphere "crossed-aphasia" in strongly lateralized right-handers is actually quite small. A further special consideration is the presence of bilingualism or multilingualism. Individuals who speak more than one language have different lexicons (vocabularies): "L1" for the first language, which is acquired directly from concepts, and "L2", which is most commonly a later, sequentially learned language that may be acquired by translational equivalents from L1. Aphasic disorders in these patients may result in differential patterns or impairment and recovery, with L1 generally being the more robust.

SPOKEN LANGUAGE EXAMINATION

The examiner systematically evaluates the four basic elements of the spoken language examination: fluency, comprehension, repetition, and naming. The examination begins with determining the presence of elements of nonfluency. As part of the "spontaneous fluency" determination, the examiner also listens for prosody, or intonation and rhythm, and lexical stress. Testing "verbal fluency," or word-list generation, further clarifies overall language fluency ability. The language examination continues with an assessment of auditory comprehension of both words and sentences. The examiner also listens for linguistic content and the presence of paraphasias or word errors. The spoken language examiner proceeds to an evaluation of the patient's ability to repeat sentences and to name on confrontation a series of items, pictures, or drawings. Finally, the language examination is not complete without additionally assessing for speech disorders. Other related aspects, such the nonlinguistic content of verbal output and pragmatics or the effects of context, are usually manifestations of thought processes as discussed in Chapter 14.

Fluency. Language fluency is the ability to produce words, phrases, and sentences proficiently and smoothly. It is initially assessed qualitatively by listening to the patient's spontaneous speech and discourse. The best way to elicit this is with open-ended questions: "Tell me why you are seeing a doctor?" "What brought you to this clinic visit?" "Tell me about yourself, your family, and what kind of work you have done." The examiner may also have the patient describe an activity or a picture, such as the "Cookie Theft" picture from the *Boston Diagnostic Aphasia Examination* (Fig. 8.2). During this period, the examiner listens for the main elements of nonfluency.

Nonfluent speech has at least four elements (Table 8.1). First, there is sparse output, with a decreased number of words per minute (<50) and shortened phrases, typically less than four or five words. Decreased words/minute or slow verbal output are the most sensitive, but least specific, of the characteristics of dysfluency, and can result from many causes, including a simple reticence to speak. The decreased length of phrases is more specific for dysfluency and is often quantified as mean length of utterance, or the number of morphemes between a stretch of spoken language preceded and followed by silence. Even mean length of utterance, however, may vary considerably in a given patient depending on the emotional valence and complexity of the conversational topic. In addition to sparse output, nonfluent patients have an abnormal flow of speech, with frequent pauses, often to search for words, false starts and hesitations, as well as effortfulness with difficulty in word initiation, sometimes evident as an explosive onset to a word.

Nonfluent aphasics may still successfully convey information with a limited number of nouns, verbs, or substantive words. An example of the nonfluent, but understandable, response of a patient with Broca aphasia when asked why she had come to see the doctor: *"Ah, Ah, today, brought today, Ah, father prove today…come hospital for talking…bad talking…doctors for talking…words hard speeches."*

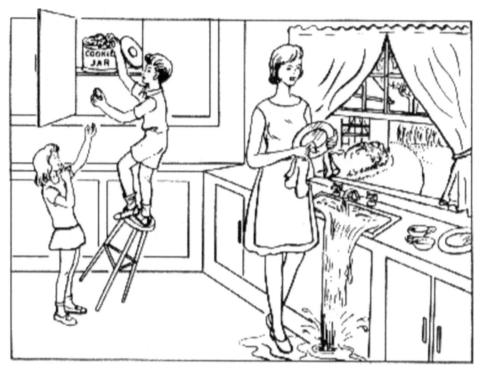

Fig. 8.2   Cookie theft picture. (Reproduced with permission from Kaplan E, Goodglass H, Barresi B. *Boston Diagnostic Aphasia Examination.* 3rd ed. Austin, TX: Psychological Assessment Resources; 2001.)

TABLE 8.1   Elements of Nonfluency
1. Quantity of verbal output
a. Decreased spontaneous words/minute (abnormal about <50; normal usually 100+) or slow output (further test for decreased word-list generation)
b. Short phrase length (abnormal 1.2; normal 4+)
2. Flow of verbal output
a. Frequent word-finding pauses, halts, choppiness, or word searches
b. Labored word production with effort/struggle, delay/hesitancy, or explosive onset/breakthrough
3. Grammar (i.e., syntax)
a. Agrammatism; both expression and comprehension of grammar (see Table 8.3)
b. Telegraphic sounding output lacking functor or grammatical words
4. Speech or word sounds
a. Phonemic paraphasic or literal errors and impaired articulatory agility
b. Abnormal lexical stress (accented syllable) and prosody (intonation, rhythm)

Agrammatism is the most specific characteristic of nonfluency, and often the most difficult to evaluate (Table 8.2). It consist of simplified sentences, at least partially stripped of the elements that serve primarily to bind the sentence together. These elements are grammatical function or "functor" words (e.g., prepositions, articles, conjunctions) and grammatical morphemes (units of meaning) or inflections (e.g., "ed" for past events, "s" for plurals, "ly" for adjectives). The resulting oversimplified sentences, often confined to a noun-verb or verb-object phrases, are "telegraphic." Other common agrammatic errors include errors of tense, of subject-verb agreement, and of word order. It is important to appreciate that in some patients agrammatism is primarily evident, not in verbal output, but in the impairment of the *comprehension* of the syntax of phrases (see auditory comprehension section).

Nonfluency also includes speech or word sound errors, especially at the phoneme level, the smallest unit of sound of a language. These primarily involve the substitution of one phoneme for another (phonemic or "literal" paraphasias). For example, on attempting

TABLE 8.2 Elements of Agrammatism

1. Difficulty with grammatical elements for syntax (sentence construction)

   a. Loss of function ("functor") words (articles, preposition, auxiliary verbs, conjunctions, pronouns, "Wh" question words)

   b. Loss of inflection morphemes ("s" for plural, tense, e.g., "ed" for past tense, gender agreement, comparisons agreement)

2. Oversimplification ("telegraphic" sounding)

   a. Preference for substantive words (nouns, verbs, adjectives, adverbs)

   b. Decreased embedding and encoding of clauses, phrases

3. Abnormal word stream

   a. Abnormal word order, such as verb-noun agreement or other word concordance

   b. Broken up and short phrases

4. Decreased syntactical comprehension

   a. Problems understanding complex sentences with noncanonical and passive grammar (e.g., The lion was killed by the tiger.)

   b. Cannot use sentence structure to derive sentence meaning; loss of ability to map syntactic structure onto semantic structure

to say "artery," patients may say "argery" or "artory." In addition, they may simply omit a syllable, for example, "arty," or missequence them, for example, "erarty." Nonfluent aphasia is often accompanied by further phonemic distortions and substitutions due to "apraxia of speech," or problems with the motor planning of phonemes. Apraxia of speech is a breakdown in the ability to coordinate the articulatory movements required for comprehensible speech and is often tested as part of the speech examination as described later. Further aspects of both nonfluency and apraxia of speech is the presence of articulatory error groping or attempts at self-correction.

Prosody. Nonfluency includes changes in prosody or intonation at the sentence level and in the stressed or accented syllable in a word (lexical stress). In addition to listening for changes in pitch (rising or falling) and stress (often increased loudness), further screening for prosody can be done with repetition of sentences in different tones and asking the patient to interpret them and then to repeat them with a certain meaning. The examiner usually combines specific testing for prosodic fluency with testing for prosodic comprehension. For example, start by saying the following sentence repeated with different emphasis on the bolded and italicized word and asking the patient the meaning: ____ I *AM* going to the other movies. ____ I am going to the *OTHER* movies. ____ *I* am going to the other movies. ____ I am going to the other *MOVIES*. ____ I am *GOING* to the other movies. For prosodic fluency, ask the patient to say the same sentence with determination, sadness, anticipation, emphasis on himself/herself, and type of place or action.

Word-List Generation (verbal fluency). The inability to produce words is a very sensitive measure of language dysfunction. Although not specific for fluency, word-list generation provides a means for rapid assessment of word production, word access, and word knowledge (semantic memory). First, ask the patient to do a category word generation task. For example, ask the patient to generate a list of as many animals as possible (or other category of items such as grocery items, articles of clothing, cities, colors) in one minute. *"I am going to ask you to name as many animals as you can in one minute. An animal is any living thing that is not a plant. Please wait until we are ready to begin."* Do not count proper nouns, plurals, and repetitions in the total correct, but do count word variations or subcategory items (e.g., include both dogs and beagles). Do not suggest subcategories (e.g., "zoo animals"). Normal subjects can list 18 ± 6 animals per minute without cueing. Second, ask the patient to generate as many words as possible that begin with the letter "F" (or it can be "A" or "S," the other letters used in the Controlled Oral Word Association Test). These letters reflect word frequencies in English and vary with the language tested (e.g., in Spanish the letters would be "P," "M," and "R"). *"I will say a letter of the alphabet. Then I want you to give me as many English words that begin with that letter as quickly as possible. I do not want you to use words that are proper names. Also do not use the same word again with a different ending such as 'eat' and 'eating' or 'sixty' and 'sixty-one.' Begin when I say the letter."* Do not count close word variations of the same word, such as "four," "foursome," "fourfold," "fourth," but do count word variations with a different meaning (e.g., "fourteen"). Normal subjects can list 15 ± 5 words per minute for each letter.

Auditory Comprehension. The examination of sentence comprehension involves a series of tasks of increasing difficulty. First, there are simple axial and one-step commands, for example, "close your eyes" and "touch your nose," followed by "show me two fingers" and "point to the floor." In evaluation of auditory comprehension with pointing commands, remember that motor weakness or apraxia may interfere with pointing. Second, ask yes-or-no questions, for example, "Are you sitting down?" "Is a hammer good for cutting wood?" "Does March come before April?" "Will a stone float in water?" Third are sequential commands, for example, "Touch your nose and then your chin," "Point to your right knee and then your left shoulder," "First point to the ceiling and then to the door," "Point to the chair, then the table, and then the door." Commands that require a body part to cross the midline are more complex than those that do not, and the handling of sequences also challenges the ability to maintain a serial order. Finally, evaluate complex grammatical sentence comprehension, for example, "If the lion was killed by the tiger, which animal is dead?" "If we were in a crowd of people and I said, 'there's my wife's brother,' would I be pointing to a man and a woman?"

The isolated impairment of comprehension of grammatical sentences suggests agrammatism, as occurs in Broca aphasia (see prior fluency section). One method to test this is with noncanonical sentence comprehension. Noncanonical examples are those with a passive voice (e.g., The cat is chased by the dog) or a clause that relates to an object (e.g., Pete saw the cat who the dog is chasing) or an object-extracted wh- question (e.g., Who is the dog chasing?). The examiner may further test the ability to comprehend grammatical relations with a series of commands using common items arrayed on a table, such as pens, keys, or coins. This is patterned after the Token Test, which presents 20 tokens of 5 colors each having 2 shapes and 2 sizes and giving commands such as "put the red circle on the green rectangle" or "before touching the yellow circle, pick up the red rectangle." Using readily available items in the environment, the examiner can ask the patient to perform a similar series of commands of increasing complexity (Table 8.3).

Additional observations of impaired auditory comprehension may be evident on simply listening and observing. In contrast to nonfluent aphasics, who

TABLE 8.3   **Modified Bedside Token Test**
Using pen, pencil, penny, and nickel or similar available objects.
1. Put the pencil on the penny.
2. Touch the nickel with the pen.
3. Touch the penny and the pencil. Pick up the nickel or the pen.
4. Put the penny between the pen and the pencil.
5. Point to the pen after pointing to the pencil.
6. Except for the penny, touch the pen.
7. Instead of the pencil, take the nickel.
8. Together with the penny, take the pencil.
9. After picking up the pen, touch the penny.
10. Before touching the nickel, pick up the pencil.

successfully convey information with a limited number of nouns or verbs, those with fluent aphasia may produce long, effortless, seemingly empty sentences. The linguistic content of spoken output may sound devoid of meaning or message consequent to paraphasias and neologisms (see later text); ambiguous, indefinite, or imprecise pronouns or object names; and a lack of clarity. Moreover, the pragmatics, or context of language, such as gestures and facial expressions, may not be congruent with verbal output.

In addition to sentence comprehension, the examiner may need to test the ability to comprehend individual words. Problems with word comprehension may be initially evident on confrontational naming tasks. When this occurs, testing should be followed-up with word recognition tests. The simplest procedure is to return to misnamed items from the prior naming test, give the patient the name, and ask him/her to identify them. They can do this by either pointing to the object or picture or by identifying (defining or describing) the item. This "two-way" naming deficit, in which the patient can neither name an item nor point to it on command (despite being able to repeat the name), represent abnormal word comprehension or "semantic anomia." Additional word comprehension tests include simply presenting a series of pictures, or a plate with multiple illustrated items, and asking him/her to point to the named item. Finally, testing for semantic anomia is basically the same as testing semantic memory with tests of semantic matching, associations, and sorting (see Chapter 9).

Paraphasias. Whereas nonfluent speech has sound-based paraphasias ("literal" or sound-based with phonemic substitutions), those with fluent aphasia have both literal and whole-word paraphasias. Word paraphasias are either meaning-related to the target word (semantic paraphasias) or totally unrelated real words (verbal paraphasias). They may also make totally new and novel words (neologisms). Fluent aphasics are often unaware of these paraphasic errors. Patients with fluent aphasia such as Wernicke aphasia may have a loquacious "empty" speech with so many unintelligible paraphasias and neologisms that it is impossible to follow their verbal output; this is termed "jargon aphasia."

Repetition. The examiner asks the patient to repeat digits, multisyllabic words, phrases, and sentences. Note that tests of repetition do not include "serial speech," which are overlearned sequences (such as counting 1, 2, 3, etc., or the reciting the alphabet) as serial speech may be preserved in all but the most severe aphasics. Begin with single word or short phrase repetitions, for example, "constitutional," "Mississippi River," "hopping hippopotamus," or "Methodist Episcopal," then proceed to longer utterances and sentences. *"I'm going to read some sentences to you. Please repeat them back to me exactly the way I say it."* Examples include "No ifs, ands, or buts," "they heard him speak on the radio last night," "the truck rolled over the stone bridge," and "the quick brown fox jumped over the lazy dog." The examiner may allow one reattempt at repetition of the sentence if the patient requests it. If the patient succeeds, the examiner may ask for repetition of more difficult sentences with many functor words, for example, "if he comes soon, we will all go away with him." Failure to repeat may be through omission, substitution, altered order, mispronunciation, or limitation of the span level.

Naming. Naming difficulty is evident from word finding pauses, the use of descriptions in lieu of names, and circumlocutions around a missing word. The examiner tests word production primarily with confrontational naming but may also use other methods such as "name-by-definition." In confrontational naming, the examiner should test a range of common and uncommon words across different word frequencies. The examiner can present at least six readily accessible items for naming; for example, key, ring, button, collar, nose, chin; and six lower frequency items, for example, earlobe, eye lashes,

lapel, shoelaces, sole or heel of shoe, and watch band, crystal or crystal. Words used less frequently, such as parts of objects, are more difficult for the patient with aphasia to retrieve and constitute a more sensitive test for anomia. Photographs or line drawings are also good for confrontational naming and permit easier testing of verbs. In addition to confrontational naming, the examiner may increase the difficulty of word production tasks by asking the patient to "name-by-definition," that is, the examiner provides a definition of an object or action, and the patient provides the appropriate name. A rough guide to normal performance on all these tasks involves correctly naming all high frequency items and at least four of six low frequency ones.

Speech Examination. The examiner independently evaluates for apraxia and for dysarthrias during the speech examination. Speech represents the mechanical act of oral expression or the neuromuscular alterations needed to produce oral communication. Testing for apraxia of speech, or disturbed speech programming, involves testing for repetition of polysyllabic phrases. The examiner asks the patient to repeat each of the syllables, /pa/, /ta/, and /ka/, individually over and over again as quickly as possible (alternating motor rates), and then to repeat the three together in the sequence /pa-ta-ka/ over and over as quickly as possible (sequencing motor rates). An alternative approach is to ask the patient to repeat the words "catastrophe," "artillery," or "articulatory" as many times as possible in 5 or 10 seconds. As noted, patients with apraxia of speech make phonemic errors, which include distortions, additions, repetitions, prolongations, omissions, and substitutions. These errors in apraxia of speech are notoriously inconsistent (Table 8.4). Alternatively, some patients with apraxia of speech have primarily segmented speech with increased pauses between syllables or words.

Dysarthria is the motoric impairment of speech caused by neurological injury. Even though dysarthrias are not strictly a cognitive dysfunction, assessing for them is necessary because they must be distinguished from aphasia or language disorders. Dysarthrias are produced by disturbances in phonation (vocal cord apposition) or voicing (onset timing of vocal cord vibration), articulation (mispronunciations at the oral level), and resonance (air flow through the pharynx). In addition to dysarthrias, speech disorders include hypophonia and festinating speech, dysfluencies such

TABLE 8.4   **Apraxia of Speech**
Impaired planning or programming of movements that prevents accurate production of sounds and syllables across words or within multisyllabic words
1. Slow speech rate; halting, effortful, with false starts and restarts
2. Distorted articulation:
a. Phonemic errors: substitutions, additions, repetitions, prolongations, distortions (predominant in type 1 apraxia of speech)
b. Syllabically segmented speech: increased intersegment lengths between syllables, words, or phrases (predominant in type 2 apraxia of speech)
3. Articulation-trial and error
4. Inconsistency in sound additions, substitutions, distortions
5. Impaired phonemic sequencing:
a. With increasing utterance length, speed, and complexity
b. With sequential motion rates (e.g., "pa-ta-ka" at maximum rates) more than with alternating motion rates (e.g., each individual syllable at maximum rates)
6. Abnormal prosody with equal word stress

as stuttering or stammering (used interchangeably), echolalia (involuntary repetition of the examiner's words), palilalia (repetition of their own words), and logoclonia (repetition of the last syllables) (also see content of speech, Chapter 14).

The evaluation for dysarthrias is usually distinct from the language fluency examination. A fairly thorough evaluation of the mechanics of vocal output can be performed rather simply. First, listen to the patient's speech for loudness, vocal cord function (strained if too apposed, breathy if too open), resonance or nasality from escape of air, articulatory disturbances from labial or lingual mispronunciation, and evidence of slurring from cerebellar system dysfunction. In addition, the examiner may ask the patient to maintain an "aah" sound loudly and for as long as possible to assess respiratory and vocal power. For more precise assessment or "voicing," or voice onset time of consonant vibration at the vocal cords, the examiner has the patient say the unvoiced syllables /pa/, /ta/, and /ka/ (similar to apraxia of speech evaluation) compared with the corresponding voiced syllables /ba/, /da/, and /ga/. These simple acts will demonstrate most motor speech disorders, and various combinations of disturbance of these qualities indicate anatomically specific varieties of dysarthria.

Part 2. Written Language and Reading

Alexia (used here interchangeably with "dyslexia") is the loss or impairment of the ability to comprehend written language. Disturbances of reading are either peripheral, that is, outside of the brain's language areas with decreased access to reading routes, or central, involving the left perisylvian language system itself (Fig. 8.3). The peripheral alexias include alexia without writing difficulty ("alexia without agraphia"), neglect alexia (hemispatial), attentional alexia (interference from the presence of other letters or words), and apperceptive alexia (decreased whole-word or phrase perception). The central alexias result from disturbances of the direct and indirect reading routes and include surface,

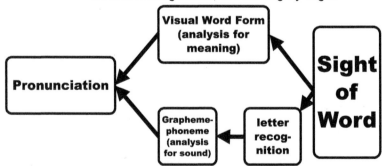

Direct Reading Route, or Reading-by-Sight

Indirect Reading Route, or Reading-by-Sound

Fig. 8.3   Written language and reading: dual-route reading model.

phonological, and deep dyslexia. Surface dyslexia is a disturbance of the direct ("whole word" or reading-by-sight) route, and phonological dyslexia is a disturbance of the indirect ("grapheme-to-phoneme" or reading-by-sound) route. Deep dyslexia is a severe impairment in both routes with reading consigned to the right hemisphere as evidenced by semantic reading errors.

Writing is disturbed in most of the aphasia syndromes and most of the alexias. Agraphia (or dysgraphia) is the loss or impairment of the ability to communicate in written language. The classification and errors in agraphia typically parallel those for the alexias. The peripheral agraphias include mechanical agraphia (often from apraxia), spatial agraphia, and transitional agraphia (integration of orthographic with graphomotor codes). The central agraphias include surface dysgraphia, phonological dysgraphia, and disorder of spelling assembly or the sequencing of letters. An isolated and probably predominantly translational agraphia, without reading difficulty, usually accompanies acalculia and other elements of Gerstmann syndrome from disturbances in the main reading and writing area in the left angular gyrus (Brodmann area 39), a region that combines perceptual and symbolic input (see Chapter 12).

READING AND WRITING EXAMINATION

Reading. The language examination is not complete without an assessment of the ability to read for comprehension and for pronunciation of words and nonsense pseudowords. The examiner starts by asking the patient to read aloud a short standard paragraph (or, for expediency, a paragraph from a newspaper or magazine). This reading material should be at the eighth grade level. For reading comprehension, the examiner can also ask patients to point to items written on a paper and to perform several written commands comparable to the verbal commands. The examiner first presents a list of written names of objects in the room, such as door, sink, table, window, telephone, and then asks the patient to read them and point to the object. If this is successful, then the examiner presents two or more sentences with commands instructing the patient to do something, for example, "Fold this paper in half and put it on the table," and "point to the source of illumination in this room." Reading comprehension may also be tested with written word-picture matching tests.

The examiner asks the patient to read a few letters then proceeds to have the patient read aloud regular words (usual grapheme-phoneme pronunciation), irregular words (irregular grapheme-phoneme pronunciation), and pseudowords (pronounceable nonsense words). An example of a word reading battery is "mint, blitor, colonel, shout, yacht, flarmic, bouquet, chrome, strotinale, quick, thartrist, pint." When the patient reads aloud, the examiner looks for differential difficulties in the ability to read 1) regularly spelled words (e.g., mint, shout, chrome, quick); 2) irregularly spelled words (e.g., colonel, yacht, bouquet, pint); or 3) pronounceable pseudowords (blitor, flarmic, strotinale, thartrist). The differential impairment in these categories of words or pseudowords differentiates the type of central alexias, including surface dyslexia, phonological dyslexia, and deep dyslexia (defined below). Finally, it is important to test comprehension for words spelled orally, particularly two or more irregular words and pronounceable pseudowords. Peripheral alexias are often able to understand a word that is spelled orally, albeit often slowly, whereas central alexias have difficulty with this task corresponding to their difficulties reading irregular words or pronounceable pseudowords.

Writing. Writing is the most vulnerable language skill and is disturbed almost any time there is a language disorder. Writing should be specially tested in the mental status examination. The ability to produce a signature is not a sufficient test of writing ability. First, the examiner asks the patient to copy single letters and a few printed words. Those with apraxic agraphia and transitional (graphomotor) agraphia may have abnormal copying even at the letter stage with distorted mechanical production. Those with spatial agraphias may have difficulty with features, crowding and spacing, and maintaining horizontal writing. Second, the examiner asks the patient to write a series of words dictated by the examiner. These words can be similar to the ones noted earlier for reading and should include regular words, irregular words, and nonsense pseudowords. Third, the examiner requests the patient to write at least two sentences, one sentence to dictation complete with punctuation and a second sentence composed by the patient. Examples of sentences to dictation are: "The children are the heirs of the earth"; "it is hard to gauge the size of a sieve"; and "the bride was taken down the aisle by the colonel." The examiner can elicit sentences for composition with a command, such as "describe what you did today in a full sentence." In all of these samples, the examiner is evaluating the patient's writing for spelling errors and paragraphic errors (written paraphasias).

CLINICAL IMPLICATIONS

Aphasias. A verbal language disorder may occur from any insult or pathologic process, including dementia, that results in damage or dysfunction of the left perisylvian language zone or surrounding area (Table 8.5). The classic aphasia syndromes of Broca, Wernicke, and conduction aphasias usually occur from dysfunction in the language zone, and the transcortical aphasias usually occur from lesions in the surrounding area outside the perisylvian region. The classical aphasia syndromes and the transcorticals differ in that the transcorticals can still repeat. Otherwise, the main characteristic of Broca and transcortical motor aphasias are nonfluency, and the main characteristic of Wernicke and transcortical sensory aphasias are fluent output with impaired comprehension. Conduction aphasia is a unique language syndrome defined by a relatively isolated impairment in repetition. Furthermore, isolated disturbances of prosody can occur from right-hemispheric abnormalities.

A number of other details distinguish these aphasia syndromes. Broca aphasia results from lesions affecting the left inferior frontal lobe and results in typical nonfluency with sparse output and agrammatism along with impaired repetition and writing. Comprehension, both verbal and written, is relatively spared except for grammatically complex speech. There is often an associated right hemiparesis reflecting injury to contiguous structures in the motor areas. Wernicke aphasia results from lesions affecting the left posterior, superior temporal gyrus and results in fluent, but somewhat "empty," output along with markedly impaired comprehension, both verbal and written. Speech is often voluminous, but meaningless, with a lack of substantive words and many paraphasic errors and neologisms. Repetition and production of written language is similarly impaired. There may not be any motor deficit with this syndrome, but there can be a right superior visual field defect. Global aphasia has the features of both Broca and Wernicke aphasias and includes deficits in all language functions. Transcortical mixed aphasia (otherwise known as "isolation of the speech area") has the features of global aphasia except, like all transcortical aphasias, has relative preservation of repetition.

The examiner needs to consider additional language and language-related syndromes. First, anomia can be the predominant feature of a language disorder. Although anomia is a common feature of most aphasia syndromes, there can be an isolated anomic aphasia from either word production (with intact phonemic cuing and intact word comprehension), word selection (with impaired phonemic cuing but intact word

TABLE 8.5 **The Principle Aphasia Syndromes**						
Aphasia	**Fluency**	**Comprehension**	**Repeat**	**Name**	**Reading Comprehension**	**Writing**
Broca	Abn	Rel Nor	Abn	Abn	Nor or Abn	Abn
Wernicke	Nor, paraphasic	Abn	Abn	Abn	Abn	Abn
Global	Abn	Abn	Abn	Abn	Abn	Abn
Conduction	Nor, paraphasic	Rel Nor	Abn	±Abn	Rel Nor	Abn
Transcortical motor	Abn	Rel Nor	Rel Nor	Abn	Rel Nor	Abn
Transcortical sensory	Nor, echolalic	Abn	Rel Nor	Abn	Abn	Abn
Anomic	Nor	Rel Nor	Nor	Abn	Nor or Abn	Nor or Abn

Abn, Abnormal; *Nor*, normal; *Rel*, relatively.
Adapted from DF Benson. *Aphasia, Alexia, and Agraphia*. New York, NY: Churchill Livingstone; 1979.

comprehension), or semantic difficulty (with impaired word comprehension). "Pure anomia" refers to a word selection anomia due to a disturbance from left hemisphere lesions classically involving the inferior, posterior temporal (Brodmann area 37) region. Second, subcortical aphasias may be due to decreased input to overlying cortex and usually have preserved repetition with initial muteness or hypophonia. Third, there are language-related syndromes with overt impairments in aspects of verbal language despite preservation of the perisylvian language network and the ability to read and write. The two main language-related syndromes are pure word deafness, with inability to comprehend spoken words, and aphemia, or dysfluency limited to speaking. Pure word deafness is a prelanguage disturbance from bilateral or unilateral lesions undercutting the Wernicke area and causing impaired comprehension of speech sounds but not of most nonspeech sounds. Aphemia is a postlanguage disturbance, a variant of apraxia of speech, from lesions typically in or around the Broca area and presenting with speech nonfluency but preserved reading and writing.

Progressive aphasias (Table 8.6). A progressive aphasia can be a manifestation of neurodegenerative disease. Primary progressive aphasia (PPA) and semantic dementia are syndromes that occur in older adults and most commonly represent frontotemporal degeneration or a variant of Alzheimer disease. Progressive nonfluent aphasia (nonfluent/agrammatic variant PPA) results from left frontotemporal atrophy and presents with gradual progression of nonfluency, agrammatism, and articulation difficulty. Most of these patients also have apraxia of speech. Semantic dementia begins with semantic variant PPA from anterior, inferolateral temporal atrophy with loss of the meaning or comprehension of words, often described as a semantic memory problem (See Chapter 9). Indeed, semantic anomia and semantic memory difficulties are the same disturbances of a semantic system that is organized and coordinated from the anterior temporal poles. On reading, these patients also have surface dyslexia. Finally, possibly the most common progressive aphasia is progressive logopenic aphasia (logopenic variant PPA) from posterior temporal-inferior parietal dysfunction most often as a consequence of Alzheimer disease. These patients have impairment of the phonological store, possibly as part of the phonological input lexicon, and cannot repeat long phrases or sentences.

TABLE 8.6 **Primary Progressive Aphasia Clinical Criteria**
Primary Progressive Aphasia: General Criteria
Inclusion criteria 1–2 must be answered positively
1. Most prominent clinical feature is difficulty with language
2. These deficits are the principal cause of impaired daily living activities
3. Aphasia should be the most prominent deficit at symptom onset and for the initial phases of the disease
Exclusion criteria 1–4 must be answered negatively for a primary progressive aphasia diagnosis
1. Pattern of deficits is better accounted for by other neurodegenerative nervous system or medical disorders
2. Cognitive disturbance is better accounted for by a psychiatric diagnosis
3. Prominent initial episodic memory, visual memory, and visuoperceptual impairments
4. Prominent initial behavioral disturbances
Nonfluent/Agrammatic Varian Primary Progressive Aphasia
At least one of the following core features must be present:
1. Agrammatism in language production
2. Effortful, halting speech with inconsistent speech sound errors and distortions (apraxia of speech)
At least 2 of 3 of the following other features must be present:
1. Impaired comprehension of syntactically complex sentences
2. Spared single-word comprehension
3. Spared object knowledge

(continued)

TABLE 8.6 **Primary Progressive Aphasia Clinical Criteria** *(cont'd)*
Semantic Variant Primary Progressive Aphasia
Both of the following core features must be present:
1. Impaired confrontational naming
2. Impaired single-word comprehension
At least 3 of the following other features must be present:
1. Impaired object knowledge, particularly for low-frequency or low-familiarity items
2. Surface dyslexia or dysgraphia
3. Spared repetition
4. Spared speech production (grammar and motor speech)
Logopenic Variant Primary Progressive Aphasia
Both of the following core features must be present:
1. Impaired single-word retrieval in spontaneous speech and naming
2. Impaired repetition of sentences and phrases
At least 3 of the following other features must be present:
1. Speech (phonologic) errors in spontaneous speech and naming
2. Spared single-word comprehension and object knowledge
3. Spared motor speech
4. Absence of frank agrammatism

From Gorno-Tempini ML, et al. Classification of primary progressive aphasia and its variants. *Neurology.* 2011;76:1006-1014.

Patients with logopenic variant PPA additionally have phonemic substitutions (literal paraphasias).

Several unusual and rare language disorders are worth mentioning, as they elicit requests for mental status assessment. First, psychotic patients may have alterations in word usage including malapropisms, neologisms, reiterative speech (palilalia and echolalia), clanging (repeating words based on the word sounds), and rhyming. These manifestations can be so frequent as to constitute an unintelligible "word salad" or "schizophasia" resembling jargon aphasia in Wernicke aphasia. Coprolalia are outbursts of obscenities or curse words not readily under the control of the speaker occurring with Tourette syndrome and psychosis. Second, glossolalia and xenolalia involve speaking in an unusual language. Xenolalia is the sudden acquisition of a foreign language that the person did not speak before, and glossolalia (speaking in tongues) refers to in an unknown or incomprehensible language over which they have no control. Finally, there is the sudden occurrence of a foreign accent with altered pronunciation of spoken vowels and consonants. This "foreign accent syndrome" can be associated with left frontal injury affecting linguistic prosody (timing, rhythm, and intonation) and word stress, and appears related, but not entirely explained by, apraxia of speech. However, there are also patients who have a psychogenic origin to their foreign accent syndrome.

Disorders of Reading and Writing. Although alexias and agraphias most commonly occur with aphasias, they can also occur as isolated disorders (Table 8.7). The classic peripheral alexia is "alexia without agraphia." In this condition, patients are unable to read, but can still write and can understand words spelled aloud. Patients with alexia without agraphia often have a right homonymous hemianopsia, color naming or recognition difficulties, and, occasionally, a visual agnosia. A common cause of this condition is a left posterior cerebral artery distribution stroke involving the left occipital lobe and the adjacent

TABLE 8.7 Important Alexia Syndromes

Alexia without Agraphia

1. Peripheral alexia from decreased visual input for reading
2. Lesion of left occipital lobe plus splenium of corpus callosum
3. Slow, letter-by-letter reading with better oral reading and preserved writing
4. Not influenced by regularity or irregularity of spelling
5. Usually have color anomia (or agnosia) and may have visual agnosia
6. Usually have right homonymous hemianopsia
7. Worse with increasing word length; normal word frequency effect

Surface Dyslexia

1. Disorder of reading-by-sight
2. Lesion at or near the left angular gyrus
3. Predominant difficulty reading irregular words
4. Better with regular and pronounceable nonsense words
5. Regularization errors (read irregular words phonetically)
6. Often associated with semantic dementia or semantic variant primary progressive aphasia
7. Worse with increased word-length; normal word-frequency effect

Phonological Dyslexia

1. Disorder of reading-by-sound
2. Lesion at left supramarginal gyrus
3. Predominant difficulty with pronounceable nonsense words
4. Better with real words
5. Lexicalization errors (read pronounceable pseudowords as if real words)
6. Visually based errors (comb → cord)
7. Worse with decreased word-frequency; normal word-length effect

Deep Dyslexia

1. Disorder of reading-by-sound and reading-by-sight
2. Large left hemisphere lesions
3. Difficulty with regular and irregular words
4. Difficulty with abstract (vs. concrete) words
5. Difficulty with grammatical elements
6. Semantic errors (substitute meaningfully related words, i.e., baby for infant)
7. Decreased word-frequency effect; decreased word-length effect

splenium of the corpus callosum. Essentially, visual information is cutoff from reaching the visual word form and language zones.

According the dual route model of reading (See Fig. 8.3), the central alexias differ depending on involvement of the direct (reading-by-sight) or indirect (reading-by-sound) pathway. In surface dyslexia there is inability to read-by-sight irregularly spelled words (or homophones) but preserved ability to sound them out. The less frequent the irregular word, the more difficult it is read, and they make "regularization" (conversion to phonetically regular words) errors. Patients with surface dyslexia most commonly have anterior temporal disease from semantic dementia (semantic variant PPA). In phonological dyslexia there is inability to read-by-sound pronounceable nonsense words (or unfamiliar, technical, or foreign words) but preserved ability to read-by-sight most real words. The longer the nonsense or unfamiliar word, the more difficult it is to read, and they make "lexicalization" (conversion to real word) errors. Patients with isolated phonological dyslexia most commonly have lesions in the left supramarginal gyrus. In deep dyslexia there is an inability to read by either direct or indirect reading route due to large left hemisphere lesions. These patients can only read through a limited right-hemisphere access to meaning or semantics. Consequently, their limited residual reading output is mostly semantic substitutions for concrete nouns, for example, reading "baby" for "infant."

Conclusions

As this chapter illustrates, the examination of spoken language and written language are among the most important aspects of the neurobehavioral status examination. Knowing how to listen and evaluate language and speech can be critical to the mental status examination, with implications for testing memory, perception, and the other cognitive domains described in subsequent chapters.

Chapter 9

Memory and Semantic Knowledge

Memory is the process of encoding, storing, and retrieving information in the brain. There are many aspects of memory. This chapter is concerned with examining the most clinically important aspects of memory, which are declarative, explicit, or conscious recollections. Patients, families, and clinicians often refer to declarative memory for recent episodic events as "short-term" memory; however, declarative memories are really long-term. Short-term (working) memory has a very different neurobiological meaning as described in this chapter. The term "amnesia," or significant memory loss, most commonly refers to declarative, episodic memory. In addition to episodic memory, this chapter discusses another clinically important form of declarative memory, that for semantic knowledge or facts.

Memory Basics

The creation of memories is a stream that includes sensory registration, short-term/working memory, and long-term storage. The memory stream starts with sensory input and finishes with stored, accessible memory traces or engrams (Fig. 9.1). After an initial brief sensory registration in the sensory organ or point of entry (auditory or echoic 10 s; visual or iconic 500 ms), there follows a period of short-term (working) memory executed in the dorsolateral frontal lobes and related areas. Short-term/working memory involves holding information online for seconds to a minute (usually 20–30 s) if unrehearsed, but much longer if the patient verbally (phonological) or visually (visuospatial) rehearses the material. Short-term/working memory is clinically difficult to differentiate from sustained attention and is usually tested as part of mental control and attentional tests such as the digit span (see Chapter 7). If short-term/working memory is impaired, it is difficult to proceed along the memory stream to the creation of long-term memories.

Long-term memory is the actual encoding and storage of information in the brain and can be either declarative (explicit) or nondeclarative (implicit). Declarative memory is consciously stored and retrieved information that is itself further divided into episodic (context, time, and place dependent) experiences or semantic (context, time, and place independent) facts, which are processed in the limbic and semantic areas, respectively. In comparison, nondeclarative memory includes procedural learning (motor and cognitive skills), which is mediated by the basal ganglia and cerebellum; priming, or the positive influence of a prior exposure on subsequent learning; and classical conditioning, which is facilitated by prefrontal cortex and other structures.

When talking about memory disorders and testing memory, clinicians are primarily concerned with declarative memory loss (circled in Fig. 9.1), often from disease affecting hippocampi or related limbic areas (Fig. 9.2). For testing purposes, these long-term memories may be divisible into those that occurred either in the recent past or the remote past. Recent memory includes the capacity to remember and learn current events and information and to be able to bring it forth after an interval ranging from minutes to days, as distinguished from the inability to retrieve remote information from years past. Episodic or time-tagged recent memory difficulty is the typical memory impairment in mild cognitive impairment, dementia, or amnestic disorders. Much rarer are disorders of semantic memory for time-independent facts/knowledge. The rest of this chapter is concerned with the testing of declarative memory, both episodic and semantic. Although this chapter does not focus on testing nondeclarative memory, when necessary, clinicians can test procedural memory by the ability to

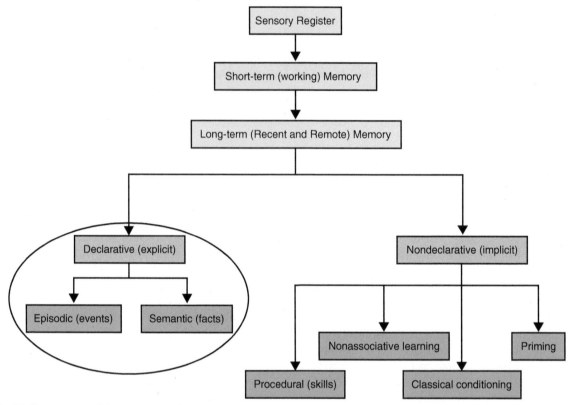

Fig. 9.1 Memory stream. This chapter emphasizes the evaluation of declarative episodic and declarative semantic memory (circled).

learn to trace an image in a mirror and priming by the speed of recognition from word fragments of previously seen words.

Declarative Episodic Memory

MEMORY HISTORY

A complaint of memory loss can mean a great many things. "Memory loss" often describes cognitive disorders of any kind, from attentional deficits, to word-finding problems, to disturbances in executive cognition. The mental status examiner's first step is to determine if the patient's "memory" complaint is actually due to a disturbance in the encoding, storage, or retrieval of information. The clarification of a memory complaint involves obtaining specific examples of their memory difficulty, either from the patient or through collateral information obtained from others. For example, complaints of forgetting what they just read or what they went into a room to get suggest

attentional or registration difficulties. They may indicate symptoms of anxiety or depression, physiological or sleep changes, medication or drug effects, or sensory impairment, such as hearing loss. However, complaints of forgetting what happened that morning or who they were recently introduced to suggest episodic recent memory difficulty.

The examination of memory requires patient effort and causes them anxiety and apprehension over their performance and its implications. Consequently, it is best to begin with a less threatening and indirect assessment of memory for their personal history. Ask the patient the reason and circumstances for their clinical encounter or hospitalization and how and when they arrived. The examiner may ask the patient what they think if an in-person clinic visit about current events that are salient and in the moment, for example, "what is going on in the news?" Ask for clarification of events that are sufficiently salient such that it would be reasonable for the patient to have been exposed to information

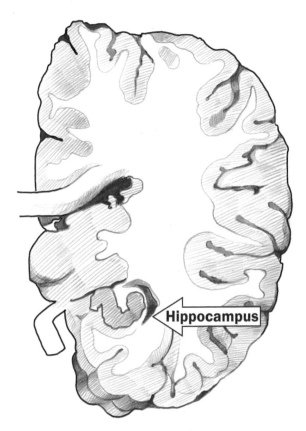

Fig. 9.2 Hippocampus. A major focus of disorders that cause declarative episodic memory loss and amnesia (outlined and arrow).

on them. Difficulty relating this "incidental" information offers insight into deficits in recent memory.

RECENT MEMORY EXAMINATION

Clinicians often begin their evaluation of memory as embedded parts of mental status scales and inventories, such as the Mini-Mental State Examination or the Montreal Cognitive Assessment (see Chapters 15 and 16). These scales include a brief 3 to 5 item word list learning task. One criticism is that the interval of delayed recall and intervening distractions may not suffice for long-term memory; if there is any ongoing rehearsal, the items have not cleared from short-term/working memory. Another consideration is the inability to analyze any memory deficits by their recall processes, as described for Verbal Learning Tests.

Verbal Learning Tests. The most detailed and widely used tests of recent memory are the Verbal Learning Tests. Clinical or bedside tests are patterned after neuropsychological tests, such as the 15-item Rey Auditory-Verbal Learning Test and the 16- or 9-item versions of the California Auditory-Verbal Learning Test. A variant of these are selective reminding tests, such as the Buschke Selective Reminding Test, in which the examiner only repeatedly presents the words that the patient failed to repeat on the prior registration trial. One of the most useful Verbal Learning Tests is the "CERAD" (Consortium to Establish a Registry for Alzheimer Disease) Memory Test. It uses 10 written words, each on a different paper or card, with three registration trials, a 5-minute delayed recall interval, and a 20 word multiple-choice recognition (10 correct and 10 incorrect words).

Verbal Learning Tests of episodic recent memory assess the three recall processes of immediate recall or registration, free delayed recall, and cued recall or recognition. First, the examiner notes the patient's registration or immediate recall of information. This process evaluates if the new information has been sufficiently attended to and held in short-term/working memory, so as to encode and store it. The ability to immediately recall and repeat back after learning trials reflects the registration process and is a prerequisite to episodic recent memory. Second, the examiner is interested in how the patient spontaneously recalls the information after a delay. Delayed recall, in which the patient must retrieve previously learned information, is the usual test for encoding and storage. Third, the examiner is interested in the retrieval of previously stored information through cuing or recognition testing. Asking the patient to recognize the previously presented items in a multiple-choice format is the usual test for retrieval. Additional processes that affect testing include visual versus verbal modality, consolidation (time needed for completion of encoding and storage), and serial processing effects ("primacy" or greater immediate recall of initial items, and "recency" or greater immediate recall of the last items).

Verbal Learning Tests involve presenting word lists for learning. The examiner can use short, bedside word list learning tasks of 3 words or up to one less than the patient's digit span, or, preferably, a longer superspan list of 8 or 10 words (Table 9.1). To prevent clustering or grouping, these word lists are composed of words that are phonemically and

TABLE 9.1 Verbal Learning Test: Registration and Delayed Recall

A. REGISTRATION/IMMEDIATE RECALL

To the patient: "I am going to give you a list of 10 words. Please listen to all of them, then, immediately afterward, give me as many as you can remember in any order. Ready?"

	TRIAL 1	TRIAL 2	TRIAL 3	TRIAL 4	TRIAL 5
	☐ Cabbage	☐ Chevrolet	☐ Ketchup	☐ Blue	☐ Hockey
	☐ Table	☐ Blue	☐ Juice	☐ Rose	☐ Juice
	☐ Horse	☐ Hockey	☐ Table	☐ Cabbage	☐ Blue
	☐ Chevrolet	☐ Cabbage	☐ Rose	☐ Horse	☐ Bell
	☐ Ketchup	☐ Horse	☐ Bell	☐ Hockey	☐ Rose
	☐ Rose	☐ Bell	☐ Horse	☐ Table	☐ Ketchup
	☐ Bell	☐ Rose	☐ Cabbage	☐ Ketchup	☐ Chevrolet
	☐ Blue	☐ Table	☐ Hockey	☐ Chevrolet	☐ Horse
	☐ Juice	☐ Juice	☐ Blue	☐ Bell	☐ Table
	☐ Hockey	☐ Ketchup	☐ Chevrolet	☐ Juice	☐ Cabbage
Correct:					
False positives:					
Perserverations:					
Total Correct (sum of all five trials):					
TOTAL NUMBER OF ERRORS:					

B. DELAYED RECALL

To be administered after a 15-minute interference interval: "Try to remember the words I asked you to remember earlier. Tell me as many of the words as you can recall."

	Remembered	Not Remembered	
Cabbage			TOTAL NUMBER CORRECT:
Table			
Horse			
Chevrolet			TOTAL NUMBER OF ERRORS:
Ketchup			
Rose			
Bell			
Blue			
Juice			
Hockey			

semantically unrelated (unless semantic clustering is of interest). As with the CERAD, the word lists can also be presented as written words, one at a time, at a regular pace in which the patient reads the word aloud. The following describes Verbal Learning Tests based on their recall processes of registration, delayed recall, and recognition.

Registration or Immediate Recall. The examiner initially presents the word lists multiple times and asks the patient to repeat them after each presentation. This "drilled" technique allows for assessment and assurance of registration of the items sufficient to allow subsequent delayed recall testing. Word lists are usually presented orally (although can be visual as well), one word at a time, in a normal voice and regular cadence. Tell the patient that you are going to repeat a list of words, "Please remember them. I will ask you to repeat the word list immediately after I finish." Specify that they may repeat the same word multiple times and in any order. Wait until the patient indicates that he or she cannot recall any more words, or a full minute, before continuing to the next reading of the same words preceded by the same instructions. On the short word list task, the presentations continue until the patient can repeat all four words in no specific order three times in a row, and the examiner records the number of trials necessary for correct repetitions. On the long 8 to 10 word list tasks, the examiner continues the presentations for 3 to 5 predetermined trials and records immediate recall over the registration trials. Some versions of the long list use "selective reminding," that is, only repeat the words missed in the prior trial in each subsequent trial, and other versions vary the word order on each presentation, as in Table 9.1. On the long lists, patients who cannot repeat two-thirds or more of the list by the fourth or fifth trial have difficulty with registration and may have a primary attentional or short-term/working memory problem. Furthermore, poor recency registration of the last items suggests short-term/working memory difficulty, whereas poor primacy registration of the initial items suggests episodic memory difficulty, and some examiners may wish to calculate a serial order recency-primacy index.

Delayed Recall. The examiner asks the examinee to recall the words after a timed delay interval. To eliminate active mental rehearsal the patient undergoes an "interference interval" with distracting tasks or other mental status tests between the last registration trial and the delayed recall. For the short form, after an interference interval of 1 to 5 minutes or more, the patient must spontaneously recall the words without hints or cuing. Normal individuals recall all the words, in no specific order. For the long form, after a predetermined interference interval of

either 10, 15, 20, or 30 minutes, the patient must spontaneously recall the 8 to 10 words without hints or cuing. The timed delay interval on the long form varies in different versions, and the longer this timed delay, the greater the "rate of forgetting"; however, this effect is mild for the 10 to 30 minute time delay interval, so that 15 minutes is acceptable for verbal word list presentations and as short as 5 minutes if presented in written format. On the long form, normal individuals recall two-thirds or more of the words, in no specific order. One valuable calculation is the "savings score." This score is the delayed recall score divided by the repetition score on the last registration trial. A savings score of less than 50% is strongly suggestive of a memory problem not due to decreased registration. Occasionally, the examiner may want to determine rates of forgetting with different interference intervals, the presence of semantic clustering or a clumping strategy, the temporal order of word recall, and the presence of intrusions (words not on the list) or perseverations (number or word repetitions).

Recognition or Cued Recall. After registration and delayed recall, the examiner asks the patient to identify the previously presented words with categorical or multiple-choice clues. On the short version, the examiner first uses categorical verbal cues (e.g., "One was the name of a vegetable") and then multiple-choice items (e.g., "It was either carrots, turnips, cabbage, or tomatoes"). If the patient is still unable to recall the word, a final cuing technique may be to provide a phonemic cue using the first syllable of the word. On the long list version, the most common recognition procedure involves multiple-choice recognition among a list composed of the memory words plus an equal number of related words that were not on the memory list (Table 9.2). For the short 4- or 5-item tasks, a normal recognition score is 3 or more, an abnormal score is 1 or less. For the long 8- to 10-item tasks, a normal recognition score maximizes true positives + true negatives (total recognition), which should be two-thirds or more of the words. A 2 or more Recognition Index (total recognition/2x delayed recall) suggests a predominant retrieval deficit, rather than a predominant encoding or storage deficit as seen

TABLE 9.2 Verbal Learning Test: Recognition/Cued Recall		
•Bolded items are true positives from Verbal Learning Test list (Table 9.1)		
Examiner: "Did you see this word before on the memory list? Please answer Yes or No."		
Stimulus	**Yes**	**No**
Rose		
Boot		
Bell		
Town		
Rope		
Blue		
Group		
Juice		
Hockey		
Chapel		
Tea		
Cabbage		
Penny		
Table		
Horse		
Four		
Chevrolet		
Hospital		
Hill		
Ketchup		
True positives (TP)	_____/10	
True negatives (TN)	_____/10	
Total recognition score (TP + TN)	_____/20	
Adjusted (for quessing) recognition score (TP + TN)-(FP + FN)	_____/20	
Recognition Index (TP + TN)/2x delayed recall	_____	

FN, false negatives; *FP*, false positives

in Alzheimer disease (Fig. 9.3). For example, "frontal-subcortical" lesions may result in poor delayed recall but "bounce back" with a good recognition score and a high Recognition Index.

Alternative Verbal Memory Tests. There are other practical ways to evaluate episodic recent memory in the verbal domain. First, the examiner can give his or her name and that of at least one other in the room, and minutes later ask the patient to recall the names. Disturbed recent memory is suggested if the patient cannot retain any names after 5 minutes. Second, the examiner can ask the patient to recall a sentence, such as the Babcock sentence: "The one thing a nation needs to be rich and strong is a large, secure supply of wood." The patient must repeat it until it is learned and is then required to recall it after 5 minutes. Third, the examiner can ask the patient to recall a story (Table 9.3). First, instruct the patient: "I am going to read you a short story. Please listen carefully because afterward I want you to tell me the story as accurately as possible." After an interference interval, say: "Tell me everything that you remember about the story." The examiner concludes by asking specific questions about the content of the short story. Finally, the examiner can ask the patient to do paired associate learning. Ask the patient to learn unrelated word pairs (e.g., chair-shovel). Give a list of four word pairs (include easy pairs and hard pairs of less related items), one word pair at a time (2 seconds). After an interference interval, ask the patient to recall one of the words in response to the word it was paired with during presentation trials (e.g., recall the word that was paired with "chair").

Visual Memory Tests. Memory should be tested in the visual, as well as verbal, modality as patient's may be differentially impaired in only one of these modalities with relative sparing of the other. One of the easiest visual memory tests involves asking the patient for delayed recall of three or four previously copied nonsense figures (Fig. 9.4). Use geometric figures that elicit minimal verbalization or verbal associations. Patients may also reproduce from memory any other drawing copied earlier during visuospatial testing (e.g., intersecting pentagons, cube). Scoring is based not on visuospatial accuracy but on the general outline and semblance of the drawing. Does it sufficiently represent the copied model? An example of grading is 2 for accuracy, 1 for recognizable semblance, and 0 for incorrect. Subsequently, they may identify the drawings from pictures of other drawings in a multiple-choice recognition task of at least twice as many nonsense geometric figures. There is a visual-visual paired associates learning version

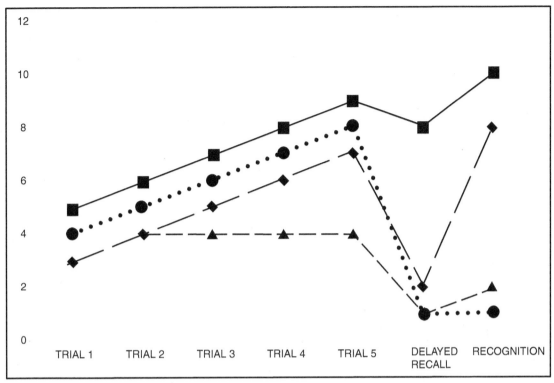

Fig. 9.3 Memory graphs. Hypothetical performance on a Verbal Learning Test for persons with normal cognition (black line; squares), Alzheimer disease (dotted line, circles), frontal-subcortical lesions or disorders (large dashes, diamonds), and delirium (small dashes, triangles).

that pairs three nonsense or geometric figures with colors and asks the patient to reproduce the figures later on presentation of the paired colors. A further related visual memory task is the reproduction from memory of a previously copied complex figure. The examiner may use the Rey-Osterrieth Complex Figure or an alternative complex figure, as described in Chapter 10. Without prior notification, the patient is asked to reproduce the figure at 3 minutes and/or at 30 minutes after the initial copy.

There are several other visual memory tasks that can be easily done in clinical encounters or at the bedside. One task involves asking the patient to recall item and location of four items previously hidden in the room. The examiner hides the items in the room while the patient observes, aware that this is a memory test, and then asks the patient to identify the object and its location after a 5-minute delay. Grading should include 2 for both item and its correct location, 1 for

correct item but incorrect location, and 1 for correct location but incorrect item. Another test is the "dot localization" test of memory using 7 tokens placed on a board of 24 empty squares (Fig. 9.5). The examiner places the tokens in 7 of the squares, shows the patient, then removes the board. After a delay of 5 minutes, the examiner reintroduces the tokens and the blank board and instructs the patient to place the tokens in the same prior squares.

REMOTE MEMORY EXAMINATION

The examination of episodic remote memory involves the retrieval of past historical or autobiographical information. Testing focuses on retrieval or recognition of established memories rather than registration and delayed recall of new information. Episodic remote memory is disproportionately preserved in contrast to impaired recent memory learning in most amnestic disorders. Another reason for testing

TABLE 9.3   **Short Three-Sentence Story Memory Test**
1. Examiner: "I am going to read you a short story. Please listen carefully because afterward I want you to tell me the story as accurately as possible."
2. The examiner reads the story aloud in a slow clear voice.
The boy went to the store with his sister. She wanted candy, so he bought her a chocolate bar. They returned home just before dinner.
3. The examiner asks the patient to repeat back as much of the story as he or she remembers immediately afterward.
4. The examiner records whether the patient described that children went to the store, bought candy, and returned home.
5. The examiner then rereads the story to the patient.
6. After an interference interval of 5 minutes, the examiner states "Now tell me everything that you remember about the story."
7. The examiner records whether the patient remembered:
a. Children went to the store
b. Boy accompanied sister
c. She wanted candy
d. The boy bought sister a chocolate bar
e. Returned home
f. Just before dinner
8. The examiner concludes by asking specific questions about the story content:
a. Did the boy go alone? (no) ___
b. Did the girl get what she wanted? (yes) ___
c. Was the candy purchased by the girl? (no) ___
d. Can you think of a reason for their mother to be angry? (yes) ___

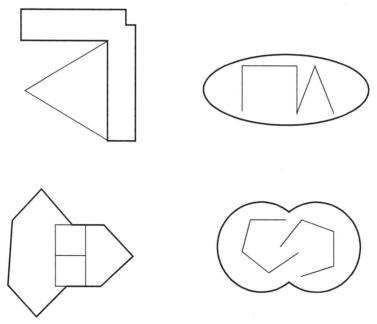

Fig. 9.4 Visual memory tests. The examiner introduces four geometric nonsense figures for the patient to copy. After a delay, the examiner asks the patient to reproduce the figures from memory. Each figure has an overall form score and an internal lines score (combined for a total of eight; normal at least six).

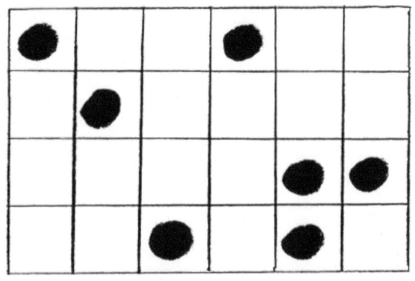

Fig. 9.5 7/24 Nonverbal memory test. The examiner introduces the board with 24 squares and places seven tokens. After a delay, the patient is provided the board and tokens and must reproduce the placement (total of seven; normal at least five).

episodic remote memory is the temporal grade of remote memory difficulty going back in time. Several amnestic disorders have characteristic temporal gradient slopes for remote memory impairment, may show "temporal disorganization" in associating event details and dates, and may even show "temporal lacunes" or discrete gaps in remote memory loss. In addition, as dementias progress, the retrieval of remote memory becomes increasingly compromised and can indicate severity of disease.

A more objective method of testing remote memory is to ask the patient to recall four or more current events or historical events that have occurred during the individual's lifetime. The main difficulty in interpreting remote historical memory is determining the extent to which the past information was acquired in the first place. The chosen events should consider the patient's age and sociocultural background and should also be sufficiently salient such that it would be reasonable for the patient to have been exposed to information about the event. The examiner may start by asking the patient to relate four major events, with some detail, in the past few months. Another example is to ask the examinee to name the prior four presidents or prime ministers in proper sequence beginning with the current leader. A further example is to ask the patient to name

major historical events from the last 2 decades, probing for details (Table 9.4). The examiner can do this by naming specific historical events and asking the patient to describe them, for example, "What was 9-11?" Finally, the examiner can determine the patient's particular interests and query him or her on them, for example, specific television shows or sports events.

The examiner asks questions concerning autobiographical history, such as the patient's family, residences, and jobs. Sample questions are: "Tell me about the home that you grew up in." "Tell me about how you met your spouse." A more formal assessment of autobiographical events asks questions similar to the Autobiographical Memory Interview. This interview asks for personal information that targets both personally experienced incidents or episodic memories and semantic memories from different eras, such as childhood, early life, and later life. Examples of potential questions are descriptions of favorite grade school or middle school memories, first remembered birthday, description of secondary school graduation, earliest memory of grandparents, and so on. Scores are calculated on the level of specificity of personal details of the experience, for example, 0 indicating no specificity and 3 indicating the ability to describe events of a discreet time and place.

TABLE 9.4	Example of Historical Test Questions
"I am going to ask you some historical questions from the last 20 years. I am checking your memory and not your knowledge or awareness of major events. Please give at least two things that you know about these events or people."	
2000–2010	
What was "9-11?"	Terrorist attack on United States Details, e.g., planes, Twin Towers, etc.
What do you know about Michael Phelps?	Swimmer Many/most Olympic gold medals
What do you know about Saddam Hossein?	Iraqi leader Toppled and executed
What was Katrina?	Hurricane New Orleans
What do you know about Michael Jackson?	Famous performer Circumstances of death
2011–2020	
What was the Sandy Hook incident?	School shooting Details, e.g., number dead, shooter, etc.
What do you know about Osama Bin Laden?	9-11 Terrorist Circumstances of death
What is Brexit?	UK's exit from the European Union Details, e.g., difficulties, politics, etc.
What happened to Crimea?	Annexed by Russia Ukrainian opposition and conflict
What do you know about COVID-19?	Viral epidemic or pandemic Causes respiratory difficulty

DECLARATIVE SEMANTIC MEMORY

Occasionally in specific situations, the examiner may need to test for deficits in semantic memory. Semantic memory is unique in that, unlike episodic memory, it is not "time or place-tagged" to personal experience, that is, it does not depend on recalling when and where an individual learned the information. Semantics, however, is more than just memory. It includes the conscious recall of facts and general knowledge about the world and an understanding of the categories and associations, such as object use, that give facts their meaning. Deficits in the access to factual knowledge that are modality-specific, that is, only inaccessible via visual, auditory, or other modality-specific inputs but not by others, are "agnosias" and are discussed with perceptual disorders in Chapter 10. In general, primary semantic deficits transcend modalities, unless they reflect unique experiences evident in only that modality, for example, face recognition is uniquely visual. Information about individual characteristics in modality-specific areas is integrated in the anterior temporal poles. Hence disease in these "convergence zones" disrupts the ability to combine unimodal representations into multimodal semantic knowledge, and semantic disturbances result from disease in the anterior temporal lobes or with advancing dementia.

Semantic knowledge most importantly involves the formation of categories. First, specific domain theories would suggest that predominant verbal categorization occurs in the left anterior region, and perceptual and animate categorization in the right anterior temporal region. Second, categories vary in hierarchical levels from the more general, or superordinate, to the more specific, or subordinate. For example, superordinate groupings, such as "animals" are less vulnerable to disease than subordinate groupings, such as "dog." Third, semantic categories have a prototypical exemplar that is most characteristic of the group. This results in a typicality effect in which the more representative members, such as "dog for animal," are less vulnerable to disease than less representative members, such as "lemur for animal." Fourth, members within categories vary depending on their semantic relatedness. Members more distant in meaning, such as "judge" to "theft," are less vulnerable to disease than members that are closer in meaning, such as "robbery" to "theft." Finally, categories vary depending on the individual's familiarity with the members of the group. Some semantic dementia patients, for example, may not know "cheese" because the lacked familiarity with varieties of cheeses. These considerations may be pertinent when interpreting someone's knowledge of a word, object, or concept.

The Examination of Semantics

The examiner can easily apply a number of tasks, which are sensitive but not specific to semantic knowledge, in clinical encounters and at the bedside. The examiner evaluates: 1) conversation (e.g., answers to "What is?" questions) and category list generation; 2) word comprehension and semantic-word picture matching; 3) object/picture semantic associations; and 4) category sorting and drawing tasks. Unlike tests of episodic memory, these observations or tasks focus less on recent memory or learning and more on retrieval of remote information.

Conversation and Category List Generation. On listening to the patient's conversation during the initial interview, look for the presence of noun omissions and compensatory circumlocutions or nonspecific pronouns or names. If significant semantic deficits are suspected, then the examiner may point to six objects that vary in familiarity, particularly parts of objects, and ask the patient to identify them by name and function. An example of available items are cuff (shirt or blouse), lapel (coat), band (wristwatch), receiver (telephone), mouse (computer), and sole (shoe). Note whether there is a hierarchical (subordinate) loss with retention of the more general term or whether the patient responds more rapidly if the items are more typical of their category, for example, a typical versus an unusual pen. In addition,

during the language examination when evaluating word-list generation per minute, ask the patient to generate word lists from multiple categories, that is, animals, fruits and vegetables, and inanimate objects such as tools or makes of cars. The patient may also generate within-class lists (Thing Categories Test), such as "all things" that are predominantly red, blue, round, and so on.

Word Comprehension and Semantic-Word Picture Matching. When semantics breaks down there are problems in word comprehension, especially with less common words. The examiner can test this by speaking word names and asking the patient to identify the word, that is, ask the patient "What is a…" Present the words one at a time and give the patient sufficient time to think of an answer. The words should range from low frequency to high frequency and cover animate and inanimate categories. The patient may show word comprehension by providing definitions, descriptions of the use or function, or common associations for the words. If the patient cannot define the word, ask the patient to describe its use or its associations, for example, "doctor" for stethoscope. If the patient is still unsuccessful, the examiner may ask the patient to demonstrate use, where possible, or to indicate an association from a multiple-choice array of four definitions to choose from. Semantic word picture matching is an alternative way to test word comprehension. This procedure requires sets of semantically related pictures (e.g., haystack, barn, chickens, plow). As before, the examiner speaks word names ("plow") and asks the patient to identify the word, but this time by choosing the picture that matches the word. The examiner can create at least four displays of four pictures each for the patient to choose from, and the patient should undergo multiple trials.

Object/Picture Semantic Associations. The examiner may want to avoid language altogether and test semantics strictly through visual-visual matching tasks. The examiner presents 10 objects/pictures one at a time and asks the patient to match them with one of an array of 10 action pictures, for example, a saw with a carpenter working and a pot with a chef cooking. The stimulus items should range from low frequency to high frequency and belong to different categories. Patients with semantic deficits may make errors in matching the correct object/picture and its semantically associated action picture. Subsequently, the examiner can reverse the order of the task. The examiner presents the action pictures and asks the patient to point to the corresponding object or picture in an array. A more sensitive nonverbal test of semantic associations involves showing the patient arrays of objects or pictures of objects and asking the patient to indicate which ones go together. So as not to overwhelm the patient, the array is best limited to four objects/pictures presented at a time (Fig. 9.6). Again, the objects or pictures should range from low frequency to high frequency and belong to different categories.

Category Sorting and Drawing Tasks. An alternative semantic task involves identifying the category or class of an item, either from words or objects/pictures. One way to do this is by asking the patient to sort an array of written words or an array of objects/pictures by predefined categories (e.g., living vs. non-living, fruits vs. vegetables, tools vs. non-tools). The examiner can also ask the patient to group 10 or more familiar objects/pictures according to use, color, material, or situation

in which they are normally found. Another useful "category" test is the "draw an animal" test in which the patient must produce a copy of specific animals, such as a dog, giraffe, or camel. This exercise is particularly useful for distinguishing subordinate deficits from relatively retained superordinate groupings, such as the outline of a generic animal (Fig. 9.7).

Clinical Implications

Clinically, amnesia is most commonly an acquired impairment in declarative episodic memory. This type of memory loss is a common concern among older people and the most common early manifestation of Alzheimer disease and mild neurocognitive disorder. This amnesia often indicates injury to the limbic system, either the hippocampi in the temporal lobes or

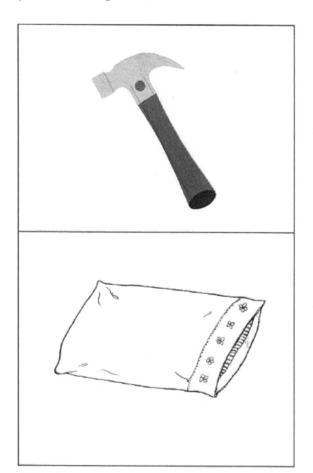 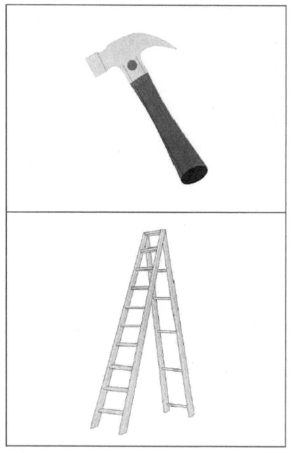

Fig. 9.6 Semantic associations. Indicate which items below go best with the item above. (Thompson, C.K., Lukic, S. King, M., Mesulam, M.M., & Weintraub, S. (2012). Verb and noun deficits in stroke-induced and primary progressive aphasia. *Aphasiology*, 26, 652-655. https://nulive.technologypublisher.com/tech/Northwestern_Naming_Battery_(NNB)).

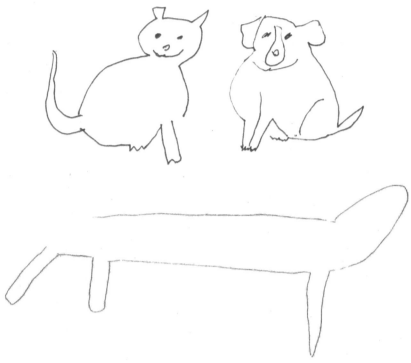

Fig. 9.7 Examples of "draw an animal" task. Top drawings indicate drawings of cat and dog from normal subject. Bottom drawing indicates drawing of both cat and dog from patient with semantic dementia. This drawing has reverted to a generic (superordinate) animal.

the midline limbic structures. A predominant verbal amnesia may result from injury in left hemispheric limbic structures, and a predominant visual amnesia may result from injury in the right hemispheric limbic structures. Amnesia also results from non-Alzheimer dementias, traumatic brain injury (TBI), strokes and other lesions involving limbic structures, anoxic encephalopathy, herpes encephalitis, limbic encephalitis, Korsakoff syndrome, transient global amnesia, epilepsy and transient epileptic amnesia, anterior communicating artery aneurysms, domoic acid from shellfish poisoning, and other lesions that affect memory-related structures.

TBI is an important source of memory impairment, particularly in the young. Patients with closed head injuries may sustain damage to the hippocampal memory structures as they are nestled in the middle cranial fossa and susceptible to the effects of rotatory acceleration during a TBI. A characteristic of TBI is "posttraumatic amnesia" (PTA), or antegrade difficulty learning new information after the brain injury. Another characteristic of TBI is retrograde amnesia, or difficulty retrieving events that occurred just before the brain

injury. The PTA, which must be distinguished from any period of loss of consciousness, is a reliable index of the severity of a TBI, whereas the retrograde amnesia is unreliable and tends to shrink with time. Hence the severity of TBI is mild if the PTA is less than 24 hours, moderate if the PTA is 24 hours to 7 days, and severe if the PTA is greater than 1 week. A permanent impairment in episodic recent memory is particularly likely if the TBI was at least moderate in severity.

Another clinical example of a memory disorder is Korsakoff syndrome from thiamine deficiency, often in poorly nourished alcoholics. The characteristics of this syndrome are severely impaired recent memory on delayed recall and impaired remote memory often with a sharp temporal gradient, that is, a distinct, linear improvement of memory going back in time over the years. The retrieval of remote information can show temporal disorganization or temporal lacunes. Because of their memory impairment, and frontal-executive impairment in monitoring, these patients may fill in the gaps in their memory with expedient misinformation, or "momentary confabulations" (see Chapter 14). This may be merely a wrong answer such as presenting an incorrect day or date, the wrong place on questions of orientation, or a recital of recent personal activities that did not occur. At times, however, confabulations can be bizarre and characterized by the spontaneous presentation of unreal or impossible activities or wish fulfillment.

Semantic dementia is one of the frontotemporal dementia syndromes. The main characteristic of semantic dementia is a multimodal loss of semantic knowledge. Early on it is also known as semantic variant primary progressive aphasia when it starts with semantic deficits in word comprehension (semantic anomia). These patients make semantic paraphasia errors, often revert to supraordinate categories, for example, animal for chipmunk, and develop surface dyslexia, or problems reading irregular words (see Chapter 8). As the disease progresses, patients with semantic dementia develop problems with person and object identification regardless of modality, that is, a loss of semantic knowledge. The patients have a much better ability to recount personal historical events and to learn new episodic material, although they lose personal semantic facts. Neuroimaging typically suggests deterioration of the anterior inferolateral temporal lobes, with the left often being more affected than the right.

Several psychiatric conditions present with memory complaints, which primarily impair memory through poor registration. These psychiatric conditions include anxiety, posttraumatic stress disorder, and depression. Additional psychiatric conditions include the Ganser syndrome, or the syndrome of approximations initially reported among prisoners, and psychogenic amnesia and fugue state, which, in sharp contrast to neurological amnesia, affects personal identity—"Who am I?"—and personal referent information—"Do I have a spouse or children?"—while often dramatically preserving episodic recent memory and the ability to learn new information.

A final clinical consideration is the phenomenon of "false memories." These are semantic or autobiographical remote memories that are factually incorrect but, nevertheless, strongly believed. The psychological mechanisms and neurological substrate of false memories are not entirely clear. Some studies suggest that they are repressed memories of real events, but others find evidence for internally generated and emotionally facilitated experiences. Alternatively, they may emerge from a need to complete and integrate disconnected memory fragments. A possible neurological substrate is altered functions in the ventromedial and other frontal regions in some patients.

Conclusions

Memory difficulty is the most common cognitive complaint. There are many things that can present as "memory difficulty," and the examiner must first distinguish whether the problem is in the memory stream. True amnesia is a problem in encoding, storing, and retrieving information and usually involves declarative episodic recent memory. Less frequently, there are patients with significant memory impairment from disease affecting declarative semantic memory or knowledge of facts. Understanding and examining these memory systems is one of the most critical aspects of mental status testing.

Chapter 10

Constructional, Perceptual, and Spatial Abilities

Constructional, perceptual, and spatial abilities are important, interrelated brain functions. This chapter discusses these abilities primarily in the visual modality; however, the principles and concepts apply to auditory and other modalities as well. Visual constructional tasks, such as figure copying or "clock" drawing, are the most common perceptual and spatial tests because they are quite sensitive to brain disease (Table 10.1). Tests of basic visual perceptual

TABLE 10.1   Testing for Visuoperceptual and Visuospatial Processing
Constructional Testing
• Simple figure copies, e.g., simple geometric, cube, Benson figure
• Complex constructions, e.g., Rey-Osterrieth
• Free drawings, e.g., "draw-a-person"
• Clock drawing
• Block assembly, picture arrangement, freehand constructions, paper folding
Basic Perceptual Testing
• Shape discrimination
• Obscured figures, e.g., cross-hatched
• Figure-ground, e.g., hidden/embedded figures or overlapping (Poppelreuter) figures
• Visual integration, e.g., incomplete or cut-up drawings
• Global-local processing, e.g., Navon figures
• Top-down gestalt, e.g., proximity, similarity, continuity, connectedness, closure
Basic Spatial Testing
• Visual search and localization, e.g., dot circling, complex drawing/picture scanning
• Hemispatial neglect, e.g., line bisection, visual search, gap test, double stimulation
• Sensory, motor, and conceptual neglect tasks
• Dressing "apraxia"
• Topographic orientation, e.g., new route, familiar route, draw route, reading map
• Balint syndrome (simultanagnosia, optic ataxia, oculomotor apraxia)
• Line orientation, e.g., Benton judgement of line orientation
• Contrast sensitivity and spatial frequencies
• Mental spatial rotation
• Movement detection (kinetopsia)
• Depth perception (stereopsis and monocular cues)

(Continued)

TABLE 10.1	Testing for Visuoperceptual and Visuospatial Processing *(Cont'd)*
Testing for Cortical Blindness and Visual Agnosias	
• Cortical blindness, e.g., Anton-Babinski syndrome, blindsight, Riddoch phenomena	
• Visual object agnosias, e.g., object/picture comprehension tasks, visual appearance and matching, drawing/copying tasks, atypical/unusual views perception tasks	
• Prosopagnosias, e.g., face recognition, face-face matching, name-to-face matching, name-identity matching	
• Topographagnosia, e.g., landmark recognition	
• Color agnosia, e.g., name, indicate, and sort colors	

disturbances include form or shape discrimination, figure-ground discrimination, and visual organization. Tests of basic spatial disturbances include visual search and location, neglect tasks, dressing ability, environmental orientation, and the unique visuospatial localization problems of Balint syndrome. In a second section, this chapter goes on to describe testing for complex visual problems including cortical blindness, visual object recognition, familiar face recognition, color recognition, and comparable auditory and olfactory difficulties. The positive perceptual and spatial phenomena, or illusions and hallucinations, are part of Chapter 14.

Visual Perceptual and Spatial Processing

Perceptual and spatial analysis occurs along a route from sensory input to a complete representational reconstruction of the visual world. A careful mental status examination can localize perceptual and spatial disturbances along this route. Visual primitives, such as line orientation and edge detection, contrast and spatial frequencies, luminance and color contrasts, and ocular dominance emerge in V1 (Brodmann area [BA] 17), the occipital striate cortex. Most importantly for mental status assessment, at this level, two cortical visual pathways, the ventral or "what" stream and the dorsal or "where stream," begin to emerge (Fig. 10.1).

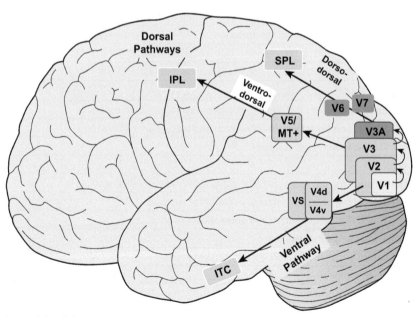

Fig. 10.1 Dorsal and ventral visual streams.

The ventral stream continues to V2 (BA18), an area involved in figure-ground analysis and other functions, through V4, an area involved in simple shape and color recognition, and ultimately to the inferior temporal cortex and object recognition. Hence ventral stream abnormalities affect basic perceptual processing and result in visual object agnosias, topographagnosia, color agnosia, and prosopagnosia. From V1, the dorsal stream continues to V2 (BA18) and dorsal V3 (BA19) involved in spatial location. A part of the dorsal stream (the "ventrodorsal" pathway to V5 [middle temporal] and inferior parietal cortex) participates in the perception of motion and the guidance of some eye movements. Dorsal stream abnormalities affect some basic perceptual processing and all spatial processing and result in hemispatial neglect, dressing "apraxia," topographic disorientation, and Balint syndrome.

Examination of Constructional Abilities

On the mental status examination, the easiest way to screen for perceptual or spatial disturbances is through paper and pencil constructional tasks. Constructional tests include simple geometric figure copies, complex figure copy, free drawing, and clock drawing. These tests are easy to administer, do not require special stimuli for the most part, and are sensitive to disorders anywhere along the ventral and dorsal streams. Right hemisphere disorders tend to result in fragmented constructions with loss of overall spatial relations and orientation, whereas left hemisphere disorders tend to result in impoverished constructions with omission of essential features or lines. Many persons have not had occasion to draw or copy figures in decades. With these subjects, it may be more accurate if they are given one practice trial, or, in some cases, have them view you as you make the figures (marked improvement in this second process may also reflect frontal lobe executive dysfunction). Finally, many clinicians describe a failure to normally copy these figures as constructional "apraxia"; however, they are best described as constructional disturbances because they are not primary disturbances of motor programming.

Simple Figure Copy. Most examiners ask the patient to copy a simple two-dimensional figure such

as a circle or a diamond, a complex two-dimensional figure such as a rectangle, or three-dimensional figures such as a box, cube, or napkin holder ("Benson figure") (Fig. 10.2). For the best constructional task performance, the examiner must be prepared beforehand. Rather than quickly drawing a stimulus on a lined progress note paper, it is best to have a preprinted design for copy, blank and unlined white sheets of paper, and a black pen or a pencil without eraser. The introductory instructions include: "Please make a copy of the picture exactly as you see it." Those who make errors and wish to start over again should be allowed to do so but keeping both copies.

There are different methods for grading the drawings. The examiner looks for abnormal or fragmented spatial relationships, absence of detail or impoverished essential features, stimulus-boundedness ("closing-in" or drawing over the master copy), loss of three-dimensional perspective, or neglect of one part of the drawing. For simpler constructions, there are suggested grading systems for the copy of a circle (closed to within 1/8" = 1; circular = 1); of a diamond (4 sides = 1; 4 closed angles = 1; sides of equal length = 1); and of a rectangle (both figures 4-sided = 1; overlaps resembles original = 1). For the cube and Benson figure, a suggested grading system is included in Fig. 10.2.

Complex Figure Copy. The Rey-Osterrieth Complex Figure is the best known complex figure test (Fig. 10.3), but there are alternative ones, such as the Taylor figure and others. These constructional tasks have the advantage of having a formal scoring system and normative data for assessing the patient's performance. The examiner gives the patient a blank piece of paper and places the stimulus figure in front of him or her. The complex figure task requires the patient to copy the entire figure as best as he or she can, and, although not given a time limit, the patient receives encouragement to complete it. To assess strategy, the examiner may change the patient's pencil or pen to different colored ones at different points in the drawing, thus indicating the sequence and strategy for copying the figure. The scoring system includes 18 specific items (Chapter 17, Fig. 17.1). As an additional visual memory task, they may reproduce the complex figure from memory (Chapter 9), and the strategy for completion can be further analyzed as an executive task (Chapter 13).

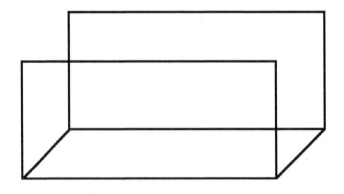

Criteria	Correct	Incorrect
1. 3-D perspective	☐	☐
2. Facing faces oriented correctly	☐	☐
3. Lines- correct number and in parallel	☐	☐
4. Number of surfaces	☐	☐

Visual construction findings:	
☐ Normal	☐ Abnormal
	Number of errors: __

Fig. 10.2 Visual constructional task, Benson figure with scoring system.

Freehand Drawing Tasks. These tasks add the element of visual imagery and remove the guide of a predetermined drawing to copy. The examiner provides the patient with a blank sheet of paper and instructs the patient to draw a house, a dog, a flower (e.g., a "daisy in a flowerpot"), or even a person (the "draw-a-person" test). The patient instructions are: "I would like you to draw simple pictures. I know that you may not be an artist, but please draw the pictures as well as you can." Evaluate the drawings in terms of the features noted for simple figural constructions. In addition to perceptual and spatial disturbances, these drawings can also reflect semantic deficits (see Chapter 9).

Clock Drawing. The freehand drawing of a clock is a sensitive measure of perceptual and spatial difficulty, but it is also affected by attention, language comprehension, numerical knowledge, and executive functions. It can be administered in a number of ways, but the best may be the presentation of a blank piece of paper with the instructions to simply "draw a clock." After the patient draws the clock circle with the numbers, the examiner then has the patient put in the hands to read "10 after 11" or, alternatively, "5 past 4." There are many scoring systems for the clock, some of which attempt to distinguish the different cognitive functions that impact on clock drawing (Table 10.2). The easiest is to evaluate for the contour of the circle, the order

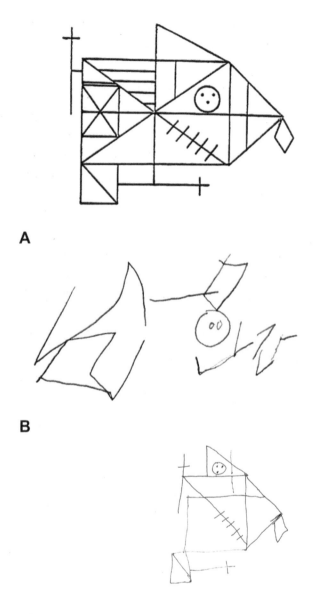

A

B

C

Fig. 10.3 Rey-Osterrieth Complex Figure tests and copies. (A) Normal template. (B) Patient with advanced posterior cortical atrophy. (C) Patient with left hemispatial neglect.

and quadrant placement of the numbers (which can be within or outside of the circle), and the presence of two hands, a short hour hand and a long minute hand, meeting near the center of the clock face (Fig. 10.4).

The examiner, where indicated, may want to test constructional ability with additional tests, such as block assembly and picture arrangement. Most of these tests, however, require special stimuli or procedures for testing and scoring performance and are highly dependent on visuomotor coordination and basic motor ability. For example, block construction can employ four Koh's blocks, which have sides that are red, white, or half red and half white. The examiner presents pictures of different four-block arrangements and asks the patient to take the blocks and make a design that looks like the pictures. Cut-up pictures can also be arranged, much like a jigsaw puzzle. The examiner can use other constructional tools, including tinker toys and readily available items such as match sticks or toothpicks, for freehand constructions. One additionally potentially useful constructional task that does not require blocks or constructional tools is paper-folding. The examiner folds the paper in different ways, for example, exactly in half, quarters, two triangles, along the diagonal, et cetera, and asks the patient to fold their paper in an identical way.

Examination of Basic Perceptual Abilities

Basic Visual Form Discrimination. If more in-depth testing is needed, the examiner evaluates basic perception. When viewing images, people must be able to recognize form at the basic, geometric level. The reconstruction and eventual recognition of basic forms and shapes is a process that underlies the ability to recognize objects, which are made up of basic forms and shapes. The easiest screen is to have the patient match two or three previous constructions with the correct choice out of a field of different geometric forms (Fig. 10.5). The examiner should note whether, in matching the figures, the patient uses a slow, feature-by-feature analysis rather than a rapid global analysis of configuration. This evaluation can also include a multiple-choice matching task using complex forms or shapes or objects in unconventional views. Each figure is presented with four other match figures varying in shape, rotation, or distortion of the figure, and the patient is asked to indicate which match figure corresponds to the stimulus figure. An alternative screening procedure, which is also easy to

TABLE 10.2 Clock Drawing Interpretation Scale (score "1" per item) Hands are placed at "10 after 11"
__ 1. There is an attempt to indicate a time in any way.
__ 2. All marks or items can be classified as either part of a closure figure, a hand, or a symbol for clock numbers.
__ 3. There is a totally closed figure without gaps (closure figure).
Score Only if Symbols for Clock Numbers are Present:
__ 4. A "2" is present and is pointed out in some way for the time.
__ 5. Most symbols are distributed as a circle without major gaps.
__ 6. Three or more clock quadrants have one or more appropriate numbers: 12–3, 3–6, 6–9, 9–12 per respective clockwise quadrant.
__ 7. Most symbols are ordered in a clockwise or rightward direction.
__ 8. All symbols are totally within a closure figure.
__ 9. An "11" is present and is pointed out in some way for the time.
__10. All numbers 1–12 are indicated.
__11. There are no repeated or duplicated number symbols.
__12. There are no substitutions for Arabic or Roman numerals.
__13. The numbers do not go beyond the number 12.
__14. All symbols lie about equally adjacent to a closure figure edge.
__15. Seven or more of the same symbol type are ordered sequentially.
Score Only if One or More Hands are Present:
__16. All hands radiate from the direction of a closure figure center.
__17. One hand is visibly longer than another hand.
__18. There are exactly two distinct and separable hands.
__19. All hands are totally within a closure figure.
__20. There is an attempt to indicate a time with one or more hands.
___ **TOTAL SCORE** (maximum score of 20)

From Mendez MF, Ala T, Underwood KL, Zander BA. Development of scoring criteria for the clock drawing task in Alzheimer's disease. *J Am Geriatr Soc*. 1992;40:1095-1099.

do in a clinical encounter, is to ask the patient to identify figures obscured by cross-hatching (Fig. 10.6A). This screen overlaps with figure-ground tests.

Figure-Ground Discrimination. When viewing images, people experience some figures projecting into the foreground, whereas others recede into the background. The brain organizes the visual field into figures that stand out from their surroundings (ground). Often "figure" and "ground" alternate or compete with each other. This figure-ground processing, which is evident at the V2 level, is a basic perceptual process that can be tested with hidden or embedded figures (Fig. 10.6B). The patients may also identify three or four overlapping figures made up of overlapping line drawings, originally popularized as the Poppelreuter figures test.

Visual Integration and Global-Local Processing. When viewing images, people automatically organize what they see into figures, objects, and scenes. This process of integration allows for the apprehension of intact figures from dilapidated or incomplete ones. The inability to apprehend and integrate at the single form or object level is sometimes called "integrative agnosia," which is related to the inability to apprehend and integrate multiple objects at a scene level. The examiner tests visual organization with incomplete or cut-up drawings (Fig. 10.6C). The Street Figures are part of

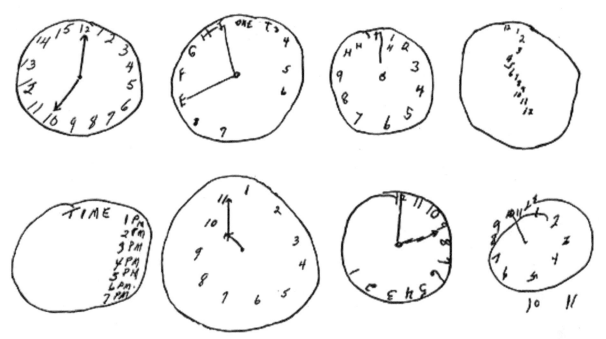

Fig. 10.4 Abnormal clock drawings among patients with Alzheimer's disease. (From Mendez MF, Ala T, Underwood KL, Zander BA. Development of scoring criteria for the clock drawing task in Alzheimer's disease. *J Am Geriatr Soc.* 1992;40:1095-1099.)

the original Street Completion Test and consist of incomplete pictures that have been used to examine perceptual integration. Alternatively, the examiner can present cut-up pictures such as compose the Hooper Visual Organization Test. The cut-up figures are fragmented objects that have to be reconstructed mentally. Global-local processing is easily tested with the "Navon" figures, which consist of letters or numbers made up of smaller letters or numbers (Fig. 10.6D). Patients may recognize the smaller numbers or letters and miss the global one. Finally, it is important to present a complex drawing to the patient (also part of visual search testing), generally representing a familiar scene (Fig. 10.7), and assess whether the patient can identify the whole theme or situation, as well as the constituent parts.

In special situations, the examiner may want to test perceptual ability with additional tests that evaluate top-down processing. In particular, perception undergoes top-down interpretation exemplified by gestalt inferences including the perception of objects or grouping from proximity, similarity, continuity, connectedness, and closure. The examiner can evaluate top-down processes, including the ability to interpret and decipher illusions.

Examination of Spatial Abilities

Visual Search and Localization. The ability to localize in visual space is a fundamental dorsal stream function usually tested with picture and dot localization or search tasks. These tasks focus on the ability to scan a picture and localize a series of random items. The examiner asks the patient to scan a complex visual scene, such as Fig. 10.7 or the Cookie Theft Picture from the language examination (See Chapter 8, Fig. 8.2), for six specific items in the two general areas of the picture. The following are the specific items that can be graded on the Cookie Theft Picture: girl, boy falling, cookie jar, mother washing, sink overflowing, and window. Alternatively, the examiner asks the patient to locate and circle 20 or 40 dots within an 11- x 17-inch field (Fig. 10.8).

Hemispatial Neglect Tasks. Each hemisphere controls the contralateral side of extra- and peripersonal space, and hemispatial neglect occurs when

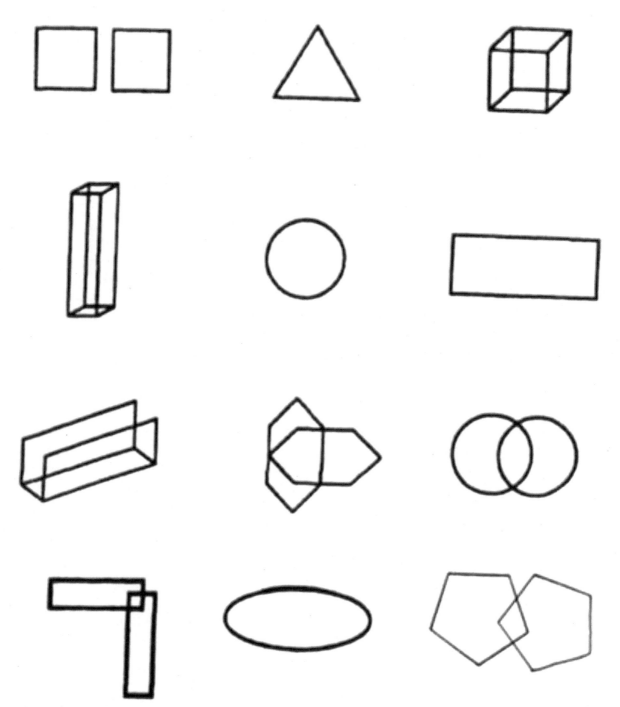

Fig. 10.5 Geometric forms for matching with previous construction. They are presented for matching with the previously copied geometric forms, such as the circle, Benson ("napkin holder"), and pentagon figures.

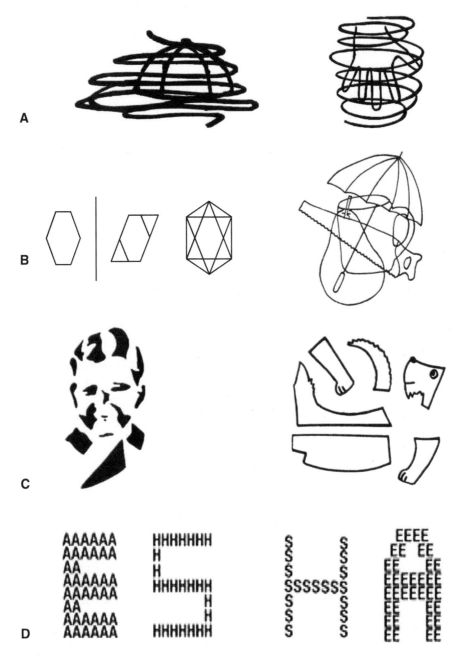

Fig. 10.6 (A) Obscured (cross-hatched) figures; (B) Embedded and overlapping (Poppelreuter) figure-ground figures; (C) Incomplete (from Street Completion Test) and cut-up pictures (from Hopper Visual Organization Test); (D) Global-local processing (Navon figures).

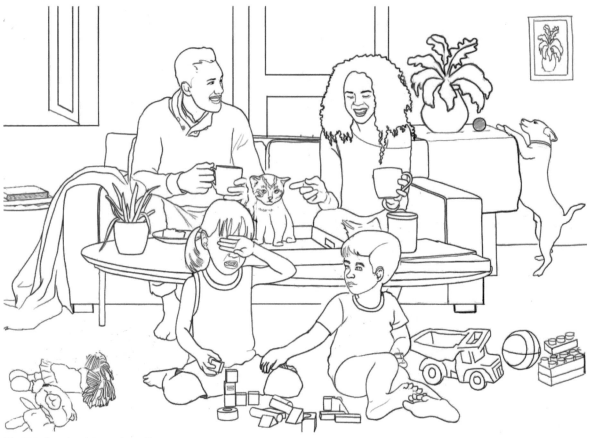

Fig. 10.7 Complex picture—domestic scene.

there is impaired spatial attention to the contralateral visual space, most commonly on the left. In this disorder, neglect may be evident if the patient tends to ignore the left side of the environment or the left side of his or her constructional drawings. Hemispatial neglect can also be detected in reading and writing (e.g., "horseradish" is seen as "radish" or "island" is seen as "land"). In addition, the examiner needs to keep in mind that hemispatial neglect itself, although usually centered to the midline of the patient's body (egocentric), is occasionally object-centered (allocentric). The predominant lesion resulting in classic left-sided hemispatial neglect involves the right inferior parietal cortex (BA29, 30), but can also occur from thalamic or other locations.

Hemispatial neglect tasks include line bisection, visual search and cancellation, the gap test, and double simultaneous stimulation. First of all, it is important

that the stimulus materials be oriented to the patient's body axis. While the patient is seated, the test sheets are placed in front of the patient, aligning the center of the sheet with the patient's midline. Second, the examiner starts with a line bisection task consisting of a test sheet with one or a series of horizontal lines differentially placed on the paper (Fig. 10.9). The examiner asks the patient to divide each line in half by placing a mark at the center of each line. The score is the mean of the percent deviation from the true center of the line. On this line bisection, the degree of displacement is directly proportional to the length of the line used. Third, the patient with suspected hemispatial neglect may undergo a cancellation test. The letter cancellation test consists of a 21.6 x 28 cm white piece of paper with different letters distributed randomly across the page (Fig. 10.10). The patient is instructed to circle the letter "A" (the target) every time they see

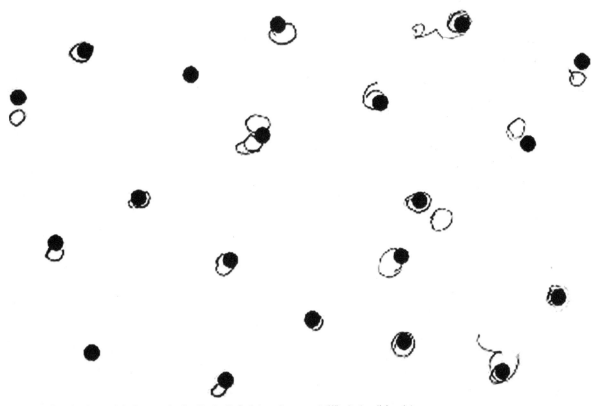

Fig. 10.8 Dot visual search task example of patient with Balint syndrome and difficulty localizing dots.

that letter, and the patient's score is determined by the number of correct targets cancelled. Fourth, the examiner may use a complex picture as a hemispatial neglect task by asking the patient to name as many objects as he or she sees in the picture. The examiner can operationalize this test by choosing 5 to 10 items in each half of the picture. Fifth, an excellent test of both egocentric allocentric neglect is the gap

Fig. 10.9 Line bisection task. (Modified from Schenkenberg T, Bradford DC, Ajax ET. Line bisection and unilateral visual neglect in patients with neurological impairment. *Neurology*. 1980;30:509-517.)

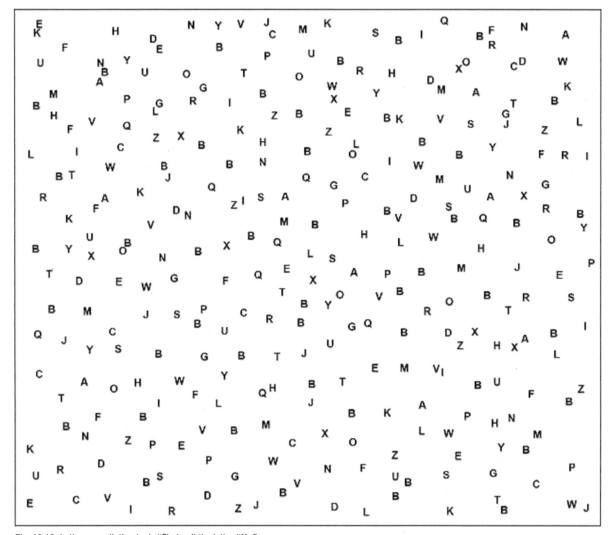

Fig. 10.10 Letter cancellation task: "Circle all the letter "A's.""

test (Fig. 10.11). The patient must indicate (circle or cross out) all the circles with a gap. Failure to cross out all gaps on one side of the page indicates egocentric neglect, whereas failure to cross out all gaps facing either left or facing right indicates allosteric neglect. Finally, in double simultaneous stimulation, stimuli, such as fingers, are simultaneously presented or held up in each hemifield, and the examiner asks the patients to report the number of objects or fingers while maintaining their gaze fixed on the examiner. Unilateral extinction occurs when the patients fail to detect the stimuli on one side.

There are other forms of neglect, including sensory, motor, and conceptual. Sensory neglect is a disturbance of the personal body map with inattention to the half of the body, such as a tendency to dress and groom one side of the body while ignoring the other. Motor neglect includes hypokinesia, motor impersistence, and inability to move one side of the body (see Chapter 11). Conceptual neglect is an inability to visualize the left-side of an imagined representation and can be considered a form of hemispatial neglect (discussed later). The examiner tests for conceptual neglect by asking patients to imagine themselves looking down from one end of a

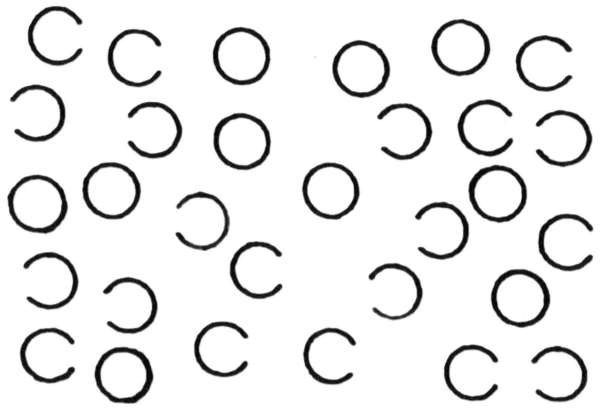

Fig. 10.11 The Gap test, indicate all the circles with a gap; count the number correct on each half of the page including those gaps facing left or facing right. (Original task in Ota H, Fujii T, Suzuki K, Fukatsu R, Yamadori A. Dissociation of body-centered and stimulus-centered representations in unilateral neglect. *Neurology.* 2001;57(11):2064-2069.)

familiar corridor or street and describe what is on each side of the corridor or street. The examiner then repeats the task by asking the patients to imagine themselves looking down from the other end of the same corridor or street. Patients with conceptual neglect may fail to report structures on the left side of their visualization, which differs depending on which end of the corridor or street they imagine themselves to be.

Dressing Disorder or "Apraxia." Spatial competence includes the ability to orient oneself in peripersonal, as well as extrapersonal or allocentric, space. The brain has different spatial maps and items within arms' reach, particularly as they relate to the person's egocentric frame of reference, can be disproportionately disturbed from right parietal lesions. One of the best ways to test this spatial map is "dressing apraxia." Although not a real apraxia in the sense of a primary disturbance in motor programming, this name has persisted. Dressing

"apraxia" is actually a dressing disorder from perispatial difficulty. Inquire whether the patient has difficulty dressing, such as correctly getting a limb through a sleeve or pant leg, or has sequential difficulty in dressing, such as putting on undergarments over street clothes. On testing, the examiner asks the patient to put on a coat several times; the examiner may provide a lab coat for testing. First, the examiner or caregiver holds the coat in an open manner with the inside facing the patient. Second, the patient must remove the hanging coat and put it on by themselves without orientation clues. In the third and fourth condition, one or both of the sleeves are inside-out. The examiner observes whether the patient gets muddled in attempting to put on the garment, inserting a limb into the wrong area, and orienting the garment incorrectly (body-garment disorientation). In addition, patients with dementia often fail to match their clothes or dress in multiple layers.

Environmental Disorientation. Spatial competence includes the ability to orient oneself in extrapersonal, as well as peripersonal, space. Patients with environmental disorientation cannot find their way in familiar and novel environments. Environmental disorientation may result from inability to form a mental map of the spatial relationships of a route (topographic disorientation) or from inability to recognize the spatial value of landmarks (topographagnosia).

In topographic disorientation, patients can recognize landmarks, but they cannot describe the route, trace or draw it (or make a floor plan), or read maps (planotopokinesia). These patients cannot find their way because they do not know how to orient themselves in relation to landmarks on a route. There are three main types of topographic disorientation: egocentric disorientation, heading disorientation, and anterograde disorientation. In egocentric disorientation, there are deficits in representing the relative location of objects with respect to self from dysfunction of the right parietal region. In heading disorientation, there is inability to derive directional information from landmarks from retrospenial or posterior cingulate lesions, especially on the right. In antegrade disorientation, there is inability to make new maps or encode information about spatial relationships, with possible loss of familiarity for old routes, from right parahippocampal dysfunction.

Classic topographagnosia is a ventral stream, category-specific visual agnosia similar to prosopagnosia. Topographagnosia is an inability to recognize salient environmental stimuli, such as buildings, as markers of a route (agnosia for landmarks). It is included here rather than with the agnosias because it is a disorder of environmental disorientation. These patients can distinguish different classes of buildings but cannot identify them as specific orienting landmarks. In topographagnosia, patients can describe the route, trace or draw it (or make a floor plan), and normally read a map. These patients may have bilateral or right-sided lesions in the medial occipital lobe involving the anterior lingual sulcus or the parahippocampal place area.

Testing for environmental orientation can include 1) orienting to a new route and its landmarks; 2) describing a familiar route and its landmarks; 3) tracing or drawing the route or a floor plan; and 4) reading a map. First, the examiner or caregiver guides the patient around a route (clinic or hospital if in-person) pointing out at least 10 landmarks along the way. The examiner instructs the patient to remember the walking route, as well as the indicated landmarks. Subsequently, after returning back to the starting point, the examiner asks the patient to guide the examiner along the same route, pointing out the previously indicated landmarks. The examiner measures the necessity for route cues and redirection and the recall of landmarks en route. Second, the examiner asks the patient to recall a familiar local route known to the examiner as well, for example, a common route to a known location or landmark. The patient must identify key intersections, roads, or buildings along the route and the correct direction from them. Third, the examiner asks the patient to draw a schematic of either the local route or the familiar route. The patient must trace one of the routes, including labeling of the landmarks or street names on the drawing. Finally, since personal topographic competence may be intact in a patient who cannot localize cities on a map, the examiner also asks the patient to read a two-dimensional map. It can be a standard road map, or one created by the examiner of the clinic, hospital, or local area. The examiner asks the patient to imagine traveling a designated route and to trace it on the map. Alternatively, planotopokinesia may be tested by asking the patient to place major cities or landmarks on a familiar map.

Balint Syndrome. The mental status examiner evaluates for the three features of Balint syndrome: dorsal simultanagnosia, optic ataxia, and oculomotor apraxia. Dorsal simultanagnosia is the inability to perceive the presence of more than one visual object or area at a time, which is distinct from ventral simultanagnosia in which everything is perceived but not integrated into a whole scene. The examiner asks the patient to look at a picture or drawing of a complex scene, such as Fig. 10.7 or the Cookie Theft Picture, and notes whether the patient reports only isolated items or segments of items in the picture. Further testing can involve drawing two adjacent circles and noting whether the patient only reports seeing one, then connecting the two circles with a "linker" that makes them glasses or a bicycle and noting whether the patient now sees the whole image (Fig. 10.12). Oculomotor apraxia is the inability to voluntarily

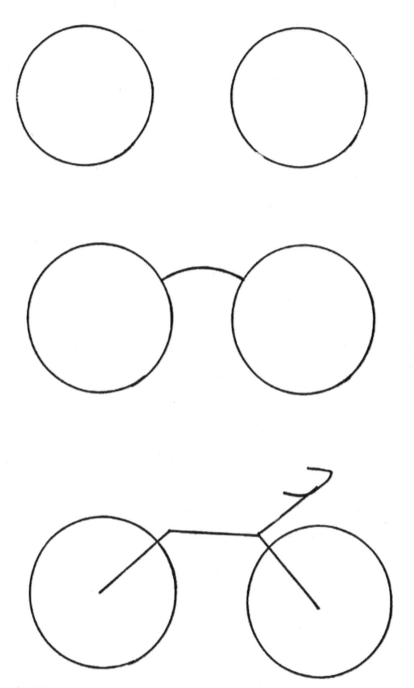

Fig. 10.12 Simultanagnosia tasks.

direct one's gaze to a particular point. For testing, the patient is seated 50 to 60 cm or approximately 2 feet from the examiner and focuses gaze on the examiner's nose. First, the examiner asks the patients to move their gaze to moving targets in each quadrant while maintaining their head straight. Second, they ask the patients to move their gaze to stationary targets in each quadrant again without moving their heads. The patients must quickly move their gaze directly to the targets in the peripheral field without evidence of undershooting, overshooting, or searching, and the maximum score is 8. A delay in the onset of eye movement on command may be the most sensitive indicator of oculomotor apraxia. Optic ataxia is the inability to voluntarily direct one's hand movements toward visually presented targets. In a similar set-up as for oculomotor apraxia, the examiner asks the patients to use the right hand to touch a moving target in each peripheral quadrant while maintaining their gaze on the examiner's nose. This is repeated with stationary targets and with the left hand. The patients must quickly reach out and touch the object without undershooting, overshooting, or searching movements. Scoring for the hand-eye coordination: 0 = total miss; 1 = near miss; 2 = accurate, with a maximum score of 16.

When needed, many other specialized tests can assess spatial abilities. These include tasks of discrimination of line orientation, contrast sensitivity and spatial frequency, mental spatial rotation (mentally rotate and visualize geometric shapes), motion detection (kinetopsia), and depth perception (relative size, interposition, perspective, texture gradient, motion parallax).

Cortical Blindness and Visual Agnosias

The examiner suspects cortical blindness when patients are unable to consciously perceive visual stimuli. For example, they cannot answer: "How many fingers do I have up?", the number of people in the room, or provide visual details about an item in front of them. The first step is to exclude primary eye disorders with an ophthalmologic examination. Patients with cortical blindness cannot fixate or track visual images but have normal pupillary reactivity and funduscopic examinations. Second, the examiner can assess select areas of vision that may be spared in cortical blindness. These include the ability to distinguish between light and dark (light on or off), movement of lights (the "Riddoch phenomena"), the presence of color, or even intermittent or unconscious responses to visual stimuli ("blindsight"). Finally, many of these patients lack insight into their visual loss and may even confabulate having a visual experience ("Anton-Babinski syndrome").

Agnosia is an inability to recognize a stimulus despite intact primary sensory functions. Clinicians may confuse agnosia with the language disorder of anomia, or inability to name a stimulus or object. In agnosia, however, there are acquired problems not only in confrontational naming but also in providing semantic knowledge or functional descriptions about objects when presented in the impaired modality. The access to factual knowledge in agnosia is restricted only in a single modality; knowledge is otherwise accessible, not only by the verbal name or associations, but also through an alternate perceptual modality. For example, in visual agnosia they can identify an object by touching it, and in auditory agnosia they can identify the source of the sound by seeing it. Some agnosias are even more limited to categories within a modality, such as face recognition (prosopagnosia) or color knowledge (color agnosia), or problems in knowing environmental sounds, music, or specific smells.

Most classifications describe two main types of agnosia: apperceptive and associative. Apperceptive agnosia results from inability to completely perceive the physical features of a stimulus, whereas associative agnosia results from inability to access the semantic knowledge of the stimulus. This section discusses the features of apperceptive and associative agnosias primarily in the visual modality. The visual object agnosias are the most common and best studied agnosias; however, the principles and concepts apply to agnosias in any modality.

Apperceptive Visual Agnosia. Patients with apperceptive visual agnosia have intact primary sensory functions, for example, visual acuity, visual fields, and elementary color vision. The problem is at a higher cortical level of perception, particularly configurational integration. Apperceptive visual agnosia is particularly evident when the stimuli or objects are the least typical or presented in unusual angles of view or directions of lighting (visual constancy), or as incomplete drawings rather than photographs or real objects. When objects are presented visually, patients with apperceptive visual agnosia cannot name, describe or pantomime use, match, copy, and sort by visual attributes. However, when allowed to touch and feel the objects, they can name and describe them. These patients most commonly have bilateral occipital (often affecting BA18 and 19) or right parietal lesions.

Associative Visual Agnosia. This disorder is due to inability of normal visual perception to access semantics such that patients are unable to name or functionally describe objects but, in contrast to apperceptive agnosia, are able to process them by their visual attributes. The presence of an intact, but meaningless, "percept" allows these patients to normally process the stimulus perceptually, for example, sort by visual features, describe visual attributes, draw a reasonable copy of the object, and even mentally rotate or manipulate the object. Moreover, their perceptual abilities are sufficiently intact such that they can discriminate and match stimuli and objects in atypical or unusual views or lighting, but they still cannot use this information to access the stimulus or object's identity. Associative visual agnosia is usually due to bilateral posterior occipitotemporal damage but can occur from left unilateral lesions (BA19, 20, 21). Finally, clinicians may confuse associative visual agnosia with optic aphasia, in which there is inability to visually name but intact visual recognition and functional descriptions, due to impaired language access through the visual modality in the left medial occipital area.

The Examination for Visual Object Agnosia

Before proceeding to visual object agnosia testing, the examiner assures that primary visual functions, acuity and visual fields, are intact. Several tasks that can diagnose and distinguish the visual agnosias are 1) object/picture comprehension tasks; 2) visual appearance and matching; 3) drawing tasks; and 4) atypical/unusual views perceptual tasks.

Object/Picture Comprehension. The examiner presents objects (preferable at least 10) visually and asks the patient to name them and, if unsuccessful, describe their function or pantomime their use. In visual agnosia, it is best to start with real objects and then, if necessary, repeat the task with photographs or line drawings. The stimulus items are presented visually only, that is, the patient must not touch, manipulate, or induce sounds from the object. There should be a sufficient number of stimulus items so as to range from low frequency to high frequency and belong to different categories. Patients with apperceptive agnosia may make errors that confuse the target with visually similar items, whereas patients with associative

agnosia make errors that confuse the target with semantically similar items. Subsequently, the examiner can reverse the order of the task, that is, the examiner names items previously missed and asks the patient to point to the corresponding object in an array. Both patients with apperceptive and associative agnosia do poorly, but those with apperceptive agnosia are more susceptible to impairment with line drawings or even photographs than with real objects. When real objects are missed, assure that the patients know what they are by having them touch (or hear) them. Finally, ask the patient "What is a…" and then present word, one at a time. Patients with visual agnosia should be able to provide definitions or functional descriptions on this last word comprehension task.

Visual Appearance and Matching. The examiner then presents the patient with a matching task involving two visual arrays of objects. The two arrays contain similar items, although not necessarily identical in all aspects. The examiner instructs the patient to "point to the two things that are the same." Once the patient has matched the items in the first array with the corresponding items in the second array, the examiner further asks the patient to describe the visual appearance or visual attributes of the items, that is, the basic shape, color, size, and so on. The patients can also sort the items by these attributes. Patients with apperceptive agnosia due poorly on this task; those with associative agnosia do well.

Drawing or Copying Tasks. One useful test is to have the patient draw or copy common visual item that the patient has not been able to identify, for example, flower, dog, whistle, or other. The examiner asks the patient to copy an object or a line drawing. Patients with apperceptive agnosia due poorly in copying the item; those with associative agnosia may be able to draw a recognizable copy but still do not recognize it.

Atypical/Unusual Perceptual Tasks. Patients with apperceptive visual agnosia, but not associative, cannot identify objects or pictures that are atypical or unusual in direction of view, lighting and shadow, size, color, or texture. This added testing requires the examiner to use unusual views tests, which may not be as readily available in a clinic encounter or at the bedside. When available, they can help establish the subtype of visual object agnosia.

Prosopagnosia

Prosopagnosia is an inability to recognize familiar or famous faces despite otherwise intact visual perceptual functions. Face recognition involves a circuit from the visual cortex to the occipital face area to the fusiform face area and ultimately to the anterior temporal semantic convergence region, primarily in the right hemisphere. Faces are unique because they occur in only the visual modality and because people can distinguish thousands of faces that differ in only minor configuration (relationship of the facial features). Patients with prosopagnosia can see faces, recognize that they are faces, and appreciate facial emotions; however, they remain unable to recognize specific faces as corresponding to known individuals. Patients with prosopagnosia often compensate with salient cues or non-face cues, such as hairstyle, glasses, facial hair, or clothes. Moreover, because prosopagnosia is specific to the visual modality, hearing someone's voice often results in immediate recognition.

Prosopagnosia can be primary due to a loss of facial feature recognition or configural patterns, or semantic due to problems accessing identifying information. In the primary form, the patients may or may not be able to form a normal percept, depending on where the lesion is. A basic apperceptive form of primary prosopagnosia may involve the occipital face area on the right and manifest with difficulties recognizing individual facial features. Those patients who have disease in the right-hemisphere fusiform face area may have damage to deposited configural or holistic patterns for known faces, exemplified by the normally greater difficulty in detecting local feature changes in a face when upside down (the "Thatcher Effect"). These patients may also have impaired ability to recognize other within-category items, such as cars, dogs, cats, and others. In contrast to primary prosopagnosias, the semantic type of prosopagnosia has deficits in semantic information about the person, usually from right anterior temporal involvement in disorders such as semantic dementia. They have problems accessing person identification "nodes," despite retaining a sense of familiarity for the faces.

Examination for Prosopagnosia

Face Recognition. Testing for prosopagnosia includes tests of face recognition, face matching, and person identification (knowledge of the person). The examiner tests familiar face recognition with photographs of famous or well-known individuals (without any salient hairstyle, glasses, etc.). For example, the examiner can present 2.5-inch square portraits of politicians or entertainers that are presumably well-known to the vast majority of people in their sociocultural and temporal cohort. The examiner asks the patient to name the person. If the patient cannot name the person, the patient should describe whether the person looks or feels familiar and the person's occupation or other salient fact. Normal is presumed to be a near perfect score.

Face-Face Matching. To exclude an apperceptive etiology, the examiner asks the patient to match photographs of unfamiliar faces with the same face among other photographs in an array. This task can include four stimuli faces, which are presented one at a time, or an array of eight other photographs laid out in front of the patient. The eight photographs in the array include the stimuli faces, in somewhat different poses or angles of view, as well as foils who are similar in appearance to the stimuli faces. The patient is asked to indicate which face in the array is the same person as the stimuli faces. Only patients with apperceptive prosopagnosia do poorly on face-face matching.

Name-to-Face Matching. To assess types of errors, the examiner shows the patient displays, each with four faces of people of the same sex. One of the four faces is the index face, and the others are a semantically related famous face (e.g., same profession or fame), a semantically unrelated famous face, and an unfamiliar but visually similar face (Fig. 10.13). For each display, the examiner names the index person and asks the patient to point to that person's picture among the four choices. The examiner determines the numbers of errors and whether visually related, suggesting primary prosopagnosia, or semantically related, suggesting a problem accessing person identity information.

Name-Identity Matching. To test for more general semantic deficits, the examiner must ask the patients for information about any familiar face that they fail to recognize in the face recognition task. After a delay, with an interference interval involving other cognitive testing, such as face-face matching and name-to-face, the patient is given the name of the missed famous person and asked to describe something about them. This can be salient facial characteristics or semantic characteristics, such as general occupation, living or dead, specific accomplishment, and so on.

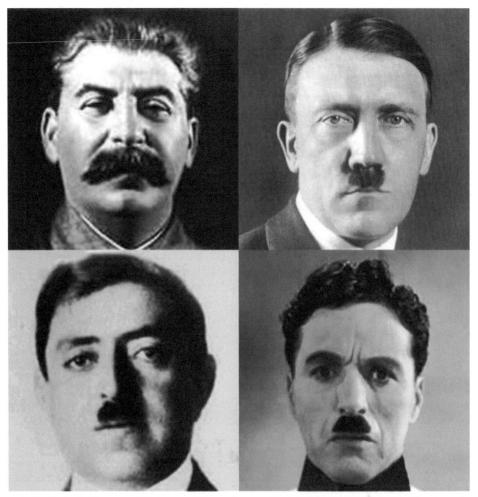

Fig. 10.13 Example of a display for face recognition by name. The examiner asks the participant, "Which one is Hitler?" and records any errors and whether they are semantically related (Stalin) or visually related (Chaplin). (From Mendez MF, Ringman JM, Shapira JS. Impairments in the face-processing network in developmental prosopagnosia and semantic dementia. *Cogn Behav Neurol.* 2015;28:188-197.)

Examination for Color Agnosia and Related Disorders

The ability to name, know, and detect color is an early function of the ventral visual stream; however, higher level color processing involves evaluating color naming for color anomia, and color knowledge for color agnosia. The examiner presents the patient with at least six different color patches (or the Ishihara Color Plates) and asks the patient to 1) name the color; 2) indicate a named color; and 3) sort the patches by the same color. In color anomia and color agnosia, patients cannot name colors on presentation, and they cannot point to named colors, but they can correctly sort them. To distinguish color agnosia from color anomia, the examiner should present the patient with a series of incorrectly colored line drawings, for example, a blue banana, a green dog, et cetera, and ask if the colors are correct. The examiner can also ask the patient to correctly color line drawings. In color agnosia, but not color anomia, the patient cannot judge the correct color for common objects and miscolors them. Color anomia and color agnosia are often associated with alexia without agraphia, a right homonymous hemianopsia, and, sometimes, associative visual agnosia. Parenthetically, if patients fail to name or point to named colors and cannot sort colors that go together, then they may have achromatopsia, or loss of color vision. For these patients, everything looks black and white or gray scale, either bilaterally or in one hemifield. Achromatopsia is usually associated with a superior quadrantanopia from a lesion in the lingual gyrus or medial occipitotemporal lobe.

Disorders of the Auditory Modality

Disorders of central auditory processing include cortical deafness, auditory sound agnosia for environmental sounds or for music (amusia), pure word deafness, aprosodia, auditory affective agnosia, and phonagnosia (Table 10.3). The auditory system is more bilateral than the visual system, making evaluation and testing more difficult. Clues to auditory processing disorders include inability to recognize speech or nonspeech sounds despite preserved basic hearing.

Cortical auditory disorders have several unique characteristics that can offer clues to the diagnosis. They evolve clinically, and there may be significant overlap between the different syndromes. These patients often fail to display "deaf" behaviors such as requests for clarification, leaning forward, requests for a louder delivery, or other attempts to understand the speaker better. They may have dysacusis (experience of sound as distorted, disagreeable, or foreign) or auditory dysesthesia or "misophonia" (experience of sound as painful). They can have paradoxical or inconsistent responses to sound suggesting a subliminal or intermittent signal reception. Finally, errors in sound recognition occur because acoustic characteristics are not deciphered. These include specific disorders of temporal ordering/sequencing with normal pitch (frequency), duration, and loudness, but abnormal sound localization and acoustic (vs. semantic) errors in auditory characteristics.

Testing the Auditory Modality

The examination of the auditory modality often requires special equipment or techniques, such as dichotic listening; however, several tests are possible in a clinic encounter at the bedside. Start by assuring that the patient does not have a primary hearing impairment before proceeding to cortical auditory processing. Then evaluate word and language comprehension

TABLE 10.3   Cortical Auditory Disorders
1. Cortical deafness
2. Generalized auditory agnosia for both verbal and nonverbal sounds
3. Selective auditory agnosia
a. Unable to recognize environmental sounds
b. Mild disturbance in temporal pattern analysis, particularly sequencing
4. Pure word deafness
a. Type 1: deficits in phonemic discrimination
b. Type 2: abnormal fine temporal resolution for auditory word
5. Amusias (receptive) (right > left temporal except left in arrhythmic amusia)
a. Affective amelodia—impaired appreciation (pleasure, affect) of music
b. Apperceptive from abnormal harmonic overtones, timbre and spectral changes, sequencing of melodic variations, or appreciating of pitch
c. Arrhythmic amusia with increased temporal thresholds
d. Melody amnesia
6. Aprosodia: The inability to express or understand the emotive content of spoken language, the variations in pitch, loudness, rate, or rhythm
7. Auditory affective agnosia (sensory aprosodia): There is selective impairment in recognizing affective information in speech despite relatively normal prosody
8. Phonagnosia: There is impaired recognition of familiar voices

as outlined in Chapter 8, followed by the examination of responses to environmental sounds. Ask the patient to identify common nonverbal sounds audible in the environment. A more formal protocol is to present prerecorded environmental sounds accompanied by four corresponding pictures. The four choices are either correct, acoustically related, semantically related, or totally unrelated. The patient must point to the corresponding picture. They can also be discriminated as same or different. If even more in-depth testing is possible, discrimination can be extended to prerecorded pure tones of varying frequency, intensity, duration, phoneme pairs, and sequences varying only in the regularity of the interstimulus interval. The ability to localize sounds in space may be evident or may requires special testing given the bilaterality of sound transmission. In the auditory modality, the examiner may give special consideration to evaluating patients for loss of prosody ("aprosodia"; see Chapter 8) or the loss of the appreciation for music ("amusias"; Table 10.2).

Olfactory Agnosia

Odor or olfactory agnosia can result from right anterior temporal disease and may present with altered dietary preferences or appreciation because much of eating involves olfaction. These patients are able to detect smells, evident with simple screens such as recognizing the presence of coffee, vanilla, lemon, or tobacco, but without recognizing what they are. Olfactory agnosia is further tested using standardized sets of common odorants, such as the University of Pennsylvania Smell Identification Test, which are embedded in "scratch and sniff" fragrance labels and administered in a multiple-choice format. Initially, the examiner evaluates the detection and intensity of the odors. Then the examiner evaluates whether they are familiar or unfamiliar.

Clinical Implications

Most perceptual and spatial difficulties occur with dysfunction involving more than just the posterior cortical regions. Patients with frontal lobe disease usually have normal constructions on simple figure copies, but they can be impaired on the complex figure copy and clock drawing as organizational deficits can impair their performance. Although both parietal lobes can disrupt perception and spatial abilities, right parietal lesions are particularly associated with difficulty with visual organization tasks and with spatial abilities, such as visual localization, dressing praxis, and environmental orientation. Patients with right hemisphere lesions may lose the basic outline of the drawing with fragmented and scattered drawings that lose spatial relationships, orientation. Those with left hemisphere lesions have the basic form, spatial relationships, and configuration but may lose the specific details and produce oversimplified copies.

Cortical blindness may occur from bilateral lesions of V1 (striate cortex), including posterior circulation strokes and anoxic encephalopathy consequent to a cardiac event. Patients with this syndrome fail visual perceptual tests, although they may show "blindsight," possibly because of an alternate, superior collicular pathway. In other words, cortically blind patients may paradoxically respond to visual stimuli that they do not consciously see, particularly moving lights but also grasping at visual stimuli or avoiding obstacles on walking. As previously noted, the Anton-Babinski syndrome refers to cortical blindness associated with a denial of blindness. A similar syndrome results from cortical deafness due to bilateral temporal lesions. Patients with cortical blindness and cortical deafness may evolve to various stages of impaired perceptual dysfunction evident on mental status testing. Among perceptual disorders, color deficits suggest left occipitotemporal lesions and the possibility of associated alexia without agraphia.

Patients with dementia, particularly those of early-onset in their 50s and 60s, may present with progressive visuoperceptual and visuospatial deficits out of proportion to other cognitive difficulties. Most of these patients have the syndrome of posterior cortical atrophy with atrophy and hypometabolism of the occipitoparietal cortex, and autopsied brains have commonly shown the neuropathology of Alzheimer disease in visual cortical areas. The clinical syndrome is most frequently dominated by visuospatial deficits, but there may be Gerstmann syndrome (agraphia, acalculia, right-left disorientation, finger agnosia) and ideomotor apraxia (see Chapters 11 and 12). When tested, patients with posterior cortical atrophy may have an apperceptive visual agnosia with abnormalities in visual matching and other perceptual tasks. A similar visual agnosia can occur later in the course of typical Alzheimer disease when memory and other cognitive impairments are prominent.

Although considered rare by some, Balint syndrome, in whole or in parts, is actually more frequent than believed, particularly as manifestations of Alzheimer disease and other dementias that result in biparietal disease. These patients present with symptoms and signs of impaired spatial navigation with difficulty scanning their environment and finding things in their drawers, closets, refrigerators, and other visually complex situations. They may walk very cautiously as if blind, bumping into door frames or sitting on the armrests of chairs. Patient's with Balint syndrome essentially are unable to move their eyes or guide their hands to visual stimuli. When looking at pictures or scenes, they see parts of the entire image and not the whole image. Testing involves documenting the presence of simultanagnosia, oculomotor apraxia, and optic ataxia.

Prosopagnosia may result from a number of different causes, suggesting different impairments in face processing. As many as 2.5% of the population are born with a selective impairment in facial processing. Although controversial, this cognitive or development prosopagnosia may result from dysfunction of a right-hemisphere fusiform face area specialized for facial configuration. Acquired prosopagnosia can result from strokes and other focal lesions, as well as neurodegenerative disease particularly affecting the right hemisphere. The most common acquired lesion for impaired face identification appears to be right anterior temporal involvement in semantic dementia. These patients may experience a sense of familiarity for faces, and may have an associative inability of a normally configured face to evoke semantic features.

Conclusions

Much of the posterior neocortex is dedicated to perceptual and spatial abilities. Visual processing, in particular, involves occipital cortex and extends into parietal and temporal lobes. The skilled mental status examiner can cover a great deal of neocortex with the application of perceptual and spatial tests. These tests range from visual constructions to specific perceptual and spatial tasks to the assessment for agnosias. The proficient mental status examiner can extend the testing to the auditory and olfactory modalities as well.

Chapter 11

Praxis and Related Cortical Movement Abnormalities

Clinicians have applied the term "praxis," and its disorder, "apraxia," to a wide number of conditions involving impaired motor performance. A strict and specific use of the term "apraxia" (or "dyspraxia"), however, is limited to disturbances in learned skilled movements due to a cognitive defect in motor programming, such as errors in pantomiming brushing one's teeth or gesturing "good-bye." Patients with apraxia have normal basic motor and sensory functions but cannot perform movements because of disturbances at a cognitive command and control level. The term "apraxia" is misapplied to visuospatial deficits, such as "constructional apraxia," "dressing apraxia," and "oculomotor apraxia" (see Chapter 10); the unique "apraxia of speech," or disorder of motor planning of speech sounds, is discussed in Chapter 8. This chapter primarily discusses the examination of apraxias of the upper extremities, with some discussion of orobuccal-facial, whole body, and gait apraxia and related cortical movement abnormalities.

Apraxia

Apraxia is not rare. It may occur in over half of patients with acute left hemisphere lesions. Causes of apraxia include strokes, tumors, multiple sclerosis, corticobasal syndrome, Alzheimer disease, Creutzfeldt-Jakob disease, Lewy body dementias, and others. In addition, apraxias cause significant dysfunction, particularly when there is difficulty with critical upper extremity and hand movements. Despite the importance of apraxia, clinicians often fail to recognize or evaluate for apraxia, particularly in the presumably spared extremity contralateral to a hemiparetic limb from stroke or other focal lesion.

The model for praxis representation in the brain is analogous to kinesthetic software programs ("praxicons") for automatized movements, which are usually localized in a left parietal hub (Fig. 11.1). This model originates with Hugo Liepmann from the early 1900s and, with elaboration, continues to be the basis for the neuroanatomy of limb praxis. These left parietal praxicons are essentially spatiotemporal movement formulas associated with the meaning of the actions (action semantics). Despite the left hemisphere lateralization, it takes both parietal lobes for automatizing effortful, unfamiliar movements, with the right parietal region contributing to spatial orientation and positioning. Through ventral and dorsal streams, the praxicons connect to the left supplementary motor area for translation into motor programs, which output to primary motor cortex for control of the contralateral limb. Finally, the motor program information traverses the corpus callosum in the frontal region for control of the ipsilateral limb. There are additional influences on praxis from frontal-subcortical motor loops in the basal ganglia, the thalami, and their white matter connections. Left-handed patients may have right parietal praxicons and apraxia from right hemisphere lesions; however, hand preference can be dissociable from the laterality of the movement formulas.

Based on this model, a useful clinical classification of the apraxias includes ideomotor (parietal or disconnection), dissociation, ideational, conceptual, limb-kinetic, and callosal types (Table 11.1). Ideomotor apraxia is the prototypical apraxia syndrome with spatiotemporal errors in performing learned motor acts from problems executing the spatiotemporal movement formulas for these acts, either from left inferior parietal disorders or from disconnection along the pathways from parietal to the ipsilateral motor areas. Dissociation apraxia results in unrecognizable movement consequent to the dissociation of the praxis network from the language commands for eliciting them. Ideational apraxia is an inability to organize

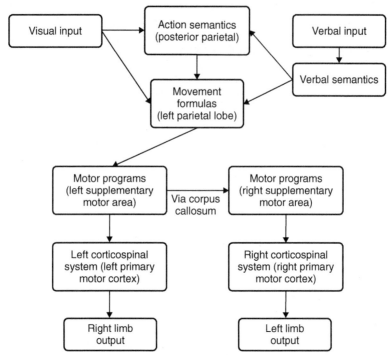

Fig. 11.1 A model of praxis. (Modified from Mendez MF, Deutsch MB. The limb apraxias and related disorders. In: Daroff RB, Fenichel GM, Jankovic MD, Mazziotta JC, Pomeroy SL, eds. *Bradley's Neurology in Clinical Practice.* 7th ed. New York, NY: Elsevier; 2016, pp. 115–121.)

and perform a series of movements in the right order. Conceptual apraxia is an incorrect, but correctly executed, choice of semantic action, such as tool use or tool selection. Clinicians often conflate ideational and conceptual apraxias because they have less specific localization and usually occur together in advanced dementias. Traditionally, the classification of apraxias also includes limb-kinetic apraxia, although this is actually a disturbance in fine finger or motor movements and not a specific disorder of praxis. Finally, the classification of apraxia includes patients with callosal lesions with limb apraxia limited to the nondominant limbs.

THE EXAMINATION OF APRAXIA

Some guidelines are useful for apraxia testing. First, the examination for apraxia and cortical motor disorders must be part of the complete mental status examination (MSX) and neurological examination. The examiner cannot characterize these disorders without excluding other deficits that might be responsible for disturbances in movement. The examiner needs to exclude other cognitive deficits, such as attentional deficits, language impairment, perceptual or spatial disturbances, or executive dysfunction. The examiner also needs to exclude primary motor or sensory problems, such as weakness, rigidity or spasticity, incoordination and dysmetria, or sensory loss. Second, note any complaints of loss of dexterity and observe for any unusual posturing or movements. Patients with apraxia may be unaware of these deficits, and the examiner needs to specifically inquire about the patient's ability to perform skilled movements. Although apraxia is not an evident dystonia or dyskinetic movement disorder, it may be evident on attempts at learned motor movements. Finally, start testing with verbal commands. The examination usually focuses on testing both upper limbs, first the dominant hand and then the nondominant hand independently, avoiding going from one hand to the other so as to avoid self-cueing. If the patient fails to perform normally on verbal commands, then the examiner can evaluate imitation, gesture comprehension, sequencing, conceptual knowledge, real object use, and imitation of meaningless gestures.

TABLE 11.1	Apraxias: Most Likely Finding on Examination					
	Ideomotor-Parietal	Ideomotor-Disconnection	Dissociation	Ideational	Conceptual	Limb-Kinetic
Pantomime to verbal command	Abnormal[1]	Abnormal[1]	Abnormal[2]	Abnormal[3]	Abnormal[4]	Abnormal[5] or Normal
Imitation of gestures	Abnormal[1]	Abnormal[1]	Normal	Normal[3]	Normal	Abnormal[5] or Normal
Gesture knowledge	Abnormal	Normal	Normal	Normal	Normal[4]	Normal
Sequential actions	Normal[1]	Normal	Abnormal	Abnormal	Normal[4]	Normal
Conceptual knowledge	Normal	Normal	Normal	Abnormal	Abnormal	Normal
Real object use	Abnormal[6]	Abnormal[6]	Normal	Abnormal[3,7]	Abnormal[4]	Abnormal[5] or Normal
Meaning-less gestures	Abnormal	Abnormal[6]	Normal	Abnormal[3,7]	Normal[7]	Abnormal[5] or Normal
Limb-kinetic	Normal	Normal	Normal	Normal	Normal	Abnormal[5]

[1]Spatiotemporal production errors on single, individual ideomotor tasks.
[2]Unrecognizable movements or attempts.
[3]For sequencing errors only, i.e., errors on multiple, serial ideomotor tasks.
[4]Abnormal if involves content of tool use/action or tool selection.
[5]For decreased dexterity in fine finger movements.
[6]Errors depend on severity of apraxia; may perform adequately.
[7]But may be abnormal from advanced dementia rather than from apraxia.
Modified from Mendez MF, Deutsch MB. The limb apraxias and related disorders. In: Daroff RB, Fenichel GM, Jankovic MD, Mazziotta JC, Pomeroy SL, eds. *Bradley's Neurology in Clinical Practice*. 7th ed. New York, NY: Elsevier; 2016, pp. 115–121.

AXIAL AND LOWER EXTREMITY APRAXIA

Before discussing limb apraxia there should be a screen for apraxia affecting the central axis of the body and the lower extremities (Table 11.2). Orobuccal-facial apraxia is associated with left inferior frontal and insular lesions. Begin evaluating for orobuccal-facial apraxia by asking the patients to pretend to suck through a straw or pretend to blow out a match. Then evaluate responses to whole body commands, such as asking the patient to stand up, bow, or assume a boxer's stance. Dementia patients with whole body apraxia may have difficulty sitting or standing from a chair or rolling over when in a supine position. Next check for gait apraxia or a "magnetic gait," reported with normal pressure hydrocephalus, vascular dementia, and other frontal lobe conditions. These patients have a hard time getting started, as if their feet are glued to the ground, with subsequent slow, shuffling gait. The examiner can videotape this whole maneuver and time it for quantification (e.g., Timed Walk or Timed Up and Go Tests). In addition to asking them to initiate a gait, evaluate for the presence of a "foot grasp," similar to a hand grasp reflex, with curling down of the toes on stroking the plantar aspect of the feet. Further evaluate for lower extremity apraxia with commands such as writing on the floor while sitting, making figure threes or eights with their legs while supine, and other activities as noted in Table 11.2.

UPPER EXTREMITY LIMB APRAXIA

The upper extremity limb apraxia syndromes differ in a series of testable maneuvers easily performed in a clinic encounter or at the bedside. These tasks include their ability to pantomime to verbal commands, imitate to visual demonstration, understand observed gestures, sequence multistep tasks, choose correct tool or object uses and actions, and perform fine finger movements (Fig. 11.2). The examination of real object use and meaningless gesture interpretation can clarify the apraxia diagnosis, when necessary. In addition, the clinician can

TABLE 11.2	**Praxis Testing of the Axis (Including Lower Extremities)**	
	Transitive Actions	**Intransitive Actions**
Orobuccal-facial	Suck on straw	Wink
	Blow out match	Blow a kiss
	Sniff flowers	Stick out tongue
	Lick icing from lips	Whistle
Whole body	Pretend to lift weights	Stand up
	Swing imaginary bat	Bow
	Pretend to walk tightrope	Roll over in bed
	Pretend to sweep floor	Assume boxer stance
Gait and lower extremities	Kick imaginary ball	Make a figures "3" or "8" with legs while supine
	Write with foot on floor	Turn around when walking
	Emulate bicycle peddling	Start and continue gait
	Put out cigarette	Timed Walk (10 meters or 30 feet) or Up and Go Test (both can videotaped)

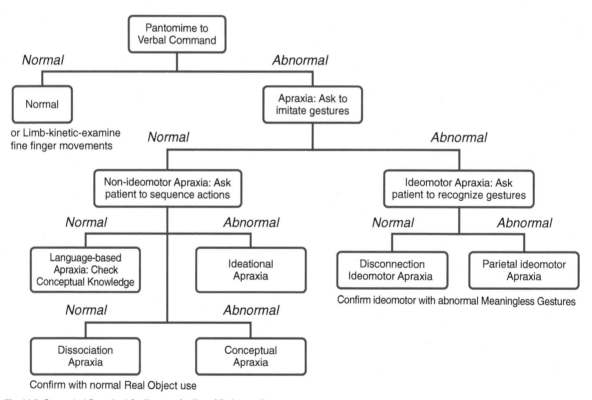

Fig. 11.2 Suggested flow chart for the examination of limb apraxia.

supplement the neurobehavioral status examination (NBSE) with instruments such as the Apraxia Battery for Adults-2, the Florida Apraxia Battery, the Cologne Apraxia Screening, the Test of Upper Limb Apraxia, the Short screening Test for Ideomotor Apraxia, the Diagnostic Instrument of Limb Apraxia, and others.

Ideomotor Apraxia. Patients with ideomotor apraxia-parietal variant and ideomotor apraxia-disconnection variant are unable to pantomime or imitate and may be differentiated in that the parietal variant has additional difficulty with the identification of gestures. The examination of ideomotor apraxia shows difficulty on both pantomime to commands and imitation of action. These patients cannot place their arm and hand in the correct space or move them at the correct speeds and trajectory. The examiner begins with both verbal "transitive" commands, that is, pretending to use an object in a task, and verbal "intransitive" commands, that is, performing symbolic gestures (Table 11.3). Common transitive commands

TABLE 11.3 The Examination for Upper Extremity Limb Apraxias	
FIRST COMPLETE WITH DOMINANT UPPER EXTREMITY, THEN NONDOMINANT	
1. Pantomime to verbal command	
a. Transitive actions	b. Intransitive actions
1. Comb hair	1. Wave good-bye
2. Brush teeth	2. Beckon someone to come
3. Flip a coin	3. Indicate someone to stop
4. Open door with key	4. Salute
5. Cut paper with scissors	5. Shake hand
6. Use a hammer	6. Show how to hitchhike
7. Use a screwdriver	7. Give the victory sign
8. Use a saw	8. Motion to go away
2. Imitation of gestures	
Demonstrate the same actions without naming them and ask patient to copy them	
3. Gesture knowledge	
Demonstrate different actions and ask patient to identify their function/purpose and how well they were performed	
4. Sequential actions	
Examiner instructs that imaginary elements for the task are laid out in front of them	
a. Pretend toothpaste, toothbrush, sink; ask to sequence actions to brush teeth	
b. Pretend paper, pen, letter, stamp; ask to sequence preparing letter for mailing	
c. Pretend bread, meat/cheese, garnish; ask to sequence making a sandwich	
5. Conceptual knowledge	
a. Show the patient either pictures or the actual tools or objects and ask the patient to pantomime or demonstrate their use or function	
b. The examiner may also show a task, such as holding a nail, and ask the patient to pantomime the correct tool use and action	
6. Real object use	
Most limb apraxias improve when using real objects for transitive actions. Dissociation apraxia should be prominently normal despite unrecognizable pantomime actions	
7. Meaningless gestures (e.g., Fig. 11.3)	
May be used to corroborate ideomotor apraxia and limb-kinetic apraxia	

include pretending to comb their hair or brush their teeth, and common intransitive commands include waving good-bye and beckoning others to approach them. If the patient has difficulty pantomiming movements, the examiner demonstrates each of the missed gestures, one at a time, and asks the patient to imitate the movements. In addition, the examiner asks the patient to identify random gestures and whether they felt that the examiner's gestures were performed correctly or poorly. Although not entirely reliable, gesture identification may be impaired with parietal ideomotor apraxia and spared in disconnection ideomotor apraxia. In summary, the sequence of testing, pantomime, imitation, and gesture identification is sufficient to characterize the ideomotor apraxias; however, other apraxias require additional testing. In addition, patients with ideomotor apraxia have difficulty with meaningless gestures because they require spatiotemporal orientation of the limbs and may not improve to normal with real object use.

Dissociation Apraxia. If the patient has difficulty pantomiming on verbal commands, the examiner proceeds to differentiate dissociation apraxia from ideomotor apraxia. Patients with dissociation apraxia, or language-motor disconnection, are unable to correctly understand and pantomime to verbal commands but can imitate them and understand gestures. These patients usually show other evidence of aphasia with decreased auditory comprehension. They may either not respond to a verbal command that they do not understand, stare at their hands, or fail to perform any related movements. However, distinct from patients with ideomotor apraxia, these patients can normally imitate the examiner's gestures and recognize their meaning because this does not require direct access through language. When dissociative apraxia is suspected, it is useful to have the patient further imitate a series of meaningless gestures. Patients with dissociation apraxia can imitate meaningless gestures and do well with real object use.

Ideational Apraxia. Ideational apraxia manifests as a disproportionate inability to correctly sequence a series of movements in a multistep action, for example, the sequence of brushing one's teeth including opening the toothpaste, putting it on the toothbrush, et cetera. Unlike patients with ideomotor apraxia, these patients can pantomime, imitate, and identify individual gestures, but cannot order them to complete a goal. Specifically, the examiner tests for ideational apraxia by telling the patient to imagine that all the items needed for a sequential task are in front of them and then asking them to pantomime the multistep tasks with the items. Other examples of tasks include making a sandwich and preparing and mailing a letter. Errors are evident as a failure to perform the tasks in the correct sequence. Isolated disturbances of ideational apraxia are most probably related to frontal lobe disease, such as in advanced dementias, and these patients may also have conceptual apraxia.

Conceptual Apraxia. Conceptual apraxia is a semantic disorder in which the patient is mistaken on the correct concept for an action. Like the ideomotor apraxias, conceptual apraxia is associated with inability to perform correctly on verbal command but for a different reason. Patients with conceptual apraxia demonstrate the wrong action to command because they are mistaken about the concept ("action semantics") behind the movement, particularly choosing the wrong tool for an action or choosing the wrong action associated with the tool. They make errors in tool-selection and tool-object knowledge with inability to indicate a tool based on its function or action. These patients, who often have advanced dementia, tend to substitute the wrong action for the tool. For example, the examiner may ask the patient to pretend to brush their teeth, and the patient may comb his or her hair instead, or, if provided a toothbrush, brush their teeth with the back and not the bristles. Patients with conceptual apraxia make these "content errors" but can otherwise normally imitate gestures and may correctly identify them. Among patients with either advanced or semantic dementia, conceptual apraxia is most evident when conceptual knowledge is tested by asking them to pantomime the action evident in pictures of tools or on presentation of actual objects.

Limb-Kinetic Apraxia. The examination for limb-kinetic apraxia focuses on fine finger movements (Table 11.4). The examiner asks the patient to do repetitive finger tapping; pick up a small coin with a pincer grasp; and rapidly twirl a coin between their fingers. Patients with limb-kinetic apraxia may have irregular tapping movements, struggle to pick up the coin without using many fingers, and drop the coin on twirling it. They may also have difficulty with meaningless

TABLE 11.4 Testing for Upper Extremity Limb-Kinetic Apraxia	
Dominant Hand	**Nondominant Hand**
____ Finger Taps	____ Finger Taps
Tap index finger in rapid succession as fast as possible	
____ Thumb-Finger Taps	____ Thumb-Finger Taps
Tap thumb with index finger in rapid succession with widest amplitude possible, each hand separately	
____ Alternate Touch	____ Alternate Touch
Touch each fingertip with thumb repeatedly and as fast as possible	
____ Snap Fingers	____ Snap Fingers
Snap thumb and middle finger several times on each hand	
____ Coin Pick-up	____ Coin Pick-up
Use thumb-index finger as pincers; no sliding of coin on surface	
____ Coin Rotations	____ Coin Rotations
Twirl coin between thumb, index, and middle fingers 10 times in a row	

gestures because of loss of dexterity. Limb-kinetic apraxia may be bilateral, particularly if it affects the preferred hand; however, these patients are more likely to have poorly coordinated finger movements in the contralateral limb. Limb-kinetic apraxia results from lesions in the left supplementary motor area or motor involvement in both the primary motor cortex and the post-Rolandic sensory cortex. Clinicians must distinguish limb-kinetic apraxia from primary motor disturbances, and, indeed, this form of apraxia may be an intermediate between limb apraxia and motor paresis.

Callosal Apraxias. Most limb apraxias are bilateral; however, strokes and other lesions in the anterior corpus callosum, where fibers cross from one motor area to the other, can result in isolated ipsilateral limb apraxia. This generally involves the nondominant, usually left, arm or hand in right-handed people. In contrast, the right limb may be affected in some left-handed individuals. Other than its isolation to one side, callosal apraxia is not a separate apraxic disorder and corresponds to one of the other apraxia mechanisms. Many have an ideomotor-disconnection apraxia confined to one extremity. These patients cannot pantomime or imitate with their nondominant limb and may show problems with meaningless gestures and real object use in that limb but can recognize and identify gestures. Others have a dissociation apraxia with inability to pantomime to command but

normal imitation, gesture comprehension, and real object use. Some patients with callosal apraxia in the nondominant limb show both ideomotor apraxia with spatiotemporal errors on imitation, and dissociation apraxia with unrecognizable movements on pantomime command. In addition, there are rare reports of patients with callosal apraxia who have had both ideomotor apraxia and limb-kinetic apraxia in the nondominant limb and who have had conceptual apraxia with action semantic difficulty when they are presented just in the right visual field. Callosal lesions can lead to alien limb phenomena and, among split-brain patients, agonistic and diagnostic apraxia; these conditions are discussed later as related cortical movement abnormalities.

SPECIAL TOPICS ON APRAXIA TESTING

Interpretation of Praxis Errors. For the examiner, it is worth emphasizing the different errors indicative of the different apraxia types. Patients with apraxia make errors in movements in their spatiotemporal configuration, sequencing, content (action semantics), and dexterity. Spatiotemporal errors, with hesitant, choppy, and effortful movements are characteristic of ideomotor apraxia. These patients have difficulty in correctly executing movements based on the spatial orientation and positioning of their hands, fingers, or limbs, particularly in relation to objects in transitive actions. They also have difficulty in correctly executing the timing of the movements and the correct trajectory of their limb through space. These errors are evident on both pantomimes to verbal command and on imitation of the examiner's gestures. These errors are most impaired with verbal commands and least impaired with real object use, and they are worse with transitive actions than with intransitive actions. The distinguishing feature of the parietal variant of ideomotor apraxia, as opposed to the disconnection variant, is further inability to recognize many gestures and their normal versus abnormal execution, presumably from damage to the praxicons themselves. Patients with dissociation apraxia do not understand the language of the verbal commands and make characteristically unrecognizable movements. Patients with ideational apraxia make errors in the sequencing of individual tasks in a multitask action, and patients with conceptual apraxia make errors in the choice of tools and their correct actions. As previously noted, patients with ideational and conceptual apraxias may have totally normal imitation and recognition of individual gestures, but they fail to either sequence actions or match them with the correct tool or object in a transitive act, respectively. Limb-kinetic apraxia is evident in the loss of finger dexterity, coordination, and speed of performance. Finally, callosal apraxia affects only one side of the body, usually the nondominant upper extremity.

An error that all apraxia patients make, as well as some normal people, is "body part substitution" or the use of a body part as a pretend object in a transitive act. On responding to a pantomime command for a transitive action, these patients may use a body part, most commonly their fingers, as the tool or object in the requested action. Examples of these "body-part-as-object" errors are using their index finger as a pretend toothbrush or their fingers as a pretend comb. This can be a normal response; hence the examiner must correct the patient and reiterate that they should not use their fingers but an imagined or "pretend" tool instead. If they persist in making body-part-as-object errors, this may be an early indicator of ideomotor apraxia. Furthermore, if body-part-as-object errors persist despite correction, then the patient may have injury to the inferior frontal cortex as part of a left parieto-fronto-temporal network.

Real Object Use, Spontaneous Performance, and Synkinesis. Patients with apraxia can improve with real objects, with their spontaneous performance, or with incorporation of the nontested extremity. The examiner may test their performance by providing them with actual tools and asking them to demonstrate their use. Because this provides additional sensory and conceptual cues, many patients with apraxia have a near normal performance; however, those with ideomotor apraxia (particularly parietal variant) or with limb-kinetic apraxia can show hesitancy or clumsiness even with the actual tools or objects. Investigators have long observed the poorly understood paradox of patients with severe apraxia on verbal command demonstrating normal performance on spontaneous initiation, for example, a normal performance on spontaneously waving good-bye as the examiner leaves the room. These patients may have normal praxicons that are accessed through other cognitive or conceptual routes, such as visuospatial input through the right hemisphere. Investigators have also observed a tendency for praxis movements in the limb being tested to improve when the movements are simultaneously done in the other, nontested extremity. Sometimes patients automatically mirror the requested movement in the opposite limb. This improvement, known as "enabling synkinesis," may be further evidence of the facilitating influence of the opposite hemisphere on movements.

Examination of Meaningless Movements. The imitation of purposeless, unfamiliar, and not yet automatized movements requires both parietal lobes and the frontal lobes. The right parietal lobe contributes through its role in spatial processing and orientation, and both parietal lobes integrate the visuospatial information with movement, hence both parietal lobes participate in learning and automatizing new movements. The prefrontal area is also required for motor sequencing. Patients with ideomotor apraxia from left parietal lesions may have difficulty imitating meaningless finger or hand gestures, and patients with limb-kinetic apraxia may have prominent difficulty with the dexterous performance of these meaningless movements. For these movements, the examiner has the patient imitate at least four unfamiliar movements, such as those illustrated in Fig. 11.3. In summary, problems imitating meaningless movements

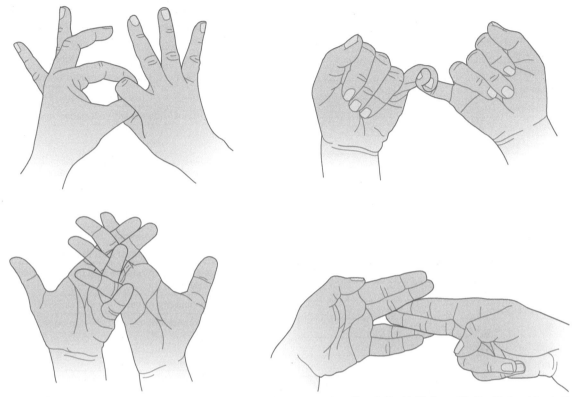

Fig. 11.3 Examples of meaningless gestures or movements for imitation. (Modified from Moo LR, Slotnick SD, Tesoro MA, Zee DS, Hart J. Interlocking finger test: a bedside screen for parietal lobe dysfunction. *J Neurol Neurosurg Psychiatry.* 2003;74:530-532.)

may be due to basic motor difficulty from limb-kinetic apraxia, ideomotor apraxia with problems integrating spatial relationships with limb movements, problems with spatial processing from the right parietal lobe, and disturbed motor sequencing from frontal dysfunction. Imitating meaningless gestures bimanually may be especially indicative of biparietal disease, as from Alzheimer disease.

RELATED CORTICAL MOVEMENT ABNORMALITIES

Disturbances of cognitive motor movements resembling apraxia include the motor neglect syndromes (Table 11.5). Motor neglect occurs when there is reluctance to either initiate movement of one part of the body or to move a part of the body into contralateral hemispace. Motor neglect occurs in the absence of hemispatial neglect or primary sensory or motor deficits. Primary motor neglect is evident when the patient fails to spontaneously move an extremity or one side of the body ("akinesia") or initiates the movement only after a notable delay ("hypokinesia"). Unilateral directional akinesia or hypokinesia is present when the patient fails or delays initiation of movement of a limb into the contralateral hemispace or in the contralateral direction. The difference between primary motor neglect and unilateral directional akinesia or hypokinesia is that the former is limb or body centered and the latter is space or direction centered. These syndromes are particularly evident in spontaneous activities and in performing bimanual actions, and they may improve when prompted to use the neglected limb or initiate the neglected movement. For detection of unilateral directional hypokinesia, the examiner additionally asks the patient to move

TABLE 11.5 Related Cortical Movement Abnormalities
1. Agonistic
2. Akinesia
3. Alien limb
4. Catalepsy
5. Compulsive-like
6. Diagnostic apraxia
7. Echopraxia
8. Hypokinesia
9. Imitation
10. Magnetic grasp and grope
11. Mitgehen
12. Mitmachen
13. Motor impersistence
14. Motor neglect
15. Perseveration
16. Stereotypies
17. Unilateral directional hypokinesia
18. Utilization

TABLE 11.6 Alien Limb Phenomena
Core features
• Sensation of an "alien limb" that feels foreign
• Limb has involuntary, semipurposeful movements
Supportive features
• Perception of not knowing limb's location in space
• Spontaneous limb levitation
Variants
• "Callosal" region with associated intermanual conflict or diagnostic dyspraxia
• "Frontal" with associated frontal release or other frontal signs
• "Posterior" or occipitoparietal
• Avoids grasping or contact with the affected limb
• Often increased with posture and decreased with posture change
• Distraction has not effect
• Movement cannot be slowed but can be stopped
Pathology
• Anteromedial corpus callosum
• Supplementary motor area or surrounding frontal area
• Occipitoparietal

the arms into contralateral hemispace. Motor neglect syndromes may result from lesions in associative motor areas in the frontal lobes or in basal ganglia and thalamus.

Alien Limb Phenomenon. Another disorder of cortical motor movements, the alien limb phenomena, often occurs in patients with apraxia but is distinguishable from any of the apraxia syndromes (Table 11.6). The "alien limb" moves, raises, or "acts on its own." In other words, this condition is a sensation of an "alien limb" because there are limb movements that the patients feel were not initiated by them or that were moved by someone else. The most common movement is spontaneous levitation of the nondominant limb, but there may be a range of semipurposeful movements. Patients with alien limb phenomena may have deficits in spatial orientation of the nondominant limb, difficulty using it for normal activities, and a need to self-restrain its "alien" actions with the normal limb. There are several variants of the alien limb phenomena. The best documented involves patients with a callosal alien limb with independent movement of the nondominant limb. It involves disconnection of the two hemispheres, either surgically or functionally, with lesions in the corpus callosum with or without involvement of the adjacent supplementary motor areas. These patients may also have nondominant limb apraxia, diagnostic apraxia, or agonistic apraxia. Another variant of alien limb phenomenon results from frontal lobe disease, with possible frontal grasp or grope reflexes, and may be associated with neurodegenerative conditions, such as corticobasal syndrome. A final variant of alien limb phenomena is a consequence of occipitoparietal damage with a tendency to avoid grasping or contact with the "alien limb."

Diagnostic and Agnostic Apraxia. Callosal lesions can partially disconnect the hemispheres and result in either "diagnostic apraxia" characterized by intermanual conflict between the actions of the two limbs acting in opposition to each other or "agonistic apraxia" characterized by automatic execution of commands with the opposite hand. This rarely occurs outside of split-brain patients who have had a corpus callosotomy. Split-brain patients may find that the left hand is unbuttoning their garment while the right one is buttoning it (diagnostic) or, conversely, that they are executing the command in the opposite limb (agonistic). There are reports of diagnostic apraxia with Marchiafava-Bignami syndrome, and callosal disconnection from multiple sclerosis.

Frontal Lobe Movements. A number of related disorders of cortical motor movements are due to frontal lesions, from frontal release signs to semipurposeful stereotypies and compulsive-like acts. These behaviors are important to note here because of the need to differentiate them from apraxia. Advanced frontal lobe disease can result in "release" signs, such as grasp reflexes, or the more extreme grope reflexes in which the patient cannot keep from actively reaching out for items in the environment or drawing over a stimulus (Chapter 13). Frontal release signs may be associated with manifestations of a more general "environmental dependency syndrome." Patients with this condition may automatically manipulate or use objects in front of them ("utilization behavior"), imitate or mimic other people's observed behavior ("imitation behavior"), and copy their motor movements ("echopraxia") or their speech ("echolalia"). Dorsolateral frontal lesions may also result in motor perseveration, which includes an inability to stop movements or an inability to keep from returning to them. Paradoxically, in some cases there is the opposite, a motor impersistence or failure to maintain a movement or posture. In some frontally impaired patients there is a tendency for a body part to be easily moved with light touch or pressure ("mitgehen"), or to be easily placed in an unusual position with gradual return ("mitmachen"), or with prolonged maintenance of the unusual position ("catalepsy" or waxy flexibility). Additional frontal origin behaviors include disinhibition and poor impulse control from orbitofrontal lesions and stereotypies and compulsive-like behaviors from fronto-limbic-striatal involvement.

Clinical Implications

Disorders of praxis and of cortical motor movements are particularly associated with disease affecting left inferior parietal, left dorsolateral frontal, and premotor or supplementary motor areas. As noted, the left hemisphere is implicated in disturbances of the "praxis circuit," including disconnection of white matter pathways involving transfer of motor information across the corpus callosum to the opposite, usually right, hemisphere (Fig. 11.1). Limb apraxias may also result from subcortical lesions affecting basal ganglia and thalamus, possibly through injury to their fronto-subcortical circuits. The apraxias are potential symptoms of focal disease, whether stroke, tumor, or other lesion in these areas, but a number of dementias or neurodegenerative diseases produce apraxias and related abnormalities, including Alzheimer disease, Creutzfeldt-Jakob disease, and corticobasal syndrome.

Corticobasal syndrome is a neurodegenerative syndrome, which is specifically characterized by limb apraxia and alien limb phenomena. Corticobasal syndrome is, perhaps, the most prototypical example of a progressive limb apraxia. This syndrome usually begins in middle-age, commonly with an asymmetric parkinsonian rigidity and other motor signs. Although the disease tends to begin on one side of the body, it becomes bilateral with progression of the disease. In addition to initial asymmetric involvement, criteria for a probable diagnosis include at least two of the following cognitive signs: apraxia (ideomotor, ideational, limb-kinetic), alien limb phenomena (beyond simple levitation), or sensory cortical deficits (graphesthesia, stereognosis), and at least two of the following motor signs: rigidity/bradykinesia, dystonia, or myoclonus. On autopsy, corticobasal syndrome may have neuropathological changes of corticobasal degeneration, Alzheimer disease, progressive supranuclear palsy, frontotemporal lobar degeneration, or dementia with Lewy bodies.

Patients with behavioral variant frontotemporal dementia have characteristic repetitive behaviors described as ritualistic, compulsive-like, or stereotypies. These movements are usually semipurposeful and performed in a repetitively stereotypical manner. They include verbal repetitions, such as palilalia, echolalia, and repetitive vocalizations, stereotypical movements of the extremities or face, and more complex compulsive-like behaviors, such as repetitive, unnecessary trips to the bathroom. These behaviors are not clearly negatively driven from anxiety or obsessions, but rather reflect a repetitive impulsivity driven by an immediate desire. These "compulsive impulses" may reflect involvement of a fronto-limbic-striatal system on the right. These behaviors are primarily detected on observations, rather than brought out with any particular testing technique.

Conclusions

The examination for apraxia is an integral part of the MSX and the NBSE. Mental status examiners sometimes neglect examining praxis because of its overtly motor nature, rather than appearing as a neurocognitive function. Nevertheless, praxis is part of the MSX and NBSE and has important localization value in neurological disease. The examination of praxis, when performed in the systematic manner with analysis of errors, can lead to valuable information. Clinicians must first distinguish apraxia from primary motor weakness, sensory deficits, or other cognitive and spatial disturbances. The systematic MSX can further distinguish the main apraxias described here, parietal-ideomotor, disconnection-ideomotor, dissociation, ideational, conceptual, limb-kinetic, and callosal apraxias. Furthermore, other related cortical motor abnormalities, such as alien limb phenomena and frontally related movements, offer additional information as to neurocognitive dysfunction. Indeed, apraxia is an important cognitive disorder evident in patients with corticobasal syndrome, Alzheimer disease, and many other conditions.

Chapter 12

Calculations and Related Functions

The ability to appreciate quantities, understand numbers, and calculate is a cognitive domain in its own right. This domain has a left inferior parietal hub involving the horizontal portion of the intraparietal sulcus, an area that appears dedicated to processing symbolic numerical information. However, many other areas and their cognitive functions can affect calculation abilities. This chapter discusses the evaluation for acalculias and includes assessment of left parietal neighborhood signs and symptoms included in the Gerstmann syndrome.

Acalculia

Acalculia is an acquired disturbance of the ability to calculate with numbers. The term "acalculia" dates to 1925 when Henschen studied impairment of computational skills from brain injury and noted the significance of the angular gyrus and intraparietal fissure for mathematical ability. The ability to calculate can be disturbed from a primary disorder of numerical ability in this region or from the secondary effects of other cognitive deficits (Table 12.1). Primary acalculia involves the loss of numerical concepts and the inability to understand or execute basic arithmetical operations, whereas secondary acalculia involves the loss of the ability to calculate from language, spatial, motor praxis, or executive impairments. Primary acalculia is often associated with the neighborhood signs of digit agnosia, right-left discrimination difficulty, and transitional agraphia in Gerstmann syndrome, discussed further in this chapter.

There are different classifications of acalculia, but one clinically useful classification presented here divides them into four primary and four secondary acalculias. The main primary acalculia, often referred to as anarithmetia, is an impairment of a "digital magnitude code" in the left inferior parietal

TABLE 12.1 An Organization of the Acalculias
Primary
1. Anarithmetia: defect in computational abilities digital magnitude code (inferior left parietal)
• Loss of numerical concepts
• Inability to understand quantities
• Defects in using syntactic rules in calculation, e.g., borrowing, carrying over
• Deficits in understanding numerical signs
2. Impaired analog magnitude code (biparietal)
3. Asymbolia for knowing arithmetic signs (left temporo-occipital junction)
4. Impaired retrieval of mathematical information
Secondary
1. Language (lexical-symbolic) difficulty
• Aphasic: Broca, Wernicke, conduction, etc.
• Alexia or agraphia for Arabic numerals
• Specific number difficulty: e.g., 7, 9, 0
• Verbal acalculia
2. Spatial difficulty
3. Motor difficulty from limb apraxia
4. Executive dysfunction, especially in working memory

area with decreased digital processing of quantity and operations. Anarithmetia is a specific disturbance of global quantification abilities and the use of syntactic rules and symbols for calculation. On testing, they fail in quantitatively comparing numbers and in doing procedures such as borrowing, carrying over, or solving successive mathematical tasks. Patients with anarithmetia have calculation defects in both oral and written operations and usually other "neighborhood" cognitive difficulties, such as Gerstmann syndrome. These patients may still be able to count aloud, perform rote numerical learning such as the multiplication tables, and conserve some numerical knowledge. Anarithmetia occurs in patients when damage affects the horizontal segment

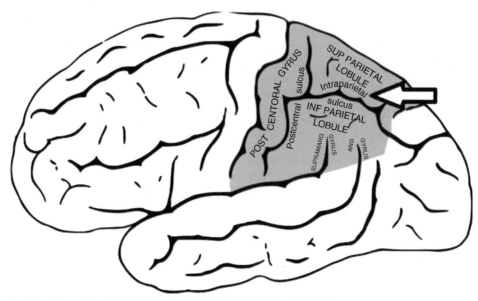

Fig. 12.1 A hub of calculation ability. Left hemisphere horizontal intraparietal sulcus indicated by arrow.

of the intraparietal sulcus, which borders the superior aspect of the inferior parietal lobule (Fig. 12.1).

Other primary acalculias include an impairment of an analog magnitude code in right and left parietal areas with decreased analog processing of position and relationships; semantic impairment of mathematical symbols ("mathematical asymbolia") in the left temporo-occipital junction with decreased knowledge of mathematical signs; and impairment of the retrieval of mathematical facts out of proportion to other executive or memory deficits. These other primary acalculias are much less common than anarithmetia. Primary acalculia from impairment of the analog code requires biparietal injury and may affect the ability to tell basic ordinal differences, for example, ordering by relative size. These patients are often very impaired and cannot be tested for acalculia in any more depth. Numerical asymbolia is a rare semantic deficit, and primary acalculia from disproportionate difficulty retrieving mathematical information, such as multiplication tables, may be a frequently missed frontal-executive deficit. In addition, there are rare and debated reports of primary acalculias that just involve difficulty with specific numbers such as 7, and other reports of acalculia limited to the verbal modality but not involving Arabic numerals and not consequent to greater language impairment.

The most common secondary acalculia is due to language impairments in appreciating the verbal names and Arabic numeral notations for numbers. This type of acalculia may accompany Broca aphasia, with impaired calculation syntax or numerical agrammatism including difficulty with number sequences. Examples of acalculia with Broca aphasia include inability to complete mathematical operations, transcoding (verbal to numerical) errors (for example, "twenty-three" to 23), and "stack" errors (for example, 27 is read as 7). Acalculia also accompanies Wernicke aphasia with lexical and semantic errors in saying, reading, and writing numbers. This is often manifest as paraphasic errors: for example, on hearing or reading 45 they may repeat 37 and write 51. In addition, they may make lexicalization errors (for example, on hearing three thousand two hundred ten they may write 300020010) and decomposition errors (for example, on reading 3210 they may say "thirty-two and ten"). Acalculia can accompany the different forms of alexia, both central and peripheral, with similar deficits for numbers as for words, including inability to read number signs with central alexias and number-by-number reading in the syndrome of alexia without agraphia (see Chapter 8).

The other secondary acalculias result from spatial, motor praxis, or executive deficits (see Chapters 10, 11, and 13). Spatial acalculia often accompanies occipitoparietal damage with perceptual impairments and right parietal damage with spatial deficits, including hemispatial neglect. Patients with spatial acalculia can count, perform successive operations, and may do somewhat better on mental calculations than on written calculations. Their main problem is in spatially organizing and placing numbers in the correct location due to visuospatial difficulty, including hemispatial neglect. Secondary acalculia may result from an inability to write numbers secondary to an ideomotor or limb-kinetic apraxia of the hands with difficulty mechanically writing numbers. Another secondary acalculia arises from prefrontal injuries with executive and working memory dysfunction in mental operations that require holding information and manipulating it, for example, multistep numerical problems and serial reversal tasks, such as counting backward from 100 by 7s. These patients are impaired in executive functions necessary for maintaining and manipulating numbers. In contrast to spatial and motor apraxic acalculia, patients with frontal acalculia do better on written calculations than on mental calculations.

The Examination for Acalculias

Calculation ability implies use of numerical concepts. Small quantities from 1 to 3 do not need to be counted, a process known as subitization and present in small children and in other animals; however, larger quantities involve the representation of quantity implicit in numbers, the numerical position within other numerical symbols, the relationships between a number and other numbers, and the relationships between numerical symbols and their verbal representations. Much of the testing for the acalculias focuses on these numerical properties. Before actual testing, however, the examiner must determine if the patient has symptoms of acalculia and whether they have the premorbid ability and education to perform calculation tests. The examiner must be aware of the many types of symptoms that can reflect difficulty with calculation abilities (Table 12.2). A good neurobehavioral history is helpful in detecting these symptoms (see Chapter 6). Some patients never learned or developed their innate mathematical abilities, and others have poor skills because of increasing reliance on calculators and other electronic devices. The examiner can

TABLE 12.2 **Acalculia Symptoms**	
Eighteen Patients with Acalculia Variant Alzheimer Disease	**N**
Difficulty with calculations, simple math, and numbers	10
Difficulty writing checks and managing checkbooks	6
Difficulty reading numbers and words	5
Word-finding problems	8
Difficulty writing and spelling	6
Inability to do finances and pay bills	4
Difficulty with depth perception AND dressing apraxia	2
Difficulty calculating the tip at restaurants	2
Inability to managing clients' bills	2
Difficulty with motor manipulation of objects or tasks	1
Difficulty counting money	1
Having trouble reading a tape measure	1
Trouble with tape and visual scales and plans	1
Difficulty with the numbers in dialing a telephone	1
Difficulty setting a timer with numbers	1
Difficulty using a measuring cup	1
Difficulty reading the time on a clock	1
Problems judging time and distance driving	1
Unable to remember how many zeros are in 10,000	1
Complaint of confusing 8 million with 8 thousand	1

From Mendez MF, Moheb N, Desarzant RE, Teng EH. The progressive acalculia presentation of parietal variant Alzheimer's disease. *J Alzheimer Dis*. 2018;63:941-948.

start by assessing if the patient has basic counting ability by asking them to count objects in the room or dots on a page (Fig. 12.2).

Examiners most frequently rely on serial subtraction tests to briefly screen for calculation difficulty. Patients must count backward from 100 by 7s or count backward from 20 by 3s, as are used for testing attention and mental control (see Chapter 7). In the first, the examiner asks the patient to subtract by 7 beginning with the number 100, for example, 93, 86, 79, 72, 65, et cetera. The number of errors are the number of incorrect subtractions; if the patient makes an incorrect subtraction at one level, the examiner corrects the patient

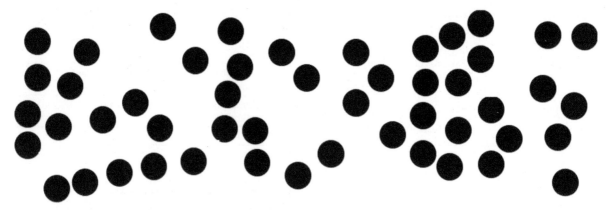

Fig. 12.2 Counting screening. Count all the black circles on the page without repeating any. Total score: (___/50)

and instructs the patient to continue subtracting from the corrected number. Alternatively, the subsequent "correct" subtractions are determined from the incorrect number, that is, if the patient subtracts 7 from 100 as 94, then the subsequent correct subtraction is 87 and not 86. Patients should be able to get three or more subtractions in a row. Counting backward from 20 by 3s is a similar, but easier, version of serial subtractions.

Some clinicians briefly screen for calculation difficulty with an oral word problem. Although able to clarify the presence or absence of calculation difficulty, these word problems do not specify the type of acalculia. One example is to ask the patient to calculate the number of books on two shelves, if there are 18 books with twice as many on one shelf as the other. Another example is to ask the patient to report the number of nickels in $1.35, or the number of quarters in $6.75. Tell the patient: "The girl went to the store with $5 to buy 2 sodas for $1.85 each. What was her change?" Individuals of limited educational background may fail formal mathematical tasks but demonstrate competence when asked to handle money.

For routine screening, it is not necessary to test all four major arithmetic operations, and problems in addition and subtraction are sufficient. The patient can perform two simple double-digit calculations such as 47 + 18 = ___ and 82 − 16 = ___. During these calculations, have the patient specifically read the arithmetic signs and describe their operation. In addition, ask the patient for items reflective of numeracy (the term is used here as the ability to apply mathematics to the real world). Start by asking the number of days

in a week and weeks in a half a year, and then follow this up with a simple word problem.

The examiner can more extensively evaluate for multiple aspects of calculation ability with a screening battery of tests (Table 12.3). The examiner can determine if there is a primary acalculia by eliminating secondary acalculias based on their mistakes and any accompanying deficits. First, ask the patient to read and transpose verbal numbers to Arabic numerals and vice versa. This assesses for a language ("lexical-symbolic") secondary acalculia. Second, ask the patient to write numbers of one, two, or more digits. This assesses for apraxia or motor deficits in writing. Third, ask them to write a dictated addition and subtraction problem with double or triple digits without performing the problem. Spatial errors in alignment may emerge. Fourth, the examiner asks a series of simple mental calculations. To test mental calculation, ask the patient to do 4 + 13, 21 − 3, 6 x 5, and 25/5 in their head. Alternatively, give the continuous additions task in which the patient must add the successive overlapping pairs as rapidly as possible: 5, 2, 7, 3, 4, et cetera (adds last to next to last for 7, 9, 10, 7). Finally, follow this up with actual performance on written calculations.

A systematic evaluation of calculation functions is indicated when a primary acalculia is suspected. Expanding on the screening battery (Table 12.3), this assessment specifically evaluates eight areas in detail: reading and transcoding, number writing, spatial alignment, mental calculations and estimates, arithmetic signs, analog and ordinal processing, and numeracy including arithmetic reasoning and

TABLE 12.3 Acalculia Battery

1. Transcoding

A. Spoken verbally	⇒ Written Arabic numeral responses
381, 495, 1405, 7643, 10280, 132406	

B. Written Arabic numerals	⇒ Read aloud responses
279, 756, 2450, 7658, 12038, 134906	

C. Written Arabic numerals	⇒ Written number word responses
316, 572, 2364, 4125, 28054, 303008	

D. Written number words	⇒ Written Arabic numeral responses
Three hundred five	Four hundred six thousand four hundred fifty three
Five thousand eight hundred seventy six	One thousand five hundred eighty one
Twelve thousand three hundred ninety	Two hundred eighty seven

2. Writing numbers

Instruct to write a series of numbers to dictation: 21 84 2,304 84 730 17,241 3 107

3. Spatial alignment

Align without calculating; one item for each operation (each with three- and two-digit numbers):

A. 376 + 25	B. 621 − 72
C. 73 x 308	D. 869 ÷ 69

4. Mental calculations and estimates ("perform in your head")

16 + 5	27 + 14	29 − 7	15 − 6
7 x 8	11 x 3	12 ÷ 4	28 ÷ 7

Estimate of 39 x 28.7: a. 600, b. 1200, c. 2300, d. 1.5

5. Written calculation performance (examples; see also Table 12.4)

A. Addition	376 + 27	495 + 51
B. Subtraction	129 − 32	621 − 73
C. Multiplication	824 x 16	417 x 325

6. Arithmetic sign recognition

Reading aloud:	1 + 2	5 x 7	9 − 3	16 ÷ 4
Writing from dictation:	6 + 2	13 x 4	25 ÷ 5	42 − 20

7. Analog-ordinal processing

A. Place numbers 57, 32, 78, 12, 93 on the following analog line:

0 _____ 100

B. Which number in each pair is larger?

6 or 5	14 or 12	24 or 27	133 or 143
782 or 872	2,142 or 1,242	6,580 or 8,650	71,142 or 72,300

8. Numerosity and arithmetic reasoning (see also Table 12.5)

How many days in a week? How many seasons in a year? How many months in a year? How many hours in a day? How many days in a year?

Estimate either weights, lengths, or number of elements: e.g., truck (weight), players on a basketball team, chair height, number of schoolchildren in a classroom, frog length.

TABLE 12.4	**More Extensive Mathematical Testing**				
A. Addition			**B. Subtraction**		
5	15	55	5	31	72
+ 3	+ 7	+ 89	− 2	− 8	− 35
C. Multiplication			**D. Division (optional)**		
5	5	14	—	—	—
x 6	x 13	x 15	2√4	3√39	13√31

TABLE 12.5	**Numeracy**
Including Math Knowledge, Arithmetic Reasoning, and Cognitive Estimations	
1.	How far is it from New York City to Paris (London, Cairo, etc.)?
2.	If it takes 4 employees 42 minutes to pack 100 boxes, how many could they pack in 1 hour?
3.	What is the height of the tallest building in the world (United States, Asia, etc.)?
4.	How many apples would it take to make 5 dozen?
5.	What is the population of North America (United States, Europe, etc.)?
6.	Each of 8 workmen are paid 128 dollars to evenly divide among themselves; how many dollars does each workman get?
7.	What is average height of U.S. men (women, etc.)?
8.	If 4 men can paint a house in 6 days; how long should it take 3 men to do it?
9.	If a house is 2400 square feet, how many rooms of 12 square feet could you fit in the house?
10.	How long would it take to walk 1 mile (kilometer, etc.)?
11.	The temperature started at 74 degrees then went down 15 degrees before rising 7 degrees. What is the temperature?
12.	How long ago was the First World War?
13.	How many people are 11 men and 4 women?
14.	How many people died in World War II?
15.	If you are 38 miles from home and drive 17 miles toward it, how far are you from home?
16.	How big is Russia (France, Japan, etc.)?
17.	At 55 miles an hour, approximately how long would it take you to drive 14 miles?
18.	Approximately how many insects are there in the world?
19.	A half a pound of sliced meat costs $3.92. How much can you get $15?
20.	What is the fastest speed of a horse (deer, wolf, etc.)?

knowledge. For this systematic evaluation, the examiner asks the patient to do more calculations, particularly written ones as this allows for a greater process interpretation of the actual steps and errors in calculation. Instruct the patient that you are going to do arithmetic problems that range from easy to hard and not to worry about missing a problem but just to complete them. There should be a wide number of both single- and double-digit problems, two or more each of addition, subtraction, and multiplication, with division being optional (Table 12.4). During this testing, the examiner evaluates several other areas in addition to the problem itself. Have the patient read the problems out loud prior to performing them. This indicates whether the patient can read and recognize individual numbers. Then assess the recognition of the basic four signs for calculation as there can be an asymbolia for these operands. Note whether the patient has knowledge of rote operations and can retrieve multiplication and other facts. During the calculations, observe for errors in borrowing, carrying over, sequencing, and spatially aligning the written calculations. If indicated, ask the patient to do analog and ordinal tasks as outlined in Table 12.3, item 7. If these functions are impaired and language is intact, the patient may have biparietal dysfunction that precludes further testing for acalculia. Finish with numeracy, evaluating mathematical knowledge, arithmetic reasoning, and cognitive estimations (Table 12.5). For example, the examiner can ask the patient to estimate the distance between New York and Paris or the height of the tallest building in the world.

Ultimately, this thorough assessment should be able to distinguish between the different acalculias (Table 12.6). If an even more thorough assessment is still required, there are a number of published batteries that can further characterize acalculia. One well-designed calculation battery widely discussed in the literature is the EC301 battery developed by Deloche et al. (1994). This acalculia battery has been standardized to age, educational level, and sex, and consists

TABLE 12.6   Acalculia Examination

Main, but Not Exclusive, Errors in Following Tasks	Lexical-Symbolic	Motor/Apraxia	Spatial	Executive	Anarithmetia	Asymbolia	Analog	Numerosity
Transcoding (stack, lexicalization, decomposition, paraphasic errors)	X							
Writing numbers		X						
Spatial alignment (placement errors)			X					
Mental calculations				X				
Calculation process (borrowing and carryover errors)					X			
Arithmetic sign recognition						X		
Analog-ordinal (number positioning and ordering errors)							X	
Numerosity and arithmetic reasoning (including cognitive estimations)								X

of 31 subtests organized in 13 sections: 1) counting: spoken verbal counting, digit counting, and written verbal counting; 2) dot enumeration; 3) transcoding; 4) arithmetical signs; 5) magnitude comparison; 6) mental calculation; 7) calculation approximations; 8) placing numbers on an analog line; 9) writing down an operation; 10) written calculations; 11) perceptual quantity estimation; 12) contextual magnitude judgment; and 13) numerical knowledge.

Gerstmann Syndrome

In 1940, Gerstmann's original description involved a constellation of symptoms from lesions in the left parietal lobe, specifically the left angular gyrus, although extending into supramarginal and adjacent parietal gyri. The greater "angular gyrus syndrome" is composed of Gerstmann syndrome with accompanying anomia and alexia. The four dissociable elements of Gerstmann syndrome itself are anarithmetic acalculia (discussed earlier), digit agnosia, right-left disorientation, and transitional agraphia. Digit agnosia in the upper extremities ("finger agnosia") is the inability to distinguish, name, or recognize fingers including on one's own hand, the examiner's hand, or in a drawing of a hand. Many investigators have postulated an evolutionary relationship between numerical knowledge, the digital or decimal system, counting, and finger knowledge reflected in digit agnosia. Patients with right-left disorientation are easily perplexed with what is the right or the left side on themselves or others, particularly when there are crossed commands, for example, "touch your right ear with your left hand." Digit agnosia and right-left disorientation are disturbances that are sometimes associated with autotopagnosia or somatotopagnosia (inability to localize on one's own or others' body) and may indicate a body map in the left inferior parietal region. Digit agnosia may be a mild form of autotopagnosia. Finally, the agraphia in Gerstmann syndrome appears to include, in part, difficulty integrating orthographic with graphomotor codes in the hand; this "transitional" agraphia can occur without any alexia or reading disturbance and without other language impairment (see Chapter 8).

TABLE 12.7	**Digit Agnosia**		
	IDENTIFICATION BY NAMING, POINTING		
	Correct	Incorrect ⇒	Response if incorrect:
Right thumb	☐	☐	
Right pointer finger	☐	☐	
Right middle finger	☐	☐	
Right ring finger	☐	☐	
Right pinky	☐	☐	
Left thumb	☐	☐	
Left pointer finger	☐	☐	
Left middle finger	☐	☐	
Left ring finger	☐	☐	
Left pinky	☐	☐	
If fail above, then additional Nonverbal Digit Agnosia tasks:			
1. Number of fingers between two touched and unseen fingers			
2. Move fingers on a hand that is out of sight and indicate corresponding finger on the contralateral hand			
3. Tasks with drawings or pictures of hands			
Digit agnosia findings:			
☐ Normal		☐ Abnormal	
		Number of errors: __	

The Examination for Gerstmann Syndrome Beyond Acalculia

Digit Agnosia. First, the examiner asks to the patient to name each of the fingers on their hands and on the examiner's hands (Table 12.7). The tests for digit agnosia particularly focus on the index, middle, and third fingers and can be extended to the toes. Second, the examiner asks the patient to point to named fingers on their own hands and on the examiner's hands. Although these tests assess naming or pointing to individual fingers on oneself and on others, the examination is really about the absence of "gnosis," or knowing the digits, rather than the absence of naming, or anomia for digit names. Both of these tasks may be failed because of aphasia or anomia, rather than because of true agnosia for digits or fingers; therefore if they fail naming and pointing tasks, a nonverbal test is indicated. The examiner can ask the patient to state, with occluded vision, the number of fingers between two fingers touched by the examiner. Alternatively, the examiner moves one of the patient's fingers on a hand held out of the patient's sight, usually above and behind their head, and asks the patient to indicate, on the contralateral hand, the correspondingly correct finger moved.

There is another good test for digit agnosia using drawings of hands. The examiner presents a drawing of the left and right hands in front of the patient. The hand drawings are with the palms down and the fingers facing the patient. On the drawing, the examiner asks the patient to point to the corresponding fingers named by the examiner. For nonverbal recognition, the examiner touches the fingers on the drawings and asks the patient to move his or her corresponding fingers. Alternatively, the examiner simultaneously touches pairs of fingers on the dorsal side of the patient's hand, unseen by the patient, and asks the patient to point to the corresponding fingers on the drawings of the hands.

Right-Left Orientation. For right-left discrimination, the examiner asks the patient to follow uncrossed and crossed right-left body commands followed by "Double-Own" and "Double-Other" commands (adapted from Goodglass et al, 2001) (Table 12.8). First, the examiner asks the patient to show his or her

TABLE 12.8   Right-Left Disorientation

UNCROSSED AND CROSSED POINTING COMMANDS

	Self		Other (person, picture of person, or doll)	
	Correct	Incorrect	Correct	Incorrect
Left ear	☐	☐	☐	☐
Left shoulder	☐	☐	☐	☐
Right ear	☐	☐	☐	☐
Right shoulde	☐	☐	☐	☐

Double-Own and Double-Other Commands

A. With Right Hand

	Self		Other (person, picture of person, doll)	
	Correct	Incorrect	Correct	Incorrect
Left ear	☐	☐	☐	☐
Left shoulder	☐	☐	☐	☐
Right ear	☐	☐	☐	☐
Right shoulder	☐	☐	☐	☐

B. With Left Hand

	Self		Other (person, picture of person, doll)	
	Correct	Incorrect	Correct	Incorrect
Left ear	☐	☐	☐	☐
Left shoulder	☐	☐	☐	☐
Right ear	☐	☐	☐	☐
Right shoulder	☐	☐	☐	☐

Right-Left Disorientation Findings

☐ Normal   ☐ Abnormal

Types of errors (check all that apply):
- ☐ Right-left "self" disorientation
- ☐ Right-left "other" disorientation
- ☐ Right-left "self" and "other" disorientation

Number of errors: ____

right and left hands. If this is correctly performed, the examiner asks the patient to identify body parts on the left and right side of both the patient's body and the examiner's body of the examiner or other person, a picture of a person, or a doll. In a right-handed patient, uncrossed commands are "point to your right ear," and crossed commands are "point to my or the other's right shoulder." Double-Own commands are "point with your left hand to your left ear," or "point with your right hand to your left shoulder." Double-Other commands are "point with your right hand to my or the other's right shoulder," or "point with your left hand to my or the other's right ear." The examiner needs to keep in mind that patients may fail these tests not because of right-left disorientation but because of hemineglect, apraxia, language comprehension, or executive disturbances.

Autotopagnosia and Somatotopagnosia. These are agnosias for localization and orientation on a body map. It is included here because of a relationship with digit agnosia and right-left disorientation.

Autotopagnosia is difficulty localizing on one's own body, whereas somatotopagnosia also includes difficulty localizing on the body parts of others or on pictures, drawings, or dolls. Both conditions are due to lesion in the left parietal lobe or to advanced dementia. For testing, the examiner asks the patient to point to individual parts of the body (neck, ankle, ear, etc.) and to name parts of the body. The examiner names a body part while asking the patients to point to the corresponding body part first on themselves and then on the other. The examiner can also point to their own body parts (or the patient's) while asking the patient to point to the corresponding body part on themselves (or on the other). The examiner evaluates for errors of localization to the surrounding body parts rather than the correct one (contiguity error) or in localization to an incorrect but semantically related body part (semantic error), for example, pointing to an eye when asked to point to an ear. Disturbance is indicative of significant brain disturbance that involves the left parietal lobe.

Transitional Agraphia. Gerstmann syndrome includes agraphia without alexia (writing without reading difficulty). This disturbance of writing manifests as lexical (spelling) difficulty, which is often consistent with a phonological agraphia (difficulty with grapheme-phoneme conversion; see Chapter 8). However, the agraphia of Gerstmann syndrome often extends to the transition between lexical elements to motor elements. The transitional components of this agraphia may affect graphemic motor (sets of motor programs for writing), including allographic (style, script, upper or lower case) elements and the actual graphic codes for their motor execution. These patients may have these problems without evidence of upper extremity limb apraxia. On obtaining a writing sample, patients make corresponding errors in the direction, relative size, and ordering of strokes, and in the correct use of script or case.

Clinical Implications

In most cases, acalculias occur in association with other cognitive deficits, and may be secondary to those deficits. Diagnosing anarithmetia and other primary acalculias requires careful exclusion of calculation difficulty because of language, spatial, motor praxis, and executive difficulty. When anarithmetia occurs, it is usually associated with other elements of Gerstmann syndrome or with additional elements of the larger angular gyrus syndrome. The secondary acalculias may result from lesions in many areas of the brain, particularly left perisylvian, right parietal, more extensive left parietal, and dorsolateral frontal. In addition, lesions in the left thalamus and basal ganglia may result in secondary acalculias. Both primary or secondary acalculia can be progressive from some forms of neurodegenerative disease, such as Alzheimer disease, particularly the early-onset variants, as well as tumors and other progressive lesions of the brain.

Gerstmann syndrome remains a controversial association of anarithmetia, digit agnosia, right-left disorientation, and agraphia. This syndrome occurs in whole or in part from damage in the left angular or inferior parietal area regardless of cause. Stimulation studies of the left inferior parietal cortex have shown dissociation of the four components of Gerstmann syndrome. Other patients, with larger lesions in that area, have anomia, conduction or other aphasias, alexia, and other cognitive impairments indicating that the left inferior parietal region may be a crossroads for relating language and visual and other cognitive abilities. Additional reports describe a developmental form of Gerstmann syndrome of unknown etiology in children who have inordinate problems with arithmetic on entering school. There is no specific treatment for Gerstmann syndrome, except for occupational and rehabilitation therapy; however, most adults improve over time, and are particularly helped by the use of calculators and other modern devices.

Conclusions

Testing the ability to calculate can have great localizing value in the mental status examination. Calculation ability in humans is a unique cognitive domain that has developed beyond simple counting or ordinal judgments, but to more complex, relational mathematical processing localized in the horizontal intraparietal sulcus, particularly on the left. The ability to test for acalculias and related disturbances of the body map should be part of the armamentarium of any mental status examiner.

Chapter 13

Executive Operations and Abilities

Executive operations refer to cognitive processes that underlie goal-directed behavior, and executive attributes refer to decision-making abilities such as abstraction, judgment, and problem solving. They are what a chief executive of a company does: formulate a strategic plan toward a goal and implement it. This executive process involves steps, which can be broken down into the following: reflecting on different options and deciding on a goal, formulating the strategic plan and steps toward the goal, initiating and maintaining action to the goal, recognizing changes in pattern and altering course when necessary, inhibiting contradictory impulses or responses along the way, and preventing dependency on immediate, external stimuli versus the internal strategic plan. The mental status examiner can test executive processes with techniques that either underlie these steps or indirectly reflect decision-making.

Executive operations and attributes are, for the most part, localized to the prefrontal cortex and their connections. The prefrontal cortex has at least six major behavioral divisions, which can vary depending on how neurobiologists divide them (Fig. 13.1). One division is the dorsolateral prefrontal cortex involved in working memory and other executive operations, the ventromedial prefrontal cortex engaged in affective valuation, and the anterior cingulate cortex where they come together for motivation for action choice. Additional contributing regions are ventrolateral involved in reconciling stimuli with stored representations, orbitofrontal involved in rapid stimulus-response assessment, and the dorsomedial/frontal pole for reflection on delayed or as-if outcomes, as well as the self. These regional distinctions are useful for mental status testing and brain-behavior localization; however, these regions are involved in a number

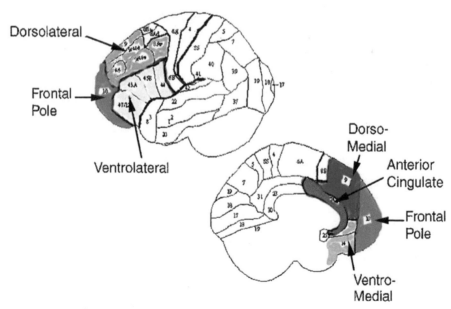

Fig. 13.1 The prefrontal cortex. Behaviorally relevant areas of the prefrontal cortex are designated.

of other subprocesses, and these functions are not as discrete as suggested in this summary. Moreover, brain disorders usually do not result in sharp separation of these manifestations, and most patients have mixtures of disturbances in executive operations and attributes.

Perhaps the most important aspect of assessing the brain's chief executive is determining the person's effectiveness in the real world. Ultimately, disturbances in both executive operations and attributes are most evident in how patients actually perform. On interview, these patients may give a very good verbal strategic plan, but then have poor initiation ("abulia") and never implement their plan ("verbal-action dissociation"). Alternatively, if they do initiate or implement, they can be disorganized, impersistent, or disinhibited.

Executive Operations

Working memory is arguably the most important executive operation (Table 13.1). Working memory involves maintaining information "online" in the brain while it is manipulated or processed. Working memory also involves phonological and visuospatial rehearsal and buffer systems, which may be located outside the dorsolateral prefrontal cortex. Patients with disturbed working memory fail in holding information online in the brain and cannot use it for planning or learning from errors. A measure of working memory is the span of apprehension, or the maximum number of objects that can be held after a brief presentation. Typically, people can only report approximately four or five items from a briefly presented array of alphanumeric sequences. As discussed in Chapter 7 on fundamental functions, working memory is a main aspect of "mental control" when combined with various aspects of complex attention, particularly the ability to sustain, shift, and divide attention.

Beyond mental control, executive operations involve a number of other processes that may be impaired with frontal-executive dysfunction. They are task setting and monitoring such as with fluency tasks, set-change detection and set-shifting, sequencing or alternating, response inhibition, and environmental independence tasks. In addition to impaired verbal fluency during language testing, patients with frontal injury may have a decline in visual design fluency, or the number of freeform designs per minute. These patients may fail to easily shift from one task to another either from problems changing set or because they cannot detect a required new pattern of responding. Patients may also fail to program a series of alternating choices and may perseverate or get stuck on a specific item or action. Frontally injured patients can be vulnerable to making in-the-moment responses to stimuli without reflection or consideration. They may be unable to avoid being drawn to environmental stimuli showing "stimulus-bound" behavior, such as the compulsion to imitate the examiner's movements or to utilize ambient objects. Conversely, they may perform better at externally driven and structured tasks than on devising and implementing an internally driven strategic plan. Finally, executive operations affect performance in other areas of cognition as well, for example, in organizing for memory retrieval especially when involving temporal-order judgments and in holding information online in the brain sufficiently for language comprehension or calculations.

The Examination of Executive Operations

When deficits are mild, mental status tasks of executive operations may be normal, despite lack of initiation and verbal-action dissociation. The history is particularly important because of this notable discrepancy between the patient's lack of effective executive or goal-oriented behavior and their often preserved performance on the MSX. Consequently, the examiner should screen with a number of tasks of executive operations as any single test can be very insensitive. Furthermore, the examiner may be able to derive much more information from reviewing the pattern and approach to task performance, that is, the organizational planning and execution, than from the actual final results or score itself.

MENTAL CONTROL

Working Memory. The common tests for working memory, such as those for attention, involve serial reversal tasks such as digits backward, spelling words backward, and serial subtraction. They are also part of the evaluation of attention described in Chapter 7, with the focus here on the "manipulation" involved in the reversal process. The first is the backward digit

TABLE 13.1 Executive Operations

Executive Operation	Task Type	Specific Task	Prefrontal Region
Mental control	Working memory	Serial reversal tasks: digit span backward, spelling backward, serial subtraction; Serial ordering tasks; N-back; Brown-Petersen; Complex/reading span	Dorsolateral
	Complex attention	Sustain (e.g., digit span); Shift (e.g., Trailmaking-A); Divide (e.g., multitask span)	Dorsolateral, anterior cingulate
Task setting and monitoring		Verbal fluency (e.g., "F"/min.); Design fluency (e.g., 5-point)	Dorsolateral
Set-change detection and set-shifting		Trailmaking-B; Alternating hand coin test	Anterior cingulate, dorsolateral
Alternating programs	Sequencing	Alternate word list generation; AZ-BY-CX-DW, etc.; Alphanumeric sequencing; Letter-number sequencing	Dorsolateral, anterior cingulate
	Motor programming	Finger opposition tapping; Alternate tapping; Shape or letter repetition; 0+00++000+++, etc.; Luria hand program	
Response inhibition		Spiral loops; Crossed response inhibition; Antisaccades test; Go-No-Go test; Color-word interference; Big-Little test; Sentence completions; Commands vs. gestures	Orbitofrontal, ventrolateral, dorsolateral
Environmental dependency		Echolalia/echopraxia; Stimulus-bound and closing-in; Imitation and utilization behavior; Grasp reflexes	Dorsolateral, orbitofrontal

span in which the patient must repeat digits in reverse order, beginning with the last number. The examiner continues to administer series of digits until the patient incorrectly repeats two strings of digits backward at the same series level. A normal performance is correct backward recitation of two less than the maximum forward digit span. The ability to spell "world" (or other words) backward is another commonly used serial reversal task that overlaps with attention testing. The patient must give the letters placed in the correct place, that is, "d-l-r-o-w." The serial subtraction tasks include counting backward by 3s from 20, or 7s from 100. For example, the examiner asks the patient to subtract by 7 beginning from 100, for example, 93,

86, 79, 72, 65, et cetera. The number of errors are the number of incorrect subtractions from the prior response. The examiner can also ask the patient to recite the days of the week backward or the months of the year backward beginning with December. Patients should be able to obtain a normal score on these last two serial reversal tasks.

If greater assessment of working memory is needed, there are at least four other tasks that are readily applicable in clinical encounters or at the bedside. These tasks involve greater maintenance or manipulation of online information in the brain. First, there are serial ordering tasks. The simplest is to have the patient rearrange digits in ascending order from smallest to largest. For example, if given the series "2-1-3," the correct answer would be "1-2-3." Most people can serially order up to five or more digits. Second is a clinical variation of the classic N-back test of working memory. In the classical test, the participant hears a series of digits or letters and is asked to indicate if a letter was previously presented a set number of places back, e.g., for N-3, the participant would indicate the ones shown in capital letters: n t s j o a **J** p q s t u **S**. In a simpler clinical variation, the examiner recites a long series of digits and, once the examiner stops, asks the patient to repeat the next to last digit in the sequence ("N-1") or, for more challenging testing, two or three back from the last digit in the sequence ("N-2" and "N-3"). A third task is a variation of the Brown-Petersen procedure, which aims to test working memory divorced from the effects of rehearsal. The examiner spells aloud a random, three-letter consonant syllable ("trigram") that the patient must remember. Immediately afterward, the patient is asked to count backward by threes from a random number. After 10 seconds, the examiner interrupts the counting backward and asks the patient to recall the consonant trigrams. The examiner repeats this procedure at least four times. Fourth are complex span paradigms that require remembering a set of items in order and combined with a concurrent secondary task. One version is the reading span task in which patients read two to six sentences and must remember the last word of each sentence, which they have to repeat back in order at the end of the task.

Complex Attention. Additional mental control tasks involve the ability to sustain, shift, and divide attention. The ability to sustain attention is reflected in many of the fundamental attentional tasks, such as forward digit span, and the ability to shift attention is reflected in tests such as Trailmaking-A (see Chapter 7). The ability to divide attention is effectively tested during dual-task or multitasking procedures. One example is the performance of simultaneous tasks, such as having the patient do a forward digit span while manually tracking the examiner's moving finger with their index finger. The examiner compares the results of this divided attention task to the results from the single task forward digit span. One old task, the face-hands test, may further reflect difficulty dividing attention. In this test, the examiner touches the patient on the hands and cheek simultaneously in 10 trials (4 contralateral, 4 ipsilateral, 2 symmetric). On the last four nonsymmetric trials, any error in recognizing where the patient was touched suggests impairment, most often from dementia or frontal lobe disease.

TASK SETTING AND MONITORING

Verbal Fluency. Word list generation, which declines with language (see Chapter 8), is also compromised with executive impairment as it requires setting and maintaining a task. The examiner instructs the patient to name, as quickly as possible, as many English words that begin with the letter "F" (or "A" or "S") and as many names of animals (or some other category) as they can in 1 minute. Ask the patient to avoid proper names or multiple versions or variations of the same word. Do not count close word variations of the same word, such as "six," "sixth," "sixtieth," but do count word variations with a different meaning, e.g., "sixteen." In a timed performance, normal subjects can list 15 ± 5 "F" words per minute and 18 ± 6 animals per minute without cueing. When the patient is impaired due to language, both lexical (letter) and category (e.g., animals) word generation declines, but when the patient is impaired due to executive operations, there is a discrepancy between impairment on the more effortful lexical word generation and an often normal performance on the more visualizable category list. A discrepancy of less than three between lexical versus category word lists can be a major clue to executive dysfunction.

Design Fluency. A further measure of executive task performance is design fluency, or the number of

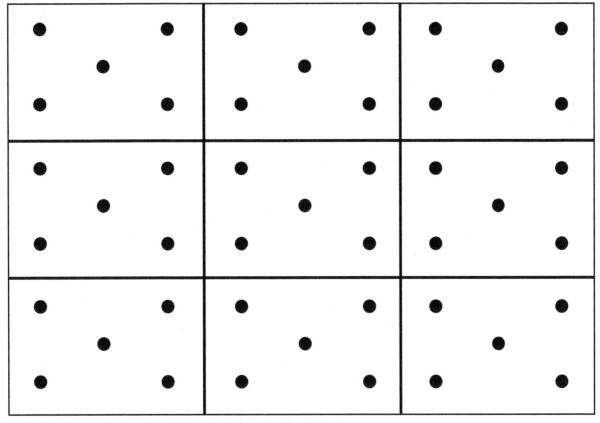

Fig. 13.2 Five-point design fluency. See text for instructions on how to make designs.

freeform designs generated in 1 minute. One easily administered version is the Five-Point test (Fig. 13.2). This test measures the ability to inhibit previously drawn responses and the ability to generate and create different visual patterns. The examiner presents the patient with squares (typically 40) containing five dots and asks the patient to make as many unique designs as possible in 1 minute by connecting the dots within each square with straight lines. The patient does not need to use all the dots in the designs. The lines must be straight ones that connect dots, and the designs should not be repeated. The examiner can start with two examples. There are several variations of this design fluency test. One counts the number of unique designs in five minutes. Another restricts the total number of lines/squares to four. A third version restricts to continuously connected straight lines. The examiner scores the total number of correct designs,

the number of rule violations, and the number of repeated designs.

SET-CHANGE DETECTION AND SET-SHIFTING

The Trailmaking-B test is a classic measure of set-shifting, which is heavily dependent on the anterior cingulate cortex. The Trailmaking tests are timed tests that measure the time required to draw a line between scattered items. On part A of the Trailmaking test, the patient must draw a line connecting a series of randomly arrayed numbers in numerical sequence (1-2-3, etc.). Part A is more of an attentional task and is described in Chapter 7. On part B of the Trailmaking test, the patient must draw a line connecting numbers and letters in alternating sequence, that is, 1 to A then A to 2 then 2 to B, et cetera. Begin by demonstrating the test to the patient using an abbreviated sample. There are more difficult

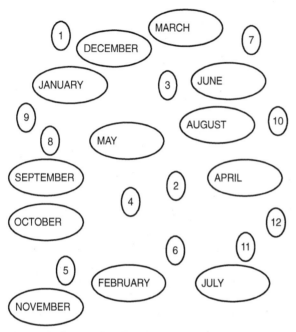

Fig. 13.3 Trailmaking-B variant with months. This variant of the classical Trailmaking-B test alternates numbers and months of the year.

variations of the Trailmaking-B, which change letters into Roman numerals, days of the week, or months of the year (Fig. 13.3). For the numbers-months variation, tell the patient: "On this page are both numbers and months of the year. Begin at number 1 and draw a line from 1 to January, then January to 2, then 2 to February, and so on. Remember, first you have a number, then a month, then a number, and so on. Draw the lines as fast as you can. Begin." If the patient makes a mistake on the practice sample, point to the error immediately and explain it. If the patient makes an error on the real test, point to the error and return the patient's pen to the last correct circle and continue from that point. Since these tests are formally timed, there are normative values available. One good measure of the task that accounts for attention is to look at the timing difference between Trailmaking-B and Trailmaking-A. The examiner, however, can also administer the Trailmaking-B test, or a modification of it, untimed and simply count the patient's errors in completing the alternating sequence. Performance on these Trailmaking-B tasks can be very informative. They not only measure the ability to shift response

sets among predetermined options but may also reveal problems with perseveration or even stimulus-boundedness, an environment-dependent behavior.

The Wisconsin Card Sort test is among the best set-shifting tests in neuropsychology and among the most used executive functions tests for assessing the presence of preservation errors. Mental status examiners have considered a number of clinical variations that do not risk a potential compromise of the subsequent neuropsychological administration of this test. One easy to implement alternative involves alternating a coin between the examiner's hands and having the patient guess the hand that has the coin. The examiner starts with hands held behind the back, then brings them forward and asks the patient to state which hand has the coin. Then the examiner uncovers his hands indicating the correct response. The examiner repeats this procedure, moving the location of the coin out-of-sight behind his or her back according to different strategies. The first strategy is a right hand–left hand alternation of the coin. Once the patient determines the correct alternating strategy for three times in a row, the examiner then switches to a two right-hand two left-hand strategy until the patient gets several in a row. This is followed by a three right-hand three left-hand strategy until the patient gets several in a row. The inability to get the set within the number of trials constitutes an abnormal response.

ALTERNATING PROGRAMS

Sequencing. A number of procedures involve sequencing words, letters, numbers, or symbols. Alternate word list generation overlap with verbal fluency measures. In these tests, the examiner asks the patient to give as many names as possible in 1 minute but in an alternating fashion, for example, between categories such as fruits versus vegetables, animals versus tools, colors versus countries. The examiner records the number of correct alternations per minute. A second task asks the patient to couple the first letters of the alphabet with the last letters and to continue as far as possible, for example, AZ-BY-CX-DW, and so on. The last correct coupling is the patient's score. The Alphanumeric Sequencing test is a similar verbal task in which the examiner asks the patient to count from 1 and recite the alphabet, but switching between numbers and letters, that is, "1-A-2-B-3-C-4-D-5-E-6-F-7-G-8-H-9-I-10-J." The number of errors is the number of mistakes in alternations. The Letter-Number Sequencing test is a variation of the serial ordering of digits for working memory but requires a separate ordering of letters and numbers. In this test, the examiner asks patients to repeat a mixed sequence of numbers and letters, for example, J-7-F-6-P-4, and then repeat the numbers in ascending order followed by the letters in alphabetical order. These is a more difficulty test; many patients struggle attaining more than three numbers–three letters.

Motor programming. These tests involve the ability to perform motor programs independent of primary motor or sensory deficits. First is simple finger opposition tapping; patients tap their thumb to each of their other four fingers and continuously repeat the series. Although this task is affected by motor dexterity and coordination, it can indicate motor programming difficulty in the absence of other neurological disturbances. In the Alternate Tapping task, the examiner asks the patient to "tap twice when I tap once" (1), and "tap once when I tap twice" (2). After a practice run (examiner taps 1-1-1 and 2-2-2), the examiner performs a random tapping sequence (e.g., 1-1-2-1-2-2-2-1-1-2, as in the Frontal Assessment Battery described later). Alternatively, to exclude visual input, the examiner may tap out-of-sight (e.g., underneath the table) and the patient responds by raising a finger. More than two errors is clearly abnormal. A second motor programming task involves copying alternating shapes or a series of "m" and "n" letters and asking the patient to continue the pattern to the end of the page (Fig. 13.4). Disturbances include perseveration of one of the shapes or letters or impersistence in completing the task. Finally, there is a similar alternating task involving writing increasing numbers of "0" (or "–") and "+" signs, continuing the sequence to the end of the page or some other cutoff point, that is, 0+00++000+++, et cetera.

Luria Alternating Hand Program. A prominent motor programming task is the Luria Three-Step Hand Sequence (Fist-Edge-Palm) (Fig. 13.5), which requires the patient to imitate three hand motions performed by the examiner. On a table, the examiner places his hand with a fist with the knuckles down, then the edge of the hand in a cutting motion, and then palm down with fingers extended. The examiner demonstrates this hand sequence three times. Then the patient must perform the sequence three times in a row along

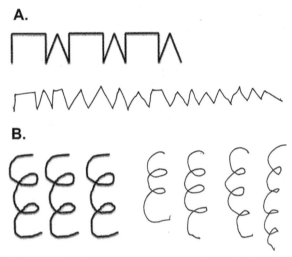

Fig. 13.4 Alternating shapes and spiral loops tasks. (A) Alternating shapes with frontally impaired patient's performance on the right. The instructions were to copy the pattern to the end of the page. (B) Spiral loops with frontally impaired patient's performance on the right. The instructions were to copy the spirals exactly as they are to the end of the page.

with the examiner. Finally, the patient must perform the hand sequence six times in a row without error, without cues, and without verbalization. A normal untimed performance is a perfect score of six correct hand sequences in a row. An alternative version demonstrates the sequence three times, then requires the patient to reproduce the sequence within five trials, and to then continue repeating the correct sequence five times in a row without error. In other variants, the hand sequence may be "cut-fist-slap" or "slap-cut-fist," and patients may say aloud the hand positions as they do them (verbal reinforcement). The test is abnormal if the hand motions differ in type or sequence from that of the examiner. Finally, a much simpler and faster motor set-change task is just to have the patient do alternate hand movements, such as alternate between one hand fisted and the other open palm down on the table, alternating simultaneously at a moderate pace.

RESPONSE INHIBITION

The goal with these tasks is to determine whether the patient is able to inhibit the continuation of a pattern. As can be seen, these tasks are not totally separable from motor programming or from set-change tasks. Nevertheless, there are some clinical tasks that are

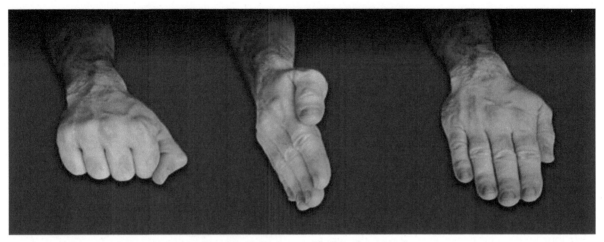

Fig. 13.5 Luria three-step hand sequence test. The original Luria steps are "fist," "cut," and "slap."

more indicative of response inhibition than others. One example is the ability to copy a set number of spirals. The patient must copy a pattern, such as spiral loops, continuing the individual spiral pattern to the end of the page without adding any additional number of loops to the spirals (Fig. 13.4). Other tests are the crossed response inhibition tasks, either the Crossed Hand or the Antisaccades tests. In the Crossed Hand test, the examiner asks the patients to close their eyes and place their hands, palm down, in front of them. The examiner then instructs the patients to lift the hand opposite to the one touched by the examiner. There are 20 trials, and errors involve initially moving the touched extremity rather than the opposite one. In the Antisaccades test, the examiner holds up index fingers in each of the patients two visual fields and randomly moves one of them. In the practice section, the examiner asks the patient to look to and from the examiner's moving index fingers and nose. Then the strategy is changed, and the examiner asks the patient to look to and from the index finger that is not moving. There are 20 trials, and errors involve initially looking at the moving finger rather than the stationary one. Finally, the Go No-Go test, in which the examiner asks the patient to alternate between tapping and not tapping, is an excellent test of response inhibition. In this test, the examiner asks the patient to "tap once when I tap once" (1) but "do not tap when I tap twice" (2). After a practice run (the examiner taps 1-1-1 and 2-2-2), the examiner performs

a random sequence (e.g., 1-1-2-1-2-2-2-1-1-2), and records the errors of commission or omission.

Four other important tests of response inhibition are included here: color-word interference, the Big-Little-Big test, unrelated sentence completion, and contradictory comments-gestures. The classic Stroop Color and Word test is one of the most important and sensitive tests for response inhibition in the neuropsychological laboratory. In this test, the patient must first read a list of color names in black and white and then name an array of colors. After this, the patient must rename the colors, but this time the colors are presented as contradictory color names (color-word interference). The patients must inhibit responses to the word color names and just name the colors that they are printed in. The examiner can time the administration, as well as record the number of errors. It is possible to administer variations of the color-word interference task in the clinic with the availability of simple stimuli, such as color words printed in different colors (Fig. 13.6), and noting the patient's errors, delays, or struggles in naming the colors. A similar test is the Big-Little-Big test in which patients have to report whether the words "big" or "little" are printed in upper- or in lowercase (Fig. 13.7). The patient must say "big" if the word is in uppercase and "little" if the word is in lowercase. The examiner records errors in correctly categorizing the case of the words. The Hayling sentence completion paradigm asks patients to complete

BLUE	BLUE	BLUE
GREEN	RED	GREEN
RED	BLUE	GREEN
RED	GREEN	RED
GREEN	BLUE	BLUE
BLUE	BLUE	RED
RED	RED	GREEN

Fig. 13.6 Color-word interference task. Patterned after the Stroop Color and Word Test, the patient must state the color and ignore the word.

sentences with totally unrelated words or endings so that the sentence does not make sense. For example, if given the phrases "Mary had a little...."; "She laughed out...."; "The dog dug a...."; Jack and Jill went up the....", the patient must give entirely different responses than "lamb," "loud," "hole," "hill," respectively. A series of this sentences can be constructed from common sayings and used to evaluate

the patient's response inhibition. Finally, a related procedure is to instruct the patient to respond to your verbal commands but not to your contradictory gestures. For example, put out an outstretched hand and say "don't shake my hand"; throw a soft object and say "don't catch it"; show your open palms and say "don't show me your hands"; beckon to stand up and say "please remain seated."

ENVIRONMENTAL DEPENDENCY

A significant executive operation is the ability to maintain personal autonomy and avoid prepotent automatic responses to the external world. The examiner can detect a number of aspects of environmental dependency on routine observations and on the patients' performance on prior tests. For example, "stimulus-bound" behavior is evident when patients tend to touch items in the environment or approach other people beyond what the context or situation requires. On the written mental status tests, such as the copy of visual figures, environmental dependency may manifest as a "closing-in" phenomena in which the patient cannot keep from making their copy either directly on the stimulus picture, connected to it, or as a continuation of it. Despite instructions to make a separate copy, the patient persists in this stimulus-bound behavior. "Imitation

Practice Line:

little little big LITTLE BIG BIG little big LITTLE LITTLE big

---

little BIG LITTLE BIG big little LITTLE BIG big LITTLE

big little BIG little LITTLE big little BIG little BIG little big

BIG BIG little big LITTLE big LITTLE little big BIG LITTLE

LITTLE little big little BIG big LITTLE little BIG big LITTLE

BIG little big big LITTLE LITTLE LITTLE BIG little big big

BIG LITTLE BIG big

Fig. 13.7 Big-little test. The examiner instructs the patient to "Say which size each of the words are, one by one, as quickly as you can. Please ignore what the word says. Say "big" for capitalized words and "little" for lowercase words."

behavior" reflects environmental dependency and manifests as the tendency for patients to imitate the examiner's (or others') movements ("echopraxia") or speech output ("echolalia"). The examiner can test imitation by making deliberate, unusual movements or postures of the hand or face, or by saying non-sense words, and observing for any imitation by the patient. "Utilization behavior" refers to the tendency for patients to touch, take, or use whatever is in front of them. The examiner can test utilization by placing items directly in front of the patient, such as paper and pencil, a stethoscope, or a reflex hammer, and observing whether the patient "utilizes" them. Finally, the presence of frontal grasp reflexes strongly indicate environmental dependency, and, although more of a motor than a cognitive finding, is included here because of its specificity for frontal-executive dysfunction. Some examiners describe three levels of grasp reflexes: prehensile, magnetic, and "grope." The prehensile grasp is a closing in of the fingers of the hand when the palms are touched or stroked. The magnetic grasp is a following of the examiner's hands when they approach the patient's outstretched hands in a palms-up position. The more severe grope is a tendency to spontaneously reach out to grasp items in the environment or the examiner.

Many of the common executive operations described earlier are incorporated in single scales or tests. One is the Frontal Assessment Battery (Table 13.2). Examiners can administer this 18-point battery in a relatively a few minutes. It screens verbal fluency, alternate programming, Go-No-Go, Fist-Edge-Palm, testing for frontal grasp reflex, and three idioms for abstractions. Many clinicians use the Clock Drawing test to screen for executive deficits and visuospatial and other difficulties. The freehand drawing of a clock is not only a sensitive measure of visuospatial and other abilities, but it also requires solving the problem of motor execution of a clock drawing with the correct time. The specific executive abnormalities on the clock test are poor planning in placing the numbers (which can also reflect visuospatial impairment) and a concrete placement of the hands. Executive dysfunction may be particularly evident on comparing the patient's spontaneous clock drawing with the degree of improvement on a clock copy made after observing the examiner draw it.

Executive Attributes

Executive attributes are those higher abilities derived or related to executive operations, but separable from them. Executive operations contribute but do not individually explain the prefrontal abilities of abstraction, judgment and reasoning, insight, and complex problem solving. Together, these attributes reflect the insertion of an analytic reflective mode that considers options and consequences. Novelty-seeking and creativity is also an emergent feature of these executive attributes.

Executive attributes are interrelated abilities whose compromise is reflected in poor decision-making. An important executive attribute is the ability for abstraction, or for recognizing and understanding relationships that are not immediately apparent and that are independent of its words and associations. In addition to executive functions from prefrontal cortex, abstracting ability is associated with semantic processing in the anterior temporal region. Judgment, another executive attribute involved in decision-making, involves a controlled mode of thinking so that intuitive responses are superseded by reasoning and logic. In everyday life, good judgment is the presence of personally and socially appropriate decisions, and the best assessment of judgment are examples or observations of the patient's behavior. One special form of judgment is insight, or the awareness and understanding of their own illness and its impact. The ability for problem solving is a critical characteristic of executive decision-making. The capacity for goal-directed and adaptive behavior depends on the ability to solve problems, adapt to new situations, and form and grasp concepts. The ability to manage increasing levels of problem complexity is the common factor for intelligence and among intelligence tests.

Tests of Executive Traits

ABSTRACTIONS

The interpretation of similarities, idioms, or proverbs challenges the ability to abstract. Although education and sociocultural background greatly affect these interpretations, the ability to abstract can be prominently impaired in frontally injured patients, as well as those with psychoses, such as schizophrenia. Additionally,

TABLE 13.2   **Frontal Assessment Battery**
1. Similarities: "In what way are they alike?"
a. Banana and orange (in the event of total failure, e.g., "they are not alike," or partial failure, e.g., "both have peel," help the patient by saying, "both a banana and an orange are…" but credit 0 for the item; do not help the patient for the two following items);
b. table and chair;
c. tulip, rose, and daisy
Score only category response (fruits, furniture, flower) correct:
3 correct = 3; 2 correct = 2; 1 correct = 1; 0 correct = 0.
2. Lexical fluency: "Say as many words as you can beginning with the letter 'S,' any word except surnames or proper nouns." If the patient gives no response during the first 5 seconds, say "for instance, snake." If the patient pauses 10 seconds, stimulate him by saying, "any word beginning with the letter 'S.'" The time allowed is 60 seconds.
Score (word repetitions or variations, surnames, proper nouns are not counted)
More than nine words = 3; six to nine = 12; three to five = 1; fewer than three = 0.
3. Motor series: "Look carefully at what I am doing." The examiner, seated in front of the patients, performs alone three times with his left hand the series of Luria "fist-edge-palm." "Now, with your right hand do the same series, first with me, then alone." The examiner performs the series three times with the patient, then says to him or her: "Now do it on your own."
Six correct consecutive series = 3; at least three correct consecutive series alone = 2; fails alone, but performs three correct consecutive series with the examiner = 1; cannot perform three correct consecutive series even with the examiner = 0.
4. Conflicting instructions: "Tap twice when I tap once." To be sure that the patient has understood the instruction, a series of three trials is run: 1-1-1. "Tap once when I tap twice." To be sure that the patient has understood the instruction, a series of three trials is run: 2-2-2. The examiner performs the following series: 1-1-2-1-2-2-2-1-1-2.
No error = 3; one or two errors = 2; more than two errors = 1; patient taps like the examiner at least four consecutive times = 0.
5. Go/No-Go: "Tap once when I tap once." To be sure that the patient has understood the instruction, a series of three trials is run: 1-1-1. "Do not tap when I tap twice." To be sure that the patient has understood the instruction, a series of three trials is run: 2-2-2. The examiner performs the following series: 1-1-2-1-2-2-2-1-1-2.
No error = 3; one or two errors = 2; more than two errors = 1; patient taps like the examiner at least four consecutive times = 0.
6. Prehensile behavior: The examiner is seated in front of the patient. Place the patient's hands palm up on his or her knees. Without saying anything or looking at the patient, the examiner brings his or her hands close to the patient's hands and touches the palms of both the patient's hands, to see if he or she will spontaneously take them. If the patient takes the hands, the examiner will try again after asking him or her: "Now do not take my hands."
Patient does not take the examiner's hands = 3; patient hesitates and asks what he or she has to do = 2; patient takes the hands without hesitation = 1; patient takes the examiner's hand even after being told not to do so = 0.
TOTAL: _____/18

Reference: Dubois B, Slachevsky A, Litvan I, Pillon B. The FAB: a frontal assessment battery at bedside. *Neurology*. 2000;55(11): 1621–1626.

these patients may have difficulties interpreting metaphors, aphorisms, euphemisms, onomatopoeia, personification, analogies, oxymorons and paradoxes, hyperbole, sarcasm, irony, allusions, and puns. The process of abstraction involves at least two general cognitive stages: a denotative stage in which the specific meaning of the individual word is retrieved from some semantic knowledge, and a connotative stage in which a coherent, abstract principle or generalizable concept is formed based on the meaning of the individual words. The denotative stage requires over-learned, fundamental language skills, and thus places fewer demands on executive functions than does the connotative stage.

The examiner should start with simple similarities and idioms and progress to proverbs that are sufficiently hard to challenge the patient. Instruct the patient as follows: "I am going to give you word pairs or sayings. Some of them you may not have ever heard before. Please tell me in your own words what these words have in common (for similarities)/are trying to say (idioms and proverbs)." For similarities, ask the patient how two objects or concepts are alike or how they converge. Examples are apple-pear, coat-shirt, talking-listening, and others (see Table 13.3 for more examples). Alternatives are to ask how two objects or concepts are different or how they diverge. The examiner may start directly with proverbs and skip similarities and idioms. Testing for proverb interpretation should include both common proverbs, whose interpretation may be recalled by memory or may reflect semantic difficulty, and rare proverbs that require the patient to actively abstract the underlying connotative meaning of the words. Ask the patient to explain the more general meaning of the proverb. If the patient gives a concrete response or is unable to interpret, give the patient the correct answer and explain that this is the expected type of response. Sometimes they give an initial concrete response but can give an abstract one if specifically asked for another way of explaining the proverb. Then continue with different proverbs until the patient fails two successive proverbs. As noted, examples of proverbs should include unfamiliar ones requiring novel ways of thinking for assessing connotative frontal-executive abilities (Table 13.4). Considering the patient's educational level and prior familiarity with proverbs, the examiner otherwise grades responses as accurate, correct but concrete (mere repetition or rephrasing of the statement given by the examiner), correct but irrelevant or bizarre, or incorrect.

JUDGMENT AND REASONING

Judgment and reasoning are reflected in successful decision-making. Testing judgment and reasoning is difficult to do in a clinical setting. Responses to questions such as "What would you do if you saw a fire in a theater?" and "What should you do if you find a stamped, addressed envelope on the street?" are unreliable and

TABLE 13.3 Examples of Similarities (and Differences) and Idioms
Similarities and Differences (also Convergence or Divergence)
1. Orange and banana
2. Lie and mistake
3. Desk and chair
4. Watch and ruler
5. Music and sculpture
6. Child and midget
7. Ballet and poetry
8. Bicycle and train
9. Shame and pride
10. Scissors and hammer
11. A dog and a wolf
12. A river and a canal
13. Thrift and avarice
14. Laziness and idleness
15. Abundance and excess
Commonly Used Idioms
1. Warm-hearted
2. Broad-minded
3. Cold-blooded
4. Level-headed
5. Head strong
6. Loud necktie
7. Give someone the cold shoulder
8. To keep a stiff upper lip
9. To thumb one's nose
10. Spill the beans
11. Seeing eye to eye
12. Throw in the towel
13. Under the weather
14. Let the cat out of the bag
15. To do it at the drop of a hat

potentially misleading. Because impaired patients may act quite differently in real situations as opposed to self-report, the best evaluation of judgment is through monitoring the patient's ability to cope with everyday problems and through specific examples or observations of daily behavior from collateral sources, such as the patient's family or friends. In particular, obtain collateral information as to whether the patient is able to function effectively within his or her environment. Additional tests of situational judgment can assess

TABLE 13.4 Examples of Proverbs Used to Assess Abstraction

1. Don't cry over spilled milk.
2. Rome wasn't built in a day.
3. Let sleeping dogs lie.
4. Don't judge a book by its cover.
5. A bird in the hand is worth two in the bush.
6. Don't change horses in the middle of the stream.
7. A stitch in time saves nine.
8. People who live in glass houses shouldn't throw stones.
9. You can't have your cake and eat it too.
10. Do not count your chickens before they are hatched.
11. Too many cooks spoil the broth.
12. Still waters run deep.
13. All that glitters is not gold.
14. No bread is without its crust.
15. The tongue is the enemy of the neck.
16. Among the blind the one-eyed man is king.
17. A good conscience is a soft pillow.
18. Barking dogs seldom bite.
19. A new broom sweeps clean.
20. Don't put the cart before the horse.
21. You show me the person and I'll show you the rule.
22. A rolling stone gathers no moss.
23. A nod is as good as a wink to a blind horse.
24. Empty bags cannot stand upright.
25. If wishes were horses, beggars would ride.
26. A golden hammer breaks an iron door.
27. Even troubled waters reflect a full moon.
28. An empty vessel makes much noise.
29. A girl with cotton stocking never sees a mouse.
30. You cannot tickle a hungry person.
31. Make sure your blanket covers your feet.
32. Mounted mendicants race their steads.

cognitive flexibility, cognitive estimations, and logical reasoning. Cognitive flexibility is exemplified by questions such as the "brick test": "Tell me all the things that you could use a brick for?" Instead of a brick, the examiner could ask about other common objects with the aim of assessing the patients flexibility in coming up with multiple common and novel uses for the particular object. Cognitive estimations are exemplified by questions such as "How far is Paris from Los Angeles?" or "How high is the tallest building in the world?" Clearly, these questions are knowledge-dependent, but they can stretch the patient's judgment. Logical reasoning is exemplified by questions such as "Why are light-colored clothes cooler in summer than dark-colored clothes?" "John, Robert, and Michael are running a race. Michael is not behind Robert. John is the slowest. Who is ahead in the race?"

Insight

Insight regarding their illness and symptoms is often impaired in patients with frontal dysfunction. These patients may have anosognosia or denial of illness, anosodiaphoria or decreased appreciation of illness, and "la belle indifference" or a flat disinterest in their illness (also present in psychiatric disorders). In some instances, the examiner can discern a total lack of emotional appreciation of their condition despite awareness of a deficit or a diagnosis. After completion of a full examination, a simple question to the patient—"And how concerned are you about your trouble?"—may demonstrate a lack of realization or a serious misinterpretation of the problem. The examiner compares the patient's responses with those of the caregiver, family, or other objective sources. Table 13.5 illustrates an example of a questionnaire used for probing insight.

COMPLEX PROBLEM SOLVING

Complex problem solving tasks are usually reserved for neuropsychological testing in a standardized setting with special testing material. Examples of neuropsychological tests of complex problem solving include the Categories test, the Raven Progressive Matrices, many of the Wechsler Adult Intelligence Scale subtests, symbol digit substitutions tasks, picture completion and absurdities, and others.

There are some mental status tests that can be used for problem solving. First, the examiner can increase calculations to reflect increasing levels of complexity (see Chapter 12). Mental calculations are particularly useful as they are disproportionately impacted by working memory. Verbal problems can substitute

TABLE 13.5 **UCLA Insight Scale**	
SECTION I. Is there collateral or objective evidence for illness?	_____
If NO, give 8 points and skip to SECTION II; If YES, give 0 points and continue:	
1. Do you have an illness or problem that requires medical attention? Very much = 2; Somewhat = 1; Not at all = 0:	_____
2. How concerned are you about having any illness? Very much = 2; Somewhat = 1; Not at all = 0:	_____
3. Do family/friends think that you have an illness or problem that requires medical attention? Very much = 2; Somewhat = 1; Not at all = 0:	_____
4. How concerned are you that family/friends worry about your having any illness? Very much = 2; Somewhat = 1; Not at all = 0:	_____
Section II. Is there collateral or objective evidence for a behavior change? If NO, give 8 points and go to SECTION III; If YES, give 0 points and continue:	_____
5. Is your behavior/personality significantly different now, compared with a few years ago? Very much = 2; Somewhat = 1; Not at all = 0:	_____
6. How concerned are you about having any behavior/personality change? Very much = 2; Somewhat = 1; Not at all = 0:	_____
7. Do family/friends think that you have had a behavior change, compared with a few years ago? Very much = 2; Somewhat = 1; Not at all = 0:	_____
8. How concerned are you that family/friends worry about your having any behavior change? Very much = 2; Somewhat = 1; Not at all = 0:	_____
SECTION III. Is there collateral or objective evidence for _____ [chief symptom(s)]? If NO, give 4 points and go to END; If YES, give 0 points and continue:	_____
9. Are you now having _____ [chief symptom(s)]? Very much = 2; Somewhat = 1; Not at all = 0:	_____
Do family/friends think that you are having _____ [chief symptom(s)]? Very much = 2; Somewhat = 1; Not at all = 0:	_____
Total score (add only scored items):	_____/20

for mathematical calculations, for example, "The girl went to the store with $5 to buy 2 sodas for $1.85 each. What was her change?" Problem solving ability is particularly reflected in solving tasks with multiple steps. For example, the Rey-Complex Figure copy, or one of the comparable complex figures, requires the patient to follow through on a series of steps to solve the visually complex problem of copying the figure (See Chapter 10). Observing their executive strategy in performing this task is facilitated if the examiner changes the patient's pencil or pen to different colored ones at different points in the drawing. Finally, the towers tests, such as the Tower of Hanoi or the Tower of London, are particularly challenging complex problem-solving tasks. These tests require the patient to solve the arrangement of colored pegs or discs in an iterative process, often in a particular order of size. For the Tower of Hanoi, there are three rods and discs of different sizes arranged from the smallest on top to the largest below. The patient must move the discs to another rod, one at a time, by taking the upper disc and placing on another rod without ever placing a larger disc on top of a smaller one. For 3 discs, a minimum number of moves is 7 and for 4 discs it is 15. Although the towers tests require special stimulus materials, a simpler clinical or bedside version is to do the Towers of Hanoi procedure using three places on the table and three or four stacked coins of different sizes on one of the places.

Clinical Implications

Patients with impairment in executive operations generally have lesions or disease affecting the frontal lobes or their connections. This part of the brain is heterogeneous. The most notably "dysexecutive" area is the dorsolateral prefrontal cortex. Generally, patients with disease in this region do poorly on tasks involving working memory and mental control, verbal and design fluency, pattern recognition and set-change, and motor programming. If severe, they may demonstrate signs of environmental dependency. These patients also have difficulty with the interpretation of idioms or proverbs. Patients with anterior cingulate involvement can be disproportionately amotivational and inattentive, with sparse behavior and relative unconcern for emotional experiences. They may have difficulty with set-change tasks and complex attentional tasks. In comparison, patients with mesial frontal lesions may perform adequately on most executive operations but do poorly on social tact and propriety with disinhibition, impulsivity, poor response inhibition, and alterations in emotional reactivity. These patients are a focus of Chapter 14. Finally, it is important to keep in mind that patients usually lack discrete lesions in these areas and commonly have mixtures of dorsolateral, anterior cingulate, and mesial frontal dysfunction.

The list of disorders that affect executive operations and the frontal lobes is very large. Dysfunction of the frontal lobes can occur from focal frontal lobe disease, its subcortical and caudate connections, diffuse neurological disorders that also affect the executive operations, and psychiatric disorders that alter cognition. Focal frontal disease includes strokes, trauma (e.g., frontotemporal contusions), tumors (e.g., butterfly glioma), surgeries (e.g., lobotomies), frontal epilepsy, or other lesions in that area, as well as dementias with a predilection for frontal dysfunction, including frontotemporal dementia, dysexecutive/behavioral variant Alzheimer disease, Huntington disease, and obstructive or normal pressure hydrocephalus with disproportionate frontal horn enlargement. Toxins and alcohol are other conditions that can target the frontal lobes and result in disturbances of executive operations. Diffuse neurological disorders that also affect frontal-executive operations include vascular dementia, anoxic encephalopathy, parkinsonian dementias such as dementia with Lewy bodies, demyelinating disorders, infectious encephalopathies (e.g., Creutzfeldt-Jakob disease, neurosyphilis, human immunodeficiency virus), and noninfectious encephalopathies (e.g., autoimmune, steroid-responsive, and paraneoplastic). Psychiatric conditions such as schizophrenia and bipolar disorder may have deficits in abstraction, judgment, and insight. In addition, autism spectrum disorder is a unique neuropsychiatric condition that can alter both executive operations and executive attributes.

Conclusions

Executive operations and abilities are the highest cognitive functions and reflect the evolutionary enlargement of the prefrontal cortex in humans. This region is heterogeneous and includes a number of operations necessary for goal-oriented behavior along with attributes such as abstracting ability, judgment, and complex problem-solving skills. As a command and control center, the frontal lobe and executive functions hold sway over much of behavior and the brain. Despite the importance of the executive operations and attributes covered here, there is still much to discuss with regard to frontal lobe functions, specifically the frontal-limbic region and its role in the ultimate task of the brain, that of mediating many of the neurological disorders discussed in the next chapter.

Chapter 14

The Neurological Behavioral Examination

This chapter is about the neurological behavioral examination. It greatly overlaps with the psychiatric interview, which is valuable in its own right. The neurological behavioral examination targets neuropsychiatric changes potentially associated with known neurological disorders or lesions. In fact, most "psychiatric behaviors" can result from neurological disorders or lesions, and a major objective of this chapter is to emphasize the need to assess for neurological disease in patients with new onset psychiatric or behavioral symptoms. This examination relies primarily on the history, an interview, and the behavioral observations discussed in Chapter 6. That chapter discussed alertness and attention, appearance and personal hygiene, psychomotor speed and movements, speech and communication, eye and facial behavior, propriety and disinhibition, social interactions and personality, and attitude and affect. This chapter expands on those observations, targeting in greater detail the following areas: motivation and emotion, social behavior, psychophysiological behaviors (including aggression), content disorders (speech and language, thought, behavior), and altered perceptions.

Neurological Behaviors

A major prerequisite for understanding how to assess for neurological behaviors is understanding how to define and operationalize them. Terms such as "emotion," "empathy," and "aggression" vary in their usage and overlap in their origin. The assessment of these behaviors requires an initial explanation of what they are and how they relate to brain disease.

MOTIVATION AND EMOTION

Motivation. Motivation describes the intensity and persistence in working toward a goal. Motivation requires emotional responsivity, executive functions, and "autoactivation" collaborating in a motivation-action-reward

loop involving prefrontal cortex (dorsolateral; anterior cingulate) and basal ganglia (dorsal caudate, internal globus pallidus, substantia nigra, ventral striatum, ventral pallidum). Apathy and abulia are disorders of diminished motivation and important manifestation of brain disease. Apathy ("without passion") is prominently decreased emotional responsivity with a lack of emotional expression or interest in activities. Clinical conditions associated with apathy include anosodiaphoria (lack of concern for an acknowledged disorder), anosognosia (lack of knowledge for a disorder), alexithymia (inability to identify one's emotions), and "stuporous" catatonia (unresponsive, mute, immobile with inappropriate or prolonged postures or body positions into which they are placed ["cataplexy"]). In contrast to apathy, abulia ("without will") is a primary loss of initiation from executive dysfunction and autoactivation (self-initiation). Clinically, examiners have difficulty distinguishing abulia from apathy. Compared with apathy, abulia appears more severe, results from frontal cognitive impairment rather than primary emotional hyporesponsivity, and melds into akinetic mutism with absent spontaneous movements or speech beyond occasional words or short phrases (see Chapter 7).

Emotion. Many definitions of emotion view it as a type of motivation aimed at promoting adaptive behavior. Emotional experiences are subjective "feelings" associated with somatic-autonomic nervous system arousal. There are much data showing that the somatic-autonomic activity for emotional experiences vary greatly. This, along with the cognitive appraisal or interpretation of emotions, challenges the view that specific emotions originate from specific brain regions. Nevertheless, there is evidence for the reconstitution of somatic states in ventromedial prefrontal cortex when exposed to certain types of experiences. There is also some support for both right hemisphere dominance for emotions and the valence theory attributing negative emotional tendencies to the right hemisphere and positive emotional tendencies to the left. Two important components of emotion that can be disturbed in patients are mood and affect. Mood is the patient's subjective feelings, whereas affect is the outward expression of emotion, such as withdrawn expression, poor eye contact, and tearfulness. Mood and affect are not necessarily congruent and can be dissociated as in pseudobulbar palsy in which excessive affect may not reflect the quality and extent of the underlying mood.

SOCIAL BEHAVIOR

A number of brain regions participate in social behavior and can be disturbed from brain disease. Social propriety and interactions can be profoundly altered with mesial frontolimbic lesions, as exemplified by John Harlow's description of Phineas Gage, perhaps neurology's most famous patient (Fig. 14.1). Gage's behavior was dramatically changed after an accident propelled an iron rod through his brain damaging his ventromedial prefrontal areas. Subsequently, he became, in the words of John Harlow, "...fitful, irreverent, indulging at times in the grossest profanity (which was not previously his custom), manifesting but little deference for his fellows, impatient of restraint or advice when it conflicts with his desires.... [with] the animal passions of a strong man..." Gage's behavioral changes illustrate how the mesial frontal lobes (ventromedial, orbitofrontal) are particularly involved in human social behavior. The ventromedial prefrontal cortex attributes meaning to social phenomena and related areas determine the socioemotional significance of percepts (anterior insulae, anterior cingulate cortex, amygdala, anterior temporal cortex). Many neurological illnesses have prominently disturbed social tact and manners, disinhibition, and inability to comply with social norms consequent to lesions or disease in these regions (Table 14.1).

The examiner assesses social cognition not only from observation of social behavior but also through tests of Theory of Mind, empathy, and social perception. Theory of Mind is the ability to represent the thoughts, beliefs, attitudes, and feelings of others. It involves the ventromedial prefrontal cortex, amygdala and anterior temporal pole, posterior superior temporal sulcus, precuneus, and the right temporoparietal junction. There are different subtypes of Theory of Mind, including cognitive understanding, affective understanding, and first- or second-order levels. With regard to empathy, there is no universally accepted definition. Most agree that empathy is the ability to identify with the emotional experience of ("feeling as") others in a prosocial way. It involves an evaluation of the experience of others, which leads to the creation of a model in one's mind of another's feelings. The experience of empathy facilitates sympathy ("feeling for") for others and prosocial behavior (responding compassionately). An aspect of "cognitive empathy" is perspective taking, which involves the dorsal mid anterior cingulate cortex, adjacent dorsomedial frontal cortex, and ventromedial prefrontal cortex. An aspect of "emotional empathy" is affect sharing, which involves the anterior insula and inferior frontal gyrus (right frontal subgenual and right temporo-limbic). Finally, social perception for faces, body, and other signals of emotion are an additional critical part of navigating the social world. Most of these overlaps with perception, as described in Chapter 10, with special emphasis on the ability to recognize facial emotions.

PSYCHOPHYSIOLOGICAL BEHAVIORS (INCLUDING AGGRESSION)

Broadly defined, psychophysiological behaviors involve the hypothalamus and related areas, which regulate the sleep-wake cycle, the sexual drive, hunger and satiety, thirst and drinking, and aggressive behavior. Inappropriate or increased sexual behavior may be manifestations of brain disease, either from primary hypersexuality or from sexual disinhibition. In primary hypersexuality, there are recurrent and intense sexual fantasies, urges, and risky behaviors, often associated with repetitive but unsuccessful efforts to reduce or control these sexual symptoms. Primary hypersexuality has occurred with strokes and surgical resections for epilepsy, tumors, or right temporal variant frontotemporal dementia from temporal-amygdalar damage and a release of sexual arousal. Far more commonly, inappropriate sexual behavior results from sexual disinhibition as part of a frontally mediated general disinhibition. These patients react impulsively and opportunistically to tempting environmental situations involving sexual or other objects of interest, without necessarily following-through or consummating their sexual behavior.

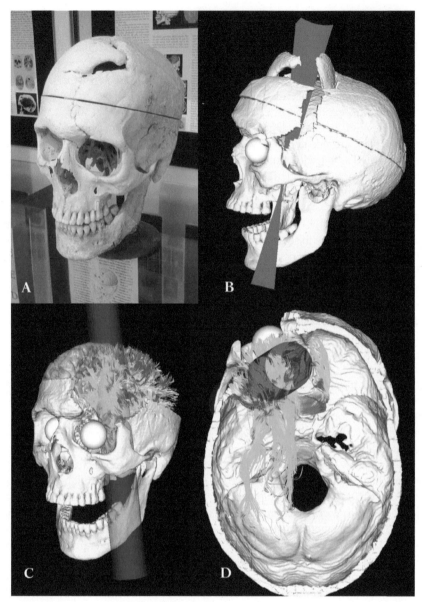

Fig. 14.1 White Matter Tracts Affected by Ventromedial Prefrontal Cortex Damage (Left worse than Right) in Phineas Gage. Modeling the path of the tamping iron through the Gage skull and its effects on white matter structure. **(A)** The skull of Phineas Gage on display at the Warren Anatomical Museum at Harvard Medical School. **(B)** CT image volumes were reconstructed, spatially aligned, and manual segmentation of the individual pieces of bone dislodged by the tamping iron (rod), top of the cranium, and mandible was performed. Surface meshes for each individual element of the skull were created. Based upon observations from previous examinations of the skull as well as upon the dimensions of the iron itself, fiducial constraint landmarks were digitally imposed and a set of possible rod trajectories were cast through the skull. This figure shows the set of possible rod trajectory centroids which satisfied each of the anatomical constraints. The trajectory nearest the mean trajectory was considered the true path of the rod and was used in all subsequent calculations. Additionally, voxels comprising the interior boundary and volume of the cranial vault were manually extracted and saved as a digital edocast of Mr. Gage's brain cavity. **(C)** A rendering of the Gage skull with the best fit rod trajectory and example fiber pathways in the left hemisphere intersected by the rod. Graph theoretical metrics for assessing brain global network integration, segregation, and efficiency were computed across each subject and averaged to emasure the changes to topological, geometrical, and wiring cost properties. **(D)** A view of the interior of the Gage skull showing the extent of fiber pathways intersected by the tamping iron in a sample subject (i.e. one having minimal spatial deformation to the Gage skull). The intersection and density of WM fibers between all possible pairs of GM parcellations was recorded, as was average fiber length and average fractional anisotropy (FA) integrated over each fiber. (From Van Horn JD, Irimia A, Torgerson CM, Chambers MC, Kikinis R, Toga AW. Mapping connectivity Damage in the Case of Phineas Gage. Plos One 7(5); 2012.)

TABLE 14.1 Neurological Disorders with Prominent Disturbances in Social Behavior
Anoxic encephalopathy
Attention deficit hyperactivity disorder
Atypical Parkinson syndromes, e.g., corticobasal syndrome, progressive supranuclear palsy
Autism spectrum disorders
Demyelinating of dysmyelinating disorders, e.g., multiple sclerosis, metachromatic leukodystrophy
Dysexecutive/behavioral variant Alzheimer disease
Epilepsy, especially of temporal limbic origin
Frontal lobotomy/leucotomy
Frontotemporal dementia syndromes
Huntington disease
Hydrocephalus
Infections: Creutzfeldt-Jakob, human immunodeficiency virus, neurosyphilis
Motor neuron disease with frontotemporal dementia
Noninfectious encephalopathies, e.g., autoimmune, paraneoplastic, Hashimoto
Other frontally predominant dementias, e.g., vascular dementia
Other inheritable disorders: Down syndrome, Prader-Willi and Angelman syndromes, Turner syndrome, fragile X syndrome
Strokes and other focal lesions in frontotemporal regions and caudate nuclei
Toxins and alcohol
Traumatic brain injury (frontotemporal contusions)
Tumors, e.g., butterfly glioma of the frontal lobes
William syndrome

Changes in dietary and eating behavior from brain disease include a spectrum from alterations of dietary preferences to the placement of nonfood or inedible items in their mouths. Basic food intake is under hypothalamic control, with a lateral region controlling feeding and a medial region controlling satiety; however, complex changes in eating behavior are more commonly associated with right frontal and temporal lobe damage rather than with hypothalamic lesions. Excessive eating (hyperphagia) is a significant feature, not only of neurological conditions, such as behavioral variant frontotemporal dementia, the Klein–Levin syndrome, and the human Klüver–Bucy syndrome, but also of developmental disorders, such as the Prader–Willi syndrome. Patients with frontotemporal dementia syndromes may have cravings for sweets or carbohydrates or obsessions for particular foods. In addition, disease in the orbitofrontal region may impair the ability to refrain from taking food or to respond to feelings of satiety.

Aggression is someone's action that intentionally delivers something unpleasant, either psychological or physical, to another. Violence is an extreme form of aggression that involves physical action. There are two major types of aggression: 1) reactive or affective aggression, which is an emotional, often explosive, response to a perceived threat or provocation; and 2) instrumental or predatory aggression, which is controlled (organized), purposeful (premeditated), and may be used to achieve an antisocial goal. The hypothalamus and periaqueductal gray of the midbrain (connected to amygdala and prefrontal cortex) control the expression of both behavioral and autonomic components of aggression. Reactive aggressive is associated with abnormalities in the hypothalamic–pituitary–adrenal axis, as well as in serotonin and catecholamine neurotransmitters. Reduced control from the prefrontal cortex, in particular its medial and orbitofrontal portions, is associated with instrumental as well as reactive aggression.

In addition, investigators have reported smaller and more hypofunctional amygdalae among chronic violent offenders.

CONTENT (SPEECH AND LANGUAGE, THOUGHT, BEHAVIOR)

Speech and Language Content. "Content" refers to subject matter expressed in speech and language, thought, and behavior. Speech and language changes reflecting disturbed content may particularly occur from frontal disease. These changes include disorganized speech, incoherence, illogicality, poverty of speech content, and the related tendencies to go off-track in their conversation or responses, such as tangentiality, circumstantiality, and frank derailment. In tangentiality, patients go from one related topic to another, each further afield from the original topic of conversation, whereas in circumstantiality, patients talk around the original topic of conversation while focusing on unnecessary but related details or facts. These patients may additionally have palilalia and echolalia, neologisms and paraphasias, word approximations, clanging and rhyming, and cataphasia or verbigeration (morbid repetition of words, phrases, or sentences).

Thought Content. Thought process describe a patient's form of thinking and expressed ideas or "themes," including false reports, such as delusions and confabulations. Delusions are false beliefs that are fixed (held with certainty), incorrigible (held against all proof to the contrary), and implausible (impossibility or falsity of content). Common themes include persecution, grandiosity, control, jealousy, guilt or sin, and content-specific delusions such as the delusion of theft in patients with Alzheimer's disease. Confabulations are false reports that are made without a conscious effort to deceive for the purpose of creating a coherent self-narrative. Most are provoked or "momentary" confabulations elicited specifically in response to questions that probe memory in patients with memory impairment, such as Korsakoff syndrome. Frontal lobe variants of confabulation, fantastic confabulations and fantastic thinking, are grandiose or impossible elaborations of internally generated ideas associated with vivid imagination and wish fulfillment. Confabulations differ from delusions in being more often provoked, inconsistent, often redirectable, and generally plausible, unless of the fantastic subtype.

Content of Behavior. Semipurposeful movements that appear goal-related reflect a type of disturbed content. These include stereotypies, compulsive-like behavior, and punding. Stereotypies are usually repetitive, rhythmic, often bilateral movements with a fixed pattern (e.g., tapping, hand posturing, head movements) and regular frequency that can usually be stopped by distraction. With stereotypies in autism or frontotemporal dementia, there appears to be striatal-thalamo-frontal neural circuit dysfunction leading to activation imbalance. In addition to traditional compulsions, similarly complex compulsive-like behaviors may also occur from frontostriatal disease. These compulsive-like behaviors are repetitive, variable, and ritualistic acts, such as repetitive trips to the bathroom or repetitive oral sounds or motor movements. Compulsive-like behaviors are an impulse-control disorder possibly from specific involvement of the right frontolimbic-striatal system rather than true compulsions, which are negatively driven by the need to relieve anxiety. Diogenes syndrome is a type of compulsive-like behavior characterized by the combination of extreme self-neglect and excessive collecting with clutter and squalor in patients with frontally predominant dementia. Punding is another related but distinct disorder characterized by even more complex, repetitive, excessive, and seemingly goal-oriented activity. First seen in amphetamine and cocaine addicts, it also occurs among patients with Parkinson disease who are receiving dopaminergic medications. The behaviors are useless, even if goal-oriented, and appear to be impulse control disturbances not driven by anxiety or the need for pleasure or gratification.

ALTERED PERCEPTIONS

Hallucinations and Illusions. Hallucinations are abnormal perceptions that occur in the absence of external sensory input, and illusions are altered perceptions that are based on a genuine sensory input. Hallucinations and illusions may involve any modality, including visual, auditory, olfactory, gustatory, or tactile. Visual hallucinations, more than auditory hallucinations, suggest neurological disease such as dementia with Lewy bodies, rather than a primary psychotic disorder. Visual hallucinations may be a "release" due to primary visual or other impairment, rapid eye movement or dream state breakthrough, or excitatory, as from seizure activity. In elderly persons, release visual hallucinations may occur in association with cognitive impairment and ophthalmological disease, that is, visual hallucinations of Bonnet, and they are often formed, animate (living), and lilliputian (small) figures. Breakthrough hallucinations may occur during transitional periods of waking (hypnopompic) or going (hypnogogic) to sleep. Illusions, in contrast to hallucinations, are due to errors in "binding" between competing basic elements of perception and require elicitation by specific perceptual stimuli. Pareidolias are visual illusions involving ambiguous forms being perceived as meaningful objects, which occur with dementia with Lewy bodies. Additionally, delusional misidentifications include Capgras (known person replaced by imposter), Fregoli (unfamiliar persons are a certain person in disguise), intermetamorphosis (people swapped identities but not appearance), and doppelgänger (a patient's double is carrying out independent action).

The general concept of body identity disorders includes a large number of conditions. These disorders refer to distortions on how people see themselves and their bodies and are associated with a visuospatial map of the body, more specifically a body-centered reference system located in the right superior parietal region. Patients with right parietal damage can have disturbances of the integrity of their body image, such as left-sided attentional neglect, asomatognosia or the loss of awareness of parts of one's body, anosognosia or loss of awareness or denial of illness, alexisomia or inability to read one's body states, anosodiaphoria or loss of concern for illness, somatoparaphrenia or the denial of ownership of a limb or one half of the body, misoplegia or hatred of the left side, and even xenomelia or the desire for the amputation of a limb. In addition, derealization and depersonalization are part of the spectrum of these disturbed body perceptions. Derealization is a feeling that the environment is unreal, strange, or alien, and depersonalization is the same feeling about oneself. These conditions should not be confused with somatotopagnosia and autotopagnosia, which are left parietal origin errors in localization on one's or another's body (see Chapter 12). Finally, phantom limbs are a phenomenon of persistent experiencing the presence, or pain from, an amputated limb, possibly from remapping of deafferented neurons unto adjacent cortex.

Elements of the Neurological Behavioral Examination

Much of the assessment for neurological behaviors is from the history, with targeted questions, and behavioral observations. There are some tests and scales, but not as many or as readily available for use in the clinical evaluation of other areas of the mental status examination.

MOTIVATION AND EMOTION

Motivation. The examiner investigates for apathy and abulia using a checklist of critical items on history and on behavioral observation. First, there should be collateral history as to whether the patient has ceased engaging in his or her usual activities. Second, the examiner determines what the patient actually does during the day, and whether the patient performs activities of daily living, from dressing to toileting, without prompting. On examination, support for a disorder of motivation include the following:

1. Inertia, or the absence of spontaneous verbal and motor behavior;
2. Detachment, or the absence of engagement with others and surroundings;
3. Lack of affect, or the presence of flat or apathetic expressions;
4. Impaired response initiation, or the presence of minimal, brief, or slow responses to command or to events;
5. Impersistence, or the need for significant prompting to continue any activity.

One of the most widely used measurement scales for apathy is the Apathy Evaluation Scale and its variations, which takes approximately 10 to 20 minutes to complete. It is included here for reference and as a guide for evaluating these patients (Table 14.2).

Emotion. The history probes whether the patient has expressed emotion to personal events or has emotional hyporesponsivity or emotional lability. Collateral history can provide information as to whether the patient has expressed specific feelings (e.g., depression, anxiety) or has had periods of tearfulness or laughter. Affect is behavior that is judged primarily by observation and, as such, is more readily recorded. On examination, support for disturbed emotion includes the following:

1. **Abnormal Mood:** Ask the patient specific questions concerning feelings, including questions related to depression and sadness, anxiety or

TABLE 14.2 Apathy Evaluation Scale, Clinician Version (AES-C)			
Name:		Date:	
Rater:			
Rate each item based on an interview of the subject. The interview should begin with a description of the subject's interest, activities, and daily routine. Base your ratings on both verbal and nonverbal information. Ratings should be based on the past 4 weeks. For each item ratings should be judged:			
Not at All Characteristic 1	Slightly Characteristic 1	Somewhat Characteristic 3	A Lot Characteristic 4
_____1.	S/he is interested in things.		+C Q
_____2.	S/he gets things done during the day.		+B Q
_____3.	Getting things started on his/her own is important to her/him.		+C SE
_____4.	S/he is interested in having new experiences.		+C Q
_____5.	S/he is interested in learning new things.		+C Q
_____6.	S/he puts little effort into anything.		−B
_____7.	S/he approaches life with intensity.		+E
_____8.	Seeing a job through to the end is important to her/him.		+C SE
_____9.	He/she spends time doing things that interest her/him.		+B
_____10.	Someone has to tell her/him what to do each day.		−B
_____11.	S/he is less concerned about his/her problems than she/he should be.		−C
_____12.	S/he has friends.		+B Q
_____13.	Getting together with friends is important to her/him.		+C SE
_____14.	When something good happens, he/she gets excited.		+E
_____15.	S/he has an accurate understanding of her/his problems.		+O
_____16.	Getting things done during the day is important to her/him.		+C SE
_____17.	S/he has initiative.		+O
_____18.	S/he has motivation.		+O

Note: Items that have positive versus negative syntax are identified by +/−. Type of item: C = cognitive; B = behavior; E = emotional; O = other. The definitions of self-evaluation (SE) and quantifiable (Q) items are discussed in the administration guidelines [see Syllabus] (Marin, 1991). For self-rated and informant-rated versions of AES, the response options are Not at all true, Slightly true, etc. The Apathy Evaluation Scale was developed by Robert S. Marin, M.D. Development and validation studies and are described in Marin et al., 1991. Supplementary administration guidelines available from author.
Reprinted with permission from Elsevier from Marin RS. Apathy: concept, syndrome, neural mechanisms, and treatment. *Semin Clin Neuropsychiatry.* 1996;1(4)304-314.

apprehension, anger or disgust, or other prevailing emotions. Statements about the patient's mood should include depth, intensity, duration, and fluctuations. The examiner may ask the patient at each visit to rate mood from 1 to 10 (with 1 being sad, and 10 being happy).

2. **Emotional Lability or Dyscontrol:** Assess whether the patient has periods of provoked or unprovoked emotional outbursts and how quickly they resolve. Specifically consider pseudobulbar affect with incontinent crying or laughing from bilateral pyramidal tract disease, Witzelsucht with facetious humor from orbitofrontal disease, or moria with childlike excitement from frontal disease.

3. **Emotional Hyporesponsivity:** Infer responsivity from the patient's facial expression, eye contact, general behavior (e.g., presence of psychomotor retardation), and responses to questions. Include the amount and lability of expressive behavior.

4. **Impaired Range of Emotion:** Specifically assess range of variation in facial expression, tone of voice, use of hands, and body movements. Determine whether the range or variability reflects a constricted, blunted, or flat affect.

5. **Incongruency of Mood and Affect:** Assess whether the patient's perceived affect corresponds to his or her underlying mood. Assess for dysphoria or euphoria and whether it is congruent with the context or situation.

There are a number of inventories or scales that can screen for emotion, including mood and affect (Table 14.3).

SOCIAL BEHAVIOR

Social Observation. Similar to motivation and emotion, the evaluation of social behavior primarily involves a careful history and behavioral observation. As before, the examiner needs collateral history from the family or caregiver for an accurate witnessed picture of the patient's actual social behavior (Table 14.4). The examiner asks specific questions on a social cognitive questionnaire and observes for comparable behavior.

1. **Change in Personality:** Determine if there has been a significant change in the patient's pervasive pattern of behavior. Personality changes in mid to later life are commonly due to neurological disease.

2. **Inappropriate Social Behavior:** Determine if there has been the development of socially awkward or unacceptable behavior, such as decreased social tact and manners, personal referent comments of others, unsolicited affiliative contacts with strangers, and frank violation of social rules or norms. Some patients may have inappropriate public or sexual behavior or perform "sociopathic" acts resulting in legal trouble.

3. **Failure to Respond to Social Cues:** Determine if the patient responds to verbal, physical, or contextual cues regarding social behavior and boundaries. Violations would include frequent interrupting, violations of verbal and physical interpersonal boundaries, lack of response to communicative gestures, and "not being in the conversation."

4. **Poor Impulse Control:** These behaviors are part of the spectrum of disinhibition. Determine if the patient is impulsive, acting opportunistically and in-the-moment without reflection, performs

TABLE 14.3   Emotional Inventory
Abnormal Mood
Prevailing feelings, (e.g., depression, anxiety, anger, excitement)
Depth, intensity and fluctuation of feelings (can rate 1 to 10)
Emotional Hyporesponsivity
Decreased reactivity (e.g., withdrawn, decreased verbal output, psychomotor retardation)
Overt indifference and lack of concern or interpersonal warmth
Emotional Lability or Dyscontrol
Presence of emotional outbursts (provoked or unprovoked and resolution)
Evidence of pseudobulbar affect, moria, or Moria Witzelsucht
Impaired Range of Emotion
Constricted, blunted, flat, or vacant overall affect
Unvarying facial expressivity, voice, and/or hand and body movements
Incongruency of Mood and Affect
Perceived affect corresponds to his or her underlying mood
Dysphoric, euphoric, or other behavior out-of-context with situation

TABLE 14.4   Social Behavioral Symptoms/ Signs
Change in personality
Decreased "people awareness" and Theory of Mind
Deficits in empathy with disregard for the distress of others
Disinhibition
Disturbed social tact, manners, graces, or etiquette
Fails to respond to social cues
Frank violation of social rules or norms
Impaired understanding of irony, sarcasm, or humor
Inappropriate sexual behavior, disinhibited or public
Interpersonal boundary infringements
Lack of affective or social sharing or reciprocity
Lack of response to interlocutors ("not being in the conversation")
Neglect of personal appearance, grooming, and hygiene
Personal referent comments of others
Poor impulse control acting opportunistically and in-the-moment without reflection
Private behaviors performed in public
Rash and careless actions
Reveals private information without consideration
Social disengagement
Sociopathic acts resulting in legal trouble
Speech is self-centered
Susceptibility to solicitations
Unconventionality in behavior, dress, or manners
Unsolicited affiliative contacts with strangers
Verbally offensive or personal comments

rash and careless actions, shows susceptibility to solicitations, blurts out private information, or performs personal behavior in public.

5. **Decreased "People Awareness"**: Determine the patient's appreciation for other people. They may behave as if they do not see other human beings or recognize that their behavior affects them. This is associated with deficits in Theory of Mind and empathy (see later).

For social behavior, investigators have used a scale such as the Social Observation Inventory, which assesses not only tact and manners but also the use of other-oriented pronouns, such as "you," and is included here for reference (Table 14.5).

Theory of Mind. Theory of Mind tests evaluate the ability to disregard one's own knowledge about the world and consider that someone else might have a different belief. A classic Theory of Mind false belief task is the Sally–Anne story: "Sally has a stroller and Anne has a toy box. Sally puts her doll in her stroller and goes out for a short time. While Sally is away, Anne moves the doll to the toy box. Sally comes back to get her doll. Where will Sally look for her doll?" (Does the patient understand that Sally has an erroneous belief of where her doll is?). This is a first-order false belief task (Fig. 14.2); it can be escalated to second-order in which the patient must understand that someone else has an erroneous belief about another character's belief (Fig. 14.3). Other false belief tasks include a cartoon test of humorous situations based on false beliefs of a character in the cartoons. Non-false belief tasks of Theory of Mind assess social inference, such as faux pas tasks that interpret the hidden meanings in scenarios. In one example of a faux pas scenario, Adam, John's boss, unexpectedly visits John at his office. John has a client with him and says, "Let me introduce Mr. Baker, one of our most important clients." The client interjects, "my name is not Baker, my name is Brown." In another faux pas scenario, Katie gives her in-laws a framed picture of her wedding. On a later visit, she discovers the picture stored in a drawer. Her mother-in-law, not recalling that it was a gift, comments, "that was my least favorite of your wedding pictures." A third test of Theory of Mind is the Reading the Mind in the Eyes test in which patients must infer the mental state of someone based on photographs of just their eyes. Less commonly used tests in a clinical encounter are the Awareness of Social Inference Test which presents videos focusing on the ability to detect sarcasm, the Strange Stories Test with stories that depend on knowing someone's mental state, and the Hinting Test of brief vignettes that depend on understanding that a character dropped a hint.

Empathy. It is difficult to observe empathy in a structured setting or to get a valid self-report. The patient's descriptions of their empathic behavior are often very unreliable as they tend to report themselves as having significant empathy even when absent. The examiner evaluates specific areas:

TABLE 14.5 **Social Observation Inventory**						
Subject: _____	Interlocutor(s): _____					
Date: _____	Rater: _____					
	Never 0	Very Rarely 1	Rarely 2	Occasionally 3	Frequent 4	Very Frequent 5
Verbal Behavior						
Decreased spontaneous verbal behavior						
Generally unresponsive to others' comments, including self-repair and encouraging responses						
Lacks acceptable timing of responses – normal latency of responses and turn-taking						
Decreased elaboration of responses, e.g., brief or minimal answers						
Responses are off-topic and not engaged in conversation						
Lack of personal references: "you" Comments or questions about the other(s)						
Lacks "I" statements (implicit or explicit)						
Verbal disinhibition, e.g., inappropriate or offensive remarks						
Inappropriate vocalizations, e.g., laughter out-of-context						
Repetitive, stereotypical, or automatic verbalizations						
Nonverbal Behavior						
Decreased spontaneous nonverbal behavior						
Does not stay with social interaction, e.g., walks away or attends to other things						
Absence of joint or shared attention						
Gaze/eye contact inappropriate to interaction						
Facial expression inappropriate to interaction						
Body positioning inappropriate to interaction						
Decreased "in-phase" movements that are engaged with the others' actions and/or absence of nonverbal encouraging responses						
Decreased social tact and propriety, e.g., poor manners, propriety, or decorum						
Nonverbal disinhibition, e.g., private behaviors in public, inappropriate touching						
Repetitive, stereotypical, or automatic motor behavior						

Total verbal: _____
Total nonverbal: _____
Total (verbal plus nonverbal): _____
From: Mendez MF, Fong SS, Shapira JS, et al. Observation of social behavior in frontotemporal dementia. *Am J Alzheimer Dis Other Dis*. 2014;29:215-221.

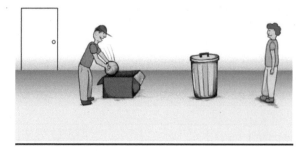

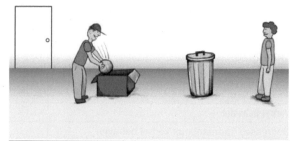

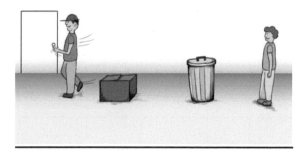

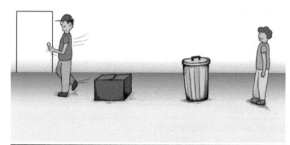

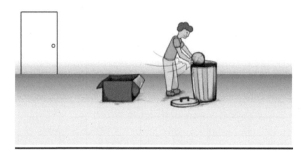

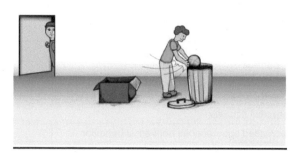

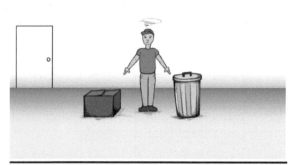

Fig. 14.2 Theory of Mind: First-Order False Belief. Panel 1: "Red puts a ball into the box." Panel 2: "Red leaves the room." Panel 3: "Green moves ball from the box to the trash can." Panel 4: "Red returns and wants his ball." 1. Where will Red look for the ball? Response: _____ 2. Where did Red put the ball before he left the room? Response: _____ 3. Where is the ball now? Response: _____

Fig. 14.3 Theory of Mind: Second-Order False Belief. Panel 1: "Red puts a ball into the box." Panel 2: "Red leaves the room." Panel 3: "Green moves ball from the box to the trash can while Red watches secretly." Panel 4: "Red returns and wants his ball." 1. Where does Green think Red will look for the ball? Response: _____ 2. Does Green think that Red saw him move it? Response: _____ 3. Did Red see Green move the ball? Response: _____ 4. Where does Red think the ball is? Response: _____

1. **Loss of Empathic Concern:** Determine if the patient is unconcerned about the feelings and emotions of others. Ask how the patient responds when their family members are in distress about a personal situation.
2. **Observed Indifference:** Often a major clue to loss of empathy in a clinical encounter or at the bedside is the observation of decreased reactivity to the family's distress when discussing the patient's condition or diagnosis.
3. **Insensitive Verbal Comments:** Overtly hurtful, thoughtless, inconsiderate, or uncaring comments are indicative of diminished empathy. Patients' comments may reflect a lack of emotional awareness of others.
4. **Reaction to Emotional Experience:** In a clinical encounter, the examiner can ask the patient about their reaction immediately after an emotional experience, for example, the birth of child, the death of a loved one, and others.
5. **Empathy-Elicitation:** In specific patients, it may be of value to test empathy by showing emotionally arousing pictures, or even videos. Pictures of people in need or in distress can be readily obtained and shown in a clinical encounter. Query the patient: "How does this picture make you feel?" The patient can also rate his or her emotional response in terms of intensity.

Studies have used validated measures such as the Interpersonal Reactivity Inventory, the Empathy Quotient, and the Multifaceted Empathy Test, which are not accessible as routine clinical screening tools.

Social Perception. For social perception, the most extensively validated stimuli assess the recognition of facial emotions, particularly the Ekman Faces, which are black and white photographs that depict six basic emotions (disgust, anger, fear, surprise, sadness, and happiness) (Fig. 14.4). The breadth and specificity of difficulties in recognizing emotions can be assessed with batteries of tests such as the Facial Expressions of Emotion: Stimuli and Tests, the Comprehensive Affect Testing System, and the Florida Affect Battery. Alternative testing involves depicting videos in which an actor portrays emotions as in the Emotions Evaluation Test part of the Awareness of Social Inference Test.

PSYCHOPHYSIOLOGICAL BEHAVIORS (INCLUDING AGGRESSION)

Sexual Behavior. Crucial information for evaluating sexuality are the following:

1. **Increased Frequency:** Determine if there has been heightened sexual behavior from premorbid levels sufficient to cause significant concern to the patient or others.
2. **Public Sexuality:** Determine if there have been known or observed public manifestations of sexual behavior, either masturbation or partner-related, and whether the sexual behavior occurred without regard to potential risk to themselves or others.
3. **Actively Seeking:** Determine if the patient is driven to go out of the way to obtain sexual gratification as opposed to just passive, opportunistic sexual behavior.
4. **Widened Sexual Interests:** Determine if there is an increased extent of the patient's sexual interests or increased ease of sexual arousal. This points to the presence of hypersexuality with increased libido.
5. **Evidence of Sexual Disinhibition:** Alternatively, there may be evidence of general disinhibition and poor impulse control that could be associated with sexual disinhibition rather than a primary increased sexual drive.

Eating Behavior. Crucial items for evaluating eating behavior are the following:

1. **Hyperphagia:** Determine if the patient's overall ingestion of food has increased, if they help themselves to more food, if it is indiscriminate, and if there has been weight gain. Record the time course of these changes.
2. **Food Preferences:** Determine if the patient's altered eating behavior is limited to carbohydrate craving, food fads, alcohol, or other specific preferences.
3. **Food Preoccupation:** Obtain information about the patient's preoccupation for food. This includes talking about food, storing or hoarding food, seeking food, and behavior if prevented from access to food.
4. **Absent Satiety:** Determine at what level the patient feels "full" or if there is no clear indication of satiety. Some patients may continue eating

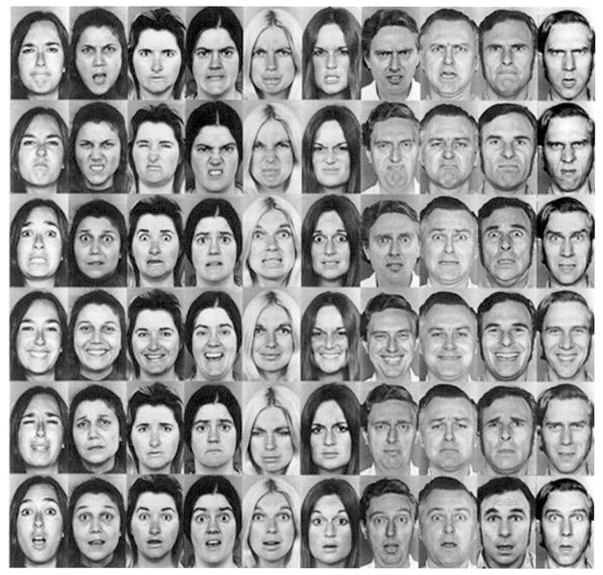

Fig. 14.4 Ekman 60 Faces Test. The Ekman faces test evaluate the ability to recognize emotion in a forced-choice paradigm where 60 individual faces are matched with one of six basic emotions: happiness, sadness, surprise, fear, disgust and anger. (From Ekman P, Friesen WV. Measuring facial movement. *J Nonverbal Behav.* 1, 56-76 (1976).)

beyond a standard meal without ever reporting being full.

5. **Hyperorality:** Determine if there is ingestion, or orality, of nonfood or inedible items. This could be other organic material, such as dog food or plants, or other objects in the environment, such as Styrofoam cups or paper towels. Hyperorality may include gum chewing, oral tobacco, smoking, and other oral activities.

Aggressive Behavior. Crucial items for evaluating aggressive behavior are the following:

1. **Verbal or Physical Aggressive Episodes:** Record the number and frequency of aggressive episodes and whether they involve physical, as well as verbal, aggression and the nature of the inflicted harm. Record if there was violence or physical harm committed against another.

2. **Reactive Aggression:** Determine if the aggression was reactive in type. Evidence for this includes an emotional reaction with anger or distress, an unpremeditated outburst with some precipitant, and possible remorse afterward.

3. **Instrumental Aggression:** Determine if the aggression was instrumental in type. Evidence for this includes an organized and planned aggressive act with a goal or purpose, which is often antisocial.

4. **Evaluate for Precipitants:** Determine if there are situational factors that facilitate aggression. For example, patients may have "pathological intoxication" with aggression related to alcohol or other drug ingestion. Others may feel threatened from someone or something in the environment and react aggressively.

5. **Psychopathy:** Evaluate for signs of psychopathic traits, such as a lack of guilt or remorse, lack of fear for punishment, risk-taking behavior, superficial charm and glibness, grandiosity, and the tendency to manipulate others.

CONTENT (SPEECH AND LANGUAGE, THOUGHT, BEHAVIOR)

Speech and Language Content. Before assessing speech and language content, the examiner must complete a language examination (See Chapter 8). The examiner must first exclude primary disorders of language or aphasia before concluding a disorder of speech content.

1. **Speech Characteristics:** Determine the rate, quantity, and loudness of speech, including whether slow or rapid and pressured, sparse or profuse, soft or loud.

2. **Speech Repetitions:** Look for repetitions of speech sounds (clanging), syllables (stuttering, logoclonia), words or phrases (palilalia), or the examiner's words or phrases (echolalia).

3. **Language Characteristics:** Determine the coherence, clarity, logicality, and overall intelligibility of language discourse. Incoherence of language may indicate a lack of coherent connections between thoughts.

4. **Disordered Relatedness:** Look for circumstantiality (circuitous answers with overinclusion of unnecessary information), tangentiality (sidetracked answers with irrelevant and digressive information), or derailment (off-topic answers that are totally unrelated to the original conversation).

5. **Idiosyncratic Language:** Look for non-aphasic neologisms (made-up words used with a specific meaning or theme) and the presence of unusual words, phrases, or grammar.

Thought Content. Before assessing thought content, the examiner must consider whether any disturbances reflect a primary psychiatric disorder, as is more commonly the case, or whether they could indicate psychiatric symptoms from neurological disorders. Manic and psychotic behavior, including delusions, can be due to brain disease or lesions, particularly if newly developed in mid or late life. The examiner records evidence of the following:

1. **Flight of Ideas:** Look for rapid speech with abrupt changes from topic to topic usually based on understandable links between topics.

2. **Loose Associations:** Evaluate whether the thoughts are illogically or loosely connected. Loose associations involve jumping from one unconnected topic to another.

3. **Delusions:** Determine if there are false reports consistent with fixed, incorrigible, and implausible beliefs. The examiner should also look for ideas of organized misinterpretations concerning self, others, or the external world.

4. **Theme:** Determine if there are beliefs of persecution, of being treated in a special way, ideas of reference or influence, or the presence of content-specific delusions.

5. **Confabulations:** Determine if there are false reports consistent with either momentary or provoked responses in an amnestic patient, or grandiose, wish fulfillment fantasies in a frontally injured patient.

Content of Behavior. The examiner records evidence for behaviors that suggest purposeful, goal-oriented acts but that are repetitive and occur on an overlapping continuum from stereotypies to punding.

1. **Stereotypies:** Inquire and look for common stereotypies such as tapping, rubbing, clapping, picking, smacking or pursing lips, and others.

2. **Compulsive-Like Behaviors:** Inquire and look for more complex perseverative or compulsive-like behaviors that could appear goal-oriented.

3. **Compulsions:** Evaluate for traditional compulsions, which can also manifest in neurological disorders, such as checking, counting, cleaning, walking, hoarding, or ordering.

4. **Punding:** Useless complex behaviors that appear goal-oriented and are repeated may constitute the impulse control behavior known as punding.

5. **Reaction to Restraint:** Determine what happens when you stop or prevent the behaviors from happening. Does the patient experience discomfort or resist? See if the patient can be diverted from the repetitive behavior.

ALTERED PERCEPTIONS

All patients should have an initial check for primary visual or hearing impairment when evaluating for altered perceptions.

Hallucinations. Critical items for hallucinations are as follows:

1. **Modality and Frequency:** The examiner determines whether hallucinations occur in the visual, auditory, or other modality and the frequency of occurrence.

2. **Features of the Hallucinations:** It is important for the examiner to note the characteristics of the hallucinations. For example, in the visual sphere, are they stereotyped or changing, animate or inanimate, Lilliputian or normal-sized, in the peripheral or central field, moving, in color, or out-of-context?

3. **Time-Period of Hallucinations:** Specifically determine when hallucinations occur and their duration. For example, they may result at peak-dose of dopaminergic medications, in periods of low light. In transitional periods of waking and going to sleep, or in drowsy states.

4. **Elicitation of Hallucinations:** Examiners are usually unable to elicit hallucinations in a clinical encounter; however, in some situations hallucinations can be brought out by holding a white piece of paper or an imaginary string between the fingers and asking the patient to describe what he or she sees.

5. **Associated Features:** Evaluate for features such as the presence of recent or worsening visual or auditory impairment, which can facilitate release hallucinations, and signs that the patient is responding to internal stimuli, such thought blocking in mid-sentence or hearing inner voices speaking to him or her. An important group of associated symptoms are those related to seizures, such as periods of altered consciousness, postictal state, or progression to generalized tonic-clonic seizures.

Illusions. Critical items for illusions are similar to those for hallucinations:

1. **Modality and Frequency:** The examiner determines whether illusions occur in the visual, auditory, or other modality and the frequency of occurrence.

2. **Features of the Illusions:** The examiner describes the characteristics of the illusions and the type of perceptual distortions experienced. Particularly important is to establish what stimuli or perceptual experience brings out the illusion. Also determine if others have shared or experienced the illusory phenomenon.

3. **Time-Period of Illusions:** Specifically determine when illusions occur and their duration. Ask if they occur in low light or other visual situations or with alterations in ambient noise. Pareidolias, for example, tend to emerge from shadows in the peripheral fields.

4. **Elicitation of Illusions:** Unlike hallucinations, examiners are frequently able to elicit hallucinations by reintroducing the sensory phenomena that is associated with the perceptual distortion.

5. **Associated Features:** Evaluate for features such as the presence of recent or worsening visual or auditory impairment. An important group of associated symptoms are the presence of primary perceptual disturbances on the mental status examination, as discussed in Chapter 10.

Misperceptions of The Body or Self

1. **Depersonalization and Derealization:** The examiner determines if the patient feels his or her thoughts and feelings are unreal, is looking

at himself or herself from outside their body, has a sense of lost identity, or feels that his or her surroundings are not real.

2. **Distortions of Self:** Determine if the patient has misperceptions of body characteristics, alterations of body sensations, or has an impaired awareness of being able to look at their own body. The patient may complain of bodily changes such as malformations.

3. **Screen for Syndromes:** The examiner specifically considers the presence of asomatognosia, anosognosia, alexisomia, anosodiaphoria, somatoparaphrenia, misoplegia, and xenomelia.

4. **Associated Features:** Evaluate for features such as the presence of primary sensory disturbances, visuospatial deficits, hemispatial or hemibody neglect, or an altered body map from associated left parietal changes (autotopagnosia and somatotopagnosia as described in Chapter 12).

5. **Amputees:** These patients may develop a phantom limb phenomenon, with the feeling of a persistent and often painful yet amputated limb. Evaluate if stimulation in adjacent intact areas elicits sensation in the phantom limb. Some patients may experience supernumerary phantom limbs.

Clinical Implications

Brain injury can result in altered emotions. Patients can have prominent persistent behavioral changes that include depression, often associated with left frontal lesions and aspects of secondary mania, often from right frontal and anterior temporal disease. Depression from left frontal stroke may persist for years after the event. Other patients can have Witzelsucht, or excessive and often inappropriate joking and facetious humor, along with a continued, lighthearted and happy affect ("Moria of Jastrowitz") from lesions involving the right orbitofrontal area and related regions. Frontal predominant injury can facilitate the emergence of mirth along with a sense of increased happiness possibly from disinhibited activation of the subcortical reward/pleasure centers of the ventral striatal limbic area.

Social behavioral changes characterize behavioral variant frontotemporal dementia, one of the most common dementias with onset in mid-life. On microscopic examination, there are microvacuoles and gliosis with or without inclusion bodies, and most patients with this disorder have either transactive response DNA binding protein-43 or hyperphosphorylated tau containing intraneuronal inclusions. In addition to apathy, these patients may present with inappropriateness, tactlessness, decreased manners, unacceptable physical contact, improper verbal comments, or unacceptable physical acts including sexual ones. Patients with behavioral variant frontotemporal dementia may even have antisocial behavior such as stealing (particularly shoplifting small objects), hit and run and other driving violations, and in-the-moment physical assaults. They also have diminished empathy, eating disorders, and stereotypies or compulsive-like behaviors. In summary, this disorder affects a social network that includes the right ventromedial region, anterior cingulate cortex, frontal insulae, the orbitofrontal cortex, and the amygdalae.

Huntington disease is a triad of dyskinetic movements (choreoathetosis), neuropsychiatric features, and dementia. Approximately one-half of patients with Huntington disease present with the movement disorder, the rest present with behavioral changes, particularly apathy or abulia. The social and other behavioral changes in Huntington disease are due to involvement of frontosubcortical tracts that traverse the caudate nuclei. Patients have a lack of behavioral initiation and initiative, decreased spontaneous speech and communication, constriction of emotional expression, and eventual self-neglect and mutism. Patients with Huntington disease may also develop disinhibition, irritability, increased suicidal behavior, compulsive-like behavior, antisocial and criminal behavior including aggressive and physically assaultive acts, and emotional lability with eruptions in response to minor provocations. Finally, hyposexuality, hypersexuality, and sexual aberrations occur in many of these patients, much of this coincident with general disinhibition.

Conclusions

Disorders of motivation and emotion, social behavior, psychophysiological behaviors (including aggression), content (speech and language, thought, behavior), and altered perceptions are important "neurological behaviors" indicative of brain disorders. Although many of these behaviors are usually thought of as psychiatric, this chapter emphasizes that they can also be manifestations of neurological disease. They are often the hardest to assess other than by history and behavioral observations as much of this behavior is episodic or lacks dedicated mental status tasks. However, a targeted interview and behavioral observation, expanding from Chapter 6, can effectively evaluate for these behaviors. Ultimately, the assessment for neurological behaviors is as much a part the neurobehavioral status examination as is the assessment for aphasia, amnesia, apraxia, or agnosia.

SCALES OR INVENTORIES, NEUROPSYCHOLOGICAL TESTS, AND COMPUTERIZED TECHNIQUES

Chapter 15

Overview of Scales and Inventories

This chapter discusses scales and inventories for mental status assessment. Scales are instruments for measuring or grading mental status attributes, and inventories are questionnaires for surveying or cataloging mental status traits. Scales and inventories are useful for screening for the presence of cognitive impairment and not for making a diagnosis. Screening is a method for determining whether there is a potential problem that could indicate a disorder. Mental status scales and inventories are indicated for identifying those patients who need more detailed and comprehensive assessment, whether an extended neurobehavioral status examination (NBSE) or referral for neuropsychological testing. In addition, they quantify or semiquantify the cognitive impairment, indicate degree of severity, allow for communication with others, and facilitate follow-up over time. This chapter on mental status scales and inventories discusses their general aspects, indications and the choice of instrument, psychometric properties, application for longitudinal assessment, and interpretation and limitations.

General Aspects

Mental status scales are brief, structured instruments with specific administration and scoring, and mental status inventories gather information by a list of questions. Some scales are combinations of mental status testing and inventories, for example, the Blessed Dementia Scale and the Alzheimer Disease Rating Scale. Mental status scales and inventories are either general instruments for cognitive deficits, or they are targeted instruments aimed at specific cognitive abilities, syndromes, or diseases. Inventories, as opposed to scales, tend to be targeted at behavioral disturbances. The purpose of general mental status scales is to distinguish patients with

impaired versus normal cognition. General scales are sensitive for identifying screening for patients with the most common cognitive impairments, but they are not for diagnosing diseases or for brain-behavior localization. No mental status scale covers all areas of cognition; therefore they cannot be entirely comprehensive screens for all possible cognitive impairments. There are over 50 mental status scales in wide use. There is no single scale that is the "gold standard", most have sufficient accuracy (sensitivity tempered by specificity) for dementia screening and share a number of advantages and deficiencies (Tables 15.1 and 15.2).

General mental status scales vary in their coverage of cognitive areas. Most scales have items for memory and orientation, as these are affected early in Alzheimer disease and other dementias. This is followed by items for mental control/attention, language, visuospatial skills, and calculations. Few extend to examination

TABLE 15.1 Major Advantages of Mental Status Scales and Inventories
Administration, relatively easy with minimal instruction
Brevity, <5–30 minutes
Cutoff screening identify impaired for further evaluation
Item heterogeneity, individual items may be sensitive to different disorders when individually inspected
Interclinician communication, facilitated
Longitudinal follow-up when using same instrument over time
Mental status screening of populations for prevalence of neurocognitive disorders
Normative data sometimes available
Quantitation of severity
Reliable, test-retest
Results, immediately available (vs. delayed report)
Targeted scales available
Valuable as a brief MSX when items include different cognitive domains

TABLE 15.2 Major Deficiencies of Mental Status Scales and Inventories
Ceiling effects or floor effects
Cognitive impairment not comprehensive
Content and comprehensiveness, variable
Heterogeneity of items affects validity
Interindividual variability
Item order or item difficulty, variable
Items per cognitive domain vary greatly
Language complexity effect (in some cases)
Specificity, absent for specific diseases or brain-behavior localization
State effects, i.e., distraction, fatigue, cooperation, etc.
Validation effects, not as applicable for different demographic groups
Versions for telephone or videoconferencing may not be available

of executive abilities, semantics, praxis, or socio-emotional changes. This is evident in the content of the Mini-Mental State Examination (MMSE) and the Montreal Cognitive Assessment (MoCA), two of the most widely used scales in the clinical setting and used as illustrative examples in this chapter (also see Chapter 16). The MMSE items include 10 for orientation, 3 for registration, 3 for memory, 8 for language, 5 for mental control/attention, and 1 for visuospatial skills. In contrast, the MoCA items include 6 for orientation, 5 for memory, 6 for language, 6 for mental control/attention, 3 for visuospatial, and 4 for executive abilities (including clock hands) (author's evaluation). Even within these content areas, there are differences in what is tested. For example, for language the MMSE, but not the MoCA, includes auditory comprehension, reading, and writing, whereas the MoCA, but not the MMSE includes verbal fluency. Of course, more than one cognitive domain may affect an individual item, but this comparison clearly shows the content variability that extends across mental status scales. Moreover, the number of items per cognitive domain, as well as the length of the instrument, can vary greatly.

The examiner should consider a number of other differences evident on both mental status scales and inventories. Although all aim for brevity, the administration times may vary between 5 minutes or less to 15–30 minutes or more. Scales may be constructed with relatively harder or easier items overall. For example,

the MMSE is much easier than the MoCA, despite a suggested average adjustment for age and education. The order of presentation of items or inventory questions can make a difference in patient responses, for example, whether easy items are presented first, when patients are less fatigued, or presented last, when they distracted when items are less challenging. Orientation items are presented first in the MMSE and last in the MoCA. Memory performance on a scale may vary with the number of intervening items between registration and delayed recall. There is one intervening item on the MMSE, and there are six on the MoCA. On the MMSE, it is conceivable to still have the registration words in working memory when asked for them on delayed recall. Finally, mental status scales differ in their sensitivity to the effects of age, education, and sociocultural and language background, and there is little adjustment for these variables on these scales. Indeed, even slight differences in the complexity of the language used by scales and inventories may affect performance.

Indications and Choice of Instrument

Examiners screening for cognitive impairment usually prefer brief instruments that can be easily and quickly administered and interpreted in the context of a clinical neurological or psychiatric examination. The choice of rating scale or inventory can vary with the specific goals of the evaluation. For example, if the goal is to administer the mental status scale over the telephone or by videoconference, the examiner needs to know what modifications to the scale, if any, may be required from the in-person administration. The choice of instrument may also depend on what is being used in the clinician's setting or institution, and whether it is in the public domain and freely accessible.

Although aimed at detecting cognitive impairment in general, most scales focus on the detection of dementia in the elderly as a surrogate for all cognitive decline (see Box 15.1). In screening for dementia, clinicians can administer general mental status scales in clinical encounters or at the bedside as part of the regular clinic visit or inpatient assessments. Clinicians use mental status scales to augment screening for early signs of dementia in the elderly as part of the Medicare Annual Wellness Visit, but they are not universally recommended unless the patient is symptomatic or there are concerns from

BOX 15.1 USES OF MENTAL STATUS SCALES

1. Proactive screening of asymptomatic individuals for identification of those needing further or more comprehensive evaluation. For screening:
   - Use liberal cut-offs for sensitivity (permits some false positives)
   - Emphasize the individual's variability over a rigid application of population cut-offs (avoids excluding potentially impaired individuals needing further evaluation)
2. Quantification of established impairment, and its stage, in an individual
3. Longitudinal follow-up of individuals in a clinic or in clinical studies
4. Brief Mental Status Examination with assessment of specifically missed content items
5. Populations studies comparing groups or disease cohorts

patients and families. If dementia is suspected in an individual patient, the examiner needs to proceed to more extensive testing with the NBSE or referral for neuropsychological assessment. In sum, mental status scales are useful and practical for screening for potential cognitive decline in a clinical setting, but not comparable to the NBSE or neuropsychological testing, which can more thoroughly establish the diagnosis. In addition, among patients who already have established dementia, these scales can provide information about dementia severity but not about the specific cause.

The major indication for scales and inventories is the need to screen for common dysfunction in a clinical setting. The evaluation for potential cognitive impairment is challenging during brief appointments that might include addressing other medical problems. Scales and inventories must be efficient and relatively easy to administer, score, and interpret. A normal screen during the clinical visit does provide some reassurance if the patient is asymptomatic; however, a more comprehensive evaluation if still necessary if the patient is symptomatic. Likewise, if the patient does not score above the designated cut-off on the scale, then a more a comprehensive evaluation is needed for diagnosis. The cut-offs should allow for a broad net and emphasize sensitivity, tolerating some false positives, over specificity. Another major indication for both scales and inventories is the need for quantification of stage and severity. Despite the effects of state factors (e.g., fatigue, discomfort, level of cooperation) at the time of testing, mental status scales and inventories can give a range of severity or impairment

at that point in time. In addition, the use of these structured instruments helps communicate the cognitive status over longitudinal clinical visits and assessments and across different clinicians and examiners.

An important aspect of scales and inventories is their brevity, with the associated benefit of having the results immediately available. The greater the instrument's brevity, the greater is its clinical utility, particularly in the midst of a busy clinical practice. Scales that are too short sacrifice cognitive content, and those that are too long are less likely to be implemented in demanding clinical settings. Some instruments take less than 5 minutes to administer (e.g., the Mini-Cog, the Six-Item screener, and the Memory Impairment Screen). Others take 5 to 15 minutes (e.g., MMSE, MoCA, and the Saint Louis University Mental State [SLUMS]). A few take 15 to 30 minutes or more (e.g., the Addenbrooke Cognitive Examination).

Targeted mental status scales and inventories have content elements felt sensitive to the specific cognitive deficits that prevail in specific conditions, such as delirium, HIV, mood and affect, and advanced dementia. General mental status scales may not help in differentiating these specific conditions from mild-moderate dementia and other cognitive disturbances. For delirium, there are the Confusion Assessment Method, the Delirium Rating Scale-Revised-98, and the Memorial Delirium Assessment Scale (see Chapter 3). Another example is HIV infection, in which the International HIV Dementia Scale is sensitive to the psychomotor slowing and other potential cognitive effects of HIV-associated neurocognitive disorder. There are many inventories that attempt to quantify mood and behavioral changes, which can be consequences of acquired brain disease. Although these inventories have at least acceptable reliability and validity, they are not as reliable or valid as cognitive rating scales. Unlike scales, inventories can be heavily dependent on the expertise of the interviewer or on the history provided by others. Some inventories are self-rated instruments, which are subject to the patient's insight and cooperation. Finally, there are also scales and inventories for more severe impairment. For example, there are scales or inventories with less difficult items applicable to patients with severe dementia, such as the Severe Impairment Rating Scale and the Severe Cognitive Impairment Scale.

Psychometrics Properties

In selecting among the different mental status scales, the clinician or investigator considers the strengths and weaknesses of the instrument. As screening instruments, mental status scales and inventories aim to maximize capture of individuals with cognitive impairment. They emphasize sensitivity over specificity, that is, increase false positives and minimize false negatives. Scales lack specificity for etiologic diagnoses but are sufficiently sensitive to identify persons with most cognitive deficits, and, as previously noted, they are not comprehensive for all cognitive deficits. This raises concerns about validity, or the degree to which an instrument actually measures what it is supposed to measure (usually determined by agreement with another measure, analysis of content, and convergent or divergent analysis). These scales are most valid at the extremes, i.e., distinguishing entirely normal patients from those with severe dementia. Validity may be particularly challenging if a scale is applied to patients with disorders that were not part of the original validation population for the scale. The examiner should know the type of patients or population on whom the instrument was validated, and whether there are normative data for them, as well as other populations. Finally, there is the issue of robustness of administration. The examiner often administers these instruments in suboptimal conditions, in clinical encounters and at the bedside. The common issues in mental status examination described in Chapter 2 are also pertinent to the administration of scales and inventories. Although most clinicians can administer these scales with a limited amount of training, some require more training than others.

Most scales have reasonable reliability, which is improved with standardized administration and with the availability of alternate forms. Reliability is the degree to which an instrument gives consistent results on repeated application (test-retest reliability) or from different examiners (interrater reliability). The issue of internal consistency, another measure of reliability, is a different matter. Internal consistency indicates the intercorrelation of items measuring a single construct, but not when the items reflect more than one construct. Most mental status scales and inventories are composed of heterogeneous items reflecting different areas. This limits internal consistency, except for specific populations or testing on the extremes (i.e., normals or the severely impaired). Nevertheless, some interitem heterogeneity is acceptable on a screening test if the intent is to screen for different disorders, for example, both typical Alzheimer disease and delirium syndrome. This places a specific burden on the examiner to look beyond just the total score, which obscures any benefits of having interitem heterogeneity. The examiner must evaluate, interpret, and report on performance on individual items within the scale and not just the total score, for example, predominantly impaired delayed recall for Alzheimer disease and impaired mental control/attention for delirium.

Longitudinal Assessment

Longitudinal assessments with mental status scales and inventories provides unique value in assessing the course of the patient over time. Mental status scales are routinely used for follow-up and monitoring in populations that are at high risk for cognitive deficits, including patients at high risk for dementia and those with specific disorders, such as multiple sclerosis, traumatic brain injuries, and psychiatric disorders.

Examiners must first establish an individual baseline for each patient. For those who perform in the unimpaired range at baseline, longitudinal follow-up testing may disclose "conversion" to cognitive decline. In addition, the changes on repeated application of mental status scales over time can disclose different paths or evolution with different disease processes. A neurodegenerative course usually has a gradually progressive decline on serial mental status scales. A more waxing and variable performance around a progressive course could suggest dementia with Lewy bodies. An improving course is consistent with a resolving delirium or encephalopathy, whereas a rapidly worsening course may suggest an intercurrent illness. There are often nonlinear rates of change during progressive stages of impairment. For example, on the MMSE, patients with dementia may decline in a sinusoidal curve faster during middle stages (Fig. 15.1).

There are potential limitations to longitudinal assessment with mental status scales. Some people

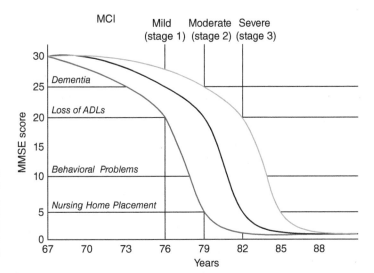

Fig. 15.1 Nonlinear longitudinal decline in Mini-Mental State Examination (MMSE) in clinically probable Alzheimer disease. *ADL,* Activities of daily living; *MCI,* mild cognitive impairment. (Reproduced from Mendez MF, Cummings JL. *Dementia: A Clinical Approach.* 3rd ed. Philadelphia, PA: Butterworth-Heinemann (Elsevier); 2003:96.)

may initially improve as they gain familiarity with the scales, particularly if alternate forms are not used. Mental status scales, including the MMSE and the MoCA, have intraindividual variance on repeated testing in normal persons. Moreover, the elderly may demonstrate a milder age-related decline, which can be confused with the cognitive decline of dementia. The extent of decline on these scales that is significant may need to be three points or more on testing from one point in time to another. There is also the use of mental status scales to monitor clinical drug trials or therapeutic responses to medications. Because of their lack of sufficient sensitivity for this use, investigators have devised specific scales for this purpose, such as the Alzheimer Disease Assessment Scale-Cognitive Subscale, which has a range of 70 items.

Interpretation and Limitations

General mental status scales and inventories screen for normal versus abnormal cognition theoretically from any disease state. However, what is normal for one person may be abnormal for another. The interindividual variability on these scales limits the generalizability of abnormal cutoffs to all persons or patients. Furthermore, the cutoffs for these scales has commonly targeted the cognitive profile of typical Alzheimer disease, limiting generalizability to all cognitive disorders. For most scales, the

test characteristics (sensitivity, specificity, accuracy) are less well defined for focal cognitive or other disorders beyond dementia, and specifically typical Alzheimer disease. All these tests have substantial false-negative rates, especially for right hemisphere focal lesions or mild impairments. In addition, the results of mental status scales and inventories should not stand by themselves in making a diagnosis. They should be interpreted in the context of the neurobehavioral history and behavioral observations, as well as further neurobehavioral or neuropsychological testing

On most mental status scales, cutoff scores are aimed at detecting all persons with cognitive impairment. Scores in the unimpaired range usually preclude the need for further testing; however, cutoff scores target the "average" normal person and not the extremes. Performance in the unimpaired range on these scales does not entirely exclude impairment. Patients with a high intellectual background may have subtle but meaningful cognitive deficits not evident on these instruments. If these patients or their families continue to complain or show concern for cognitive decline, then more sensitive and comprehensive NBSE or neuropsychological testing are indicated. Mental status scales vary in their ceiling effects (variance at higher, less impaired ranges), limiting the sensitivity for detecting deficits (e.g., the MoCA has less of a ceiling effect than the MMSE). The MoCA may have a sensitivity for mild cognitive impairment of 90% versus 18% for the MMSE. Conversely, false-positive results may occur among patients with limited education or socioeconomic status, and those of different native language or of cultural backgrounds who are unfamiliar with these tests. Mental status scales also vary in their floor effects (variance at lower, more impaired ranges), limiting their sensitivity for detecting severity of deficits (e.g., the MMSE has less of a floor effect than the MoCA). Screening mental status scale scores in the impaired range always recommend further evaluation with NBSE or neuropsychological testing.

Different populations pose additional variables that affect interpretation. It is important to know the population on which the instrument was validated. Mental status scales and inventories are most commonly aimed at patients who are between 65 and 80 years of age, have approximately 12 to 14 years of formal education, English-speaking or another native language linked to the test, Caucasian and of middle socioeconomic status. Yet, the patient's age, education, and sociocultural background can significantly affect the results of mental status assessment. The examiner should interpret with caution the screening mental status scale scores in patients from different demographic backgrounds. Some scales do adjust for some of these factors. For example, the Short Portable Mental Status Questionnaire (SPMSQ), MoCA, and SLUMS have adjusted cutoffs based on education. In general, neuropsychological testing has greater normative data across broader ranges of age, education, and other demographic variables.

Conclusions

Mental status scales and inventories are structured instruments that screen memory and other cognitive domains with quantitative scoring. They are most commonly used in older adult patients to screen for significant cognitive impairment that might reflect dementia. There are over 50 scales to choose from and countless inventories; however, the examiner should familiarize himself/herself and become proficient with just a few of them. As discussed, all mental status scales are not created equal. The best ones tend to have a broad content of cognitive areas without inordinately compromising brevity (Table 15.3). Scales with broad content in the moderate time range (5–15

TABLE 15.3 **The Ideal Mental Status Scale**
Administration easy for clinicians at all levels
Alternate forms available
Brevity, can be administered in 5–15 minutes
Minimal if any modification required for tele-neurobehavior
Cultural adaptability and free from bias
Interindividual variability low
Items include different cognitive domains allowing for use as a brief MSX
Free access without copyright restrictions
Longitudinal follow-up, consistently reliable
Normative data and validation studies available for different populations
Reliable, test-retest and interrater reliability, e.g., $r \geq 0.85$
Robust to state factors, e.g., distractions, fatigue, cooperation, etc.
Samples most major cognitive domains
Samples broad range of severity with minimal floor and ceiling effects
Sensitivity, high for common cognitive disorders, e.g., ≥ 0.9
Validation for both mild cognitive impairment and different dementias

minutes) are particularly practical, for example, the MoCA, the SLUMS, the Rowland Universal Dementia Assessment (RUDAS), and others discussed in the next chapter. The MMSE has a unique value because of its long history, which allows comparisons across a great many studies over many years, but this instrument has become less accessible because of copyright restrictions. When screening patients, consider that false positives may occur among low education and elderly patients, and false negatives may occur among high education and younger patients. In general, it is better to have false positives rather than to miss a potential, early neurocognitive disorder. If abnormal, remember that this is only the beginning; further diagnostic assessment is indicated. These scales and inventories lack specificity for diseases and for brain-behavior correlation. Abnormal mental status scores can result from dementia, delirium, aphasia or language impairment, depression with poor attention and mental controls, and many other reasons.

Chapter 16

General Mental Status Scales, Rating Instruments, and Behavior Inventories

There are over 50 general mental status scales for assessing cognition, and a large number of inventories for behavioral assessment. This does not include the many available targeted mental status scales, which focus on a particular disorder or syndrome that is not dementia or general cognitive impairment. Chapter 15 discusses general characteristics and guidelines for choosing among these instruments. This chapter expands on those guidelines and discusses individual general mental status scales, related rating instruments, and behavior inventories. The first section reviews 10 current or popular general mental status scales that can be administered under 15 minutes, plus one longer scale with an abbreviated version. These selected scales, by and large, have good sensitivity and specificity for "dementia" (although variable for "cognitive impairment") and adequate test-retest and interrater reliability. The second section surveys most general mental status scales. The third section covers information-based rating instruments, and the final section is a brief overview of behavior inventories of interest to the mental status examiner. The information presented here is primarily derived from the in-person, face-to-face administration of these instruments; Chapter 18 discusses the application or modification of these mental status scales for telemedicine, such as over the telephone or by videoconferencing.

Evaluation of Select General Mental Status Scales

General mental status scales need to be brief for practical use in clinical settings. Although clinicians use these scales to screen patients for any cognitive impairment needing further assessment, these scales are mostly validated on patients with dementia rather than those with mild or focal cognitive deficits. Many scales take 5 minutes or less to administer, but they may evaluate only memory or a limited number of cognitive areas. Among these instruments are the Clock Drawing Test (CDT), Memory Impairment Screen (MIS), Mini-Cog, Six-Item Screener (SIS), Short Portable Mental Status Questionnaire (SPMSQ), and Short Test of Mental Status (STMS) (Table 16.1). Mental status scales of somewhat longer length (>5–15 minutes) include more cognitive areas and are more sensitive to mild cognitive impairments than the brief scales. These instruments include the Mini-Mental State Examination (MMSE), Montreal Cognitive Assessment (MoCA), Rowland Universal Dementia Assessment Scale (RUDAS), and the Saint Louis University Mental Status Examination (SLUMS). Longer cognitive assessments (>15 minutes) are clearly more comprehensive but at the price of decreased brevity in administration. The Addenbrooke Cognitive Examination-III (ACE-III) is an example.

CLOCK DRAWING TEST (CDT)

Many clinicians use the drawing of the face of a clock as an "all-purpose" mental status screen. Indeed, clock drawing is incorporated into other mental status scales, from the Mini-Cog to the STMS, MoCA, RUDAS, SLUMS, and ACE-III. There are reasons for this. Drawing the face of an analog clock, with correct placement of numbers and a proscribed time, taps into multiple cognitive domains. The correct performance of the CDT requires not only visuospatial ability, but mental control (working memory), other executive functions, and numerical ability. Consequently, the CDT can be quite sensitive to cognitive impairment. The CDT is easy to administer and is less language or culture dependent than other tests. The examiner

TABLE 16.1	Select General Mental Status Scales - General Characteristics								
Abbreviation	Name	Time (minutes)	Total Score	Cutoff Scores for Dementia	Sensitivity for Dementia	Specificity for Dementia	Test-retest	Interrater	Cognitive Areas
CDT	Clock Drawing Test	1–3	10	<7	67–98	67–98	0.77–0.94	0.83–0.97	Mental control/ attention visuospatial numbers/calculation executive
MIS	Memory Impairment Screen	4–5	8	≤4	43–86	93–97	0.69	.....	Memory
Mini-Cog	Mini-Cog	2–4	5	<3	76–100	54–89	.....	0.96–0.97	Memory mental control/ attention visuospatial numbers/ calculation executive
SIS	Six-Item Screener	5	6	≤4	86–89	78–88	0.85	0.82	Memory orientation
SPMSQ	Short Portable Mental Status Questionnaire	5	10	≤7	67–74	91–100	0.82–0.83	.....	Memory orientation mental control/ attention semantic memory
STMS	Short Test of Mental Status	5	38	≤29	86–95	88–96	.....	0.82	Memory orientation mental control/ attention visuospatial numbers/calculation executive semantic memory
MMSE	Mini-Mental State Examination	8–13	30	<24	Pooled 81	Pooled 89	0.80–0.95	0.83–0.97	Memory orientation mental control/ attention language visuospatial ±numbers/calculation
MoCA	Montreal Cognitive Assessment	10–15	30	<26 vs. <23	Pooled 91	Pooled 81	0.82–0.92	0.87–0.99	Memory orientation mental control/ attention language visuospatial numbers/calculation executive

(Continued)

Abbrevia-tion	Name	Time (min-utes)	Total Score	Cutoff Scores for Dementia	Sensi-tivity for Dementia	Speci-ficity for Dementia	Test-retest	Interrater	Cognitive Areas
RUDAS	Rowland Universal Dementia Assessment Scale	10–15	30	<23	80.9–95	54–98	0.96–0.98	0.99	Memory language visuospatial right-left orientation alternating movements safety question
SLUMS	Saint Louis University Mental Status Examination	4–10	30	<20 (less than high school) <21 (high school or greater)	84–100	87–100	0.82	0.99	Memory (includes story) orientation mental control/attention language (naming) visuospatial numbers/calculation executive
ACE-III	Addenbrooke's Cognitive Examination-III	15–20	100	<82	79–100	83–100	0.91+	0.99+	Memory (more than one) orientation mental control/attention language (multiple) visuospatial (multiple) numbers/calculation executive semantic memory

Beishon LC, Batterham AP, Quinn TJ, et al. Addenbrooke's Cognitive Examination III (ACE-III) and Mini-ACE for the detection of dementia and mild cognitive impairment. *Cochrane Database Syst Rev.* 2019;12:CD013282.

Breton A, Casey D, Arnaoutoglou NA. Cognitive tests for the detection of mild cognitive impairment (MCI), the prodromal stage of dementia: meta-analysis of diagnostic accuracy studies. *Int J Geriatr Psychiatry.* 2019;34:233–242.

Cullen B, O'Neill B, Evans JJ, Coen RF, Lawlor BA. A review of screening tests for cognitive impairment. *J Neurol Neurosurg Psychiatry.* 2007;78(8):790–799.

Matias-Guiu JA, Cortés-Martínez A, Valles-Salgado M, et al. Addenbrooke's Cognitive Examination III: diagnostic utility for mild cognitive impairment and dementia and correlation with standardized neuropsychological tests. *Int Psychogeriatr.* 2017;29:105–113.

Matías-Guiu JA, Valles-Salgado M, Rognoni T, Hamre-Gil F, Moreno-Ramos T, Matías-Guiu J. Comparative diagnostic accuracy of the ACE-III, MIS, MMSE, MoCA, and RUDAS for screening of Alzheimer disease. *Dement Geriatr Cogn Disord.* 2017;43(5-6):237–246.

Tsoi KK, Chan JY, Hirai HW, et al. Cognitive tests to detect dementia: a systematic review and meta-analysis. *JAMA Intern Med.* 2015;175:1450–1458.

Wilterdink JL. Mental status scales to evaluate cognition. UpToDate Online Database.

Velayudhan L, Ryu SH, Raczek M, et al. Review of brief cognitive tests for patients with suspected dementia. *Int Psychogeriatr.* 2014;26(8):1247–1262. https://www.uptodate.com/contents/mental-status-scales-to-evaluate-cognition

usually asks the patient to draw the face of a clock, place the numbers, and indicate the time by placing the hands, most commonly at "10 after 11" or "5 past 4." Clinicians may experience variable results with the CDT in screening for dementia. One reason for this is that there are different systems for scoring and interpreting the CDT. Regardless of scoring systems, the examiner should consider exactly how the patient performed in spatial relationships, number order and location, and placement of the hands with designated time. Errors can range from left hemispatial neglect with omission of numbers on the left side to executive dysfunction with "concrete" placement of the hands, for example, the long hand on the "10" when asked to indicate "10 after 11."

MEMORY IMPAIRMENT SCREEN (MIS)

As its name suggests, the MIS is strictly a memory screen; however, this instrument has the advantage of testing both free recall and cued recall. In this way, the MIS probes in greater depth for the presence of declarative episodic verbal memory loss, the earliest impairment in typical Alzheimer disease and other dementias. The examiner asks the patient to read aloud four items presented on a sheet of paper. Then the examiner gives a different category cue for each of the four items and asks the patient to indicate which items belong to which categories. This allows for subsequent cued and free recall after 2 to 3 minutes. The patient gets two points for each item spontaneously recalled and one point if they required cuing. Given its structure, the best use of the MIS is in screening for typical Alzheimer disease; it is not a screen for nonmemory areas of cognitive decline. The MIS is relatively robust to the effects of age and education and is one of the tools recommended for use in the Medicare Annual Wellness Visit by the Alzheimer's Association.

MINI-COG

The Mini-Cog combines memory with the clock drawing task, thus combining the main elements of the CDT and MIS. Much of the earlier discussion on the CDT and the MIS applies to the Mini-Cog. Where this instrument differs from the CDT is in its simplified binary scoring system without consideration of hand length and other variables, and where it differs from the MIS is in the absence of a cued recall portion, limited only to free recall. An additional advantage of the Mini-Cog is that it has alternate word lists, which is helpful for longitudinal follow-up. An abnormal score of less than 3 occurs if the patient has an abnormal clock and misses one memory item or if the patient misses all three memory items. It is relatively robust to the effects of age and education and, like the MIS, is one of the tools recommended for use in the Medicare Annual Wellness, primarily as a screening test for Alzheimer disease.

SIX-ITEM SCREENER (SIS)

The SIS adds orientation for time (year, month, day of the week) to three memory words (free recall). The introduction of orientation items is helpful in detecting patients with dementia, who become disoriented to time from recent memory difficulty or from attentional problems. The examiner asks the orientation questions during the "interference" period between presentation of the memory words and request for recall. Each of the three memory words and three orientation questions gets one point (six total). The SIS has value in quickly screening for dementia, but it misses deficits in most cognitive domains including those involved in the clock drawing task.

SHORT PORTABLE MENTAL STATUS QUESTIONNAIRE (SPMSQ)

The SPMSQ greatly expands on testing for orientation to include orientation for place and personal information, as well as orientation for time. This instrument has 10 questions that extend to questions about the patient's telephone number, age, place of birth, and mother's maiden name. The SPMSQ does not include direct testing of episodic declarative memory, nor does it sample multiple areas of cognition. However, it has remote memory questions that ask for the names of the current and last presidents, and the last item samples mental control/attention by asking the patient to count backward from 20 by 3s. Patients must answer eight of the questions correctly for a normal score. The developers state that "One more error is allowed in the scoring if a patient has had a grade school education or less. One less error is allowed if the patient has had education beyond the high school level." Like most of the brief (≤5 minute) scales, the SPMSQ is more accurate in identifying patients with moderately or severely impaired dementia rather than detecting those with mild impairment.

THE SHORT TEST OF MENTAL STATUS (STMS)

Up to this point, the brief mental status scales have involved a limited number of cognitive areas or included the clock drawing as a vehicle to screen multiple domains. The STMS is distinctly different in this regard. It is a well-constructed test that incorporates all elements of the other tests, such as clock drawing, memory (learning and delayed recall of four items), orientation (time and place), semantic memory (presidents, weeks/year, island definition), and mental control/attention (digits forward). The STMS further adds calculations (four problems), abstractions (three similarities), and the copy of a cube. In essence, this is a much expanded "short" test, which the authors reported as still having an administration time of approximately 5 minutes. It is probable that many patients take longer to complete the STMS given all of its items. Of the brief (≤5 minute) mental status scales described here, the STMS is the most sensitive to mild impairments in cognition. One concern is that it does not have a language subtest, as language and word-finding difficulty are the second most common cognitive impairments in early dementia.

MINI-MENTAL STATE EXAMINATION (MMSE)

The most widely used and prototypical cognitive scale has been the MMSE (Table 16.2). There is extensive experience with this instrument, which has been in wide use since introduced in 1975. This 30-item instrument, which is also discussed in Chapter 15, consists of 10 orientation items followed by 8 language and 5 mental control/attention items. There are only three memory items (plus three registration) and one visuospatial task. The MMSE takes an average of 12 minutes to administer, and it has high interrater and test-retest reliability. One of the best uses of the MMSE is in measuring and following the severity of the Alzheimer clinical syndrome over time. A total score of 23 or less suggests mild dementia (<19 for moderate and <10 for severe dementia). The three-word recall is the most sensitive to dementia followed by orientation to date and the drawing of the intersecting pentagons. The MMSE is less sensitive for patients with mild cognitive impairment and cannot distinguish different types of dementia. It has a prominent ceiling effect, which results in missing many mildly impaired patients. Age and education heavily influence MMSE scores, with some normal individuals over 85 years of age and lacking a grade school education scoring as

TABLE 16.2	Select General Mental Status Scales - Advantages and Disadvantages		
Abbreviation	**Name**	**Advantages**	**Disadvantages**
CDT	Clock Drawing Test	Brief administration time Little education/language/culture effects Screens several cognitive areas	Does not target memory Many different scoring systems Misses many cognitive domains
MIS	Memory Impairment Screen	Brief administration time Little education/language/culture effects Includes both free and cued recall Alternate versions available	Only assesses memory Misses many cognitive domains Marked ceiling and floor effects
Mini-Cog	Mini-Cog	Brief administration time Little education/language/culture effects Screens several cognitive areas Alternate word lists	Misses many cognitive domains Use of different word lists may affect failure rates
SIS	Six-Item Screener	Brief administration time Little education/language/culture effects	Misses many cognitive domains Insensitive to mild impairments
SPMSQ	Short Portable Mental Status Questionnaire	Brief administration time Verbal test (no writing/drawing) Includes extensive orientation Includes semantic memory	Does not assess language Misses many cognitive domains Particularly fails to assess memory
STMS	Short Test of Mental Status	Most comprehensive among brief scales Validated in primary care Tests many separate domains	Education/language bias Studied in relatively educated May not be as applicable in others

(Continued)

TABLE 16.2 Select General Mental Status Scales - Advantages and Disadvantages (Cont'd)

Abbreviation	Name	Advantages	Disadvantages
MMSE	Mini-Mental State Examination	Widely used, Known standard reference Easy to use; no special training Valid and reliable for typical Alzheimer Longitudinal change data Can clarify severity	Few memory items Education/age/language/culture bias Many verbal items; only one visuospatial Insensitive in many cognitive areas Ceiling effect Has an either-or item Restricted by copyright
MoCA	Montreal Cognitive Assessment	Designed to test for mild impairments Tests many separate domains Examines executive abilities Alternate versions available Computerized version available	Education bias (≤12 years) Less useful in established dementia Need for certification for use Wide circulation in public mitigates validity
RUDAS	Rowland Universal Dementia Assessment Scale	Designed for multicultural populations Little education/language/culture effects More ecological valid memory item	Left-right orientation item of unclear value Judgment question of unclear value May not be as education free as believed Needs more study
SLUMS	Saint Louis University Mental Status Examination	Tests many separate domains Different cutoffs per level of education Varied cognitive items Has a story recall task	Limited use and evidence due to published data relatively new (2006) Absence of adequate psychometric data needs study, especially in different populations
ACE-III	Addenbrooke's Cognitive Examination-III	Wide range of scores Fewer ceiling and floor effects Establishes a cognitive profile Applicable for many dementias Alternate versions available Computerized version available	Length of instrument Need for more normative data

low as 18. One unique psychometric problem with the MMSE is the alternate choice of either spelling "WORLD" backward or counting backward from 100 by 7s. These tasks are not comparable or interchangeable, even when both tasks are done and the examiner takes the best score. Another concern is that memory testing is limited to brief delayed recall and may miss a disturbance in declarative episodic memory. Finally, the MMSE does not assess executive functions in any of its subtests (except serial reversals), again limiting its sensitivity for mild cognitive impairments.

A special issue with the MMSE is the emergence of a copyright restriction after many years of free access. The MMSE has served as a common language allowing clinicians and researchers to understand the stage or severity of dementia patients across different times, patients, and populations. To use the MMSE now, a clinician or researcher needs to get permission from the copyright owner and pay a fee for using MMSE forms. This has led to either withdrawal from using the MMSE or the use of alternatives that have elements of the MMSE, such as the Sweet-16 and ACE-R. Clinicians need not be limited to this scale as there are new and better alternatives and choices.

MONTREAL COGNITIVE ASSESSMENT (MOCA)

The MoCA is another widely used screening test that gained in popularity as a replacement for the MMSE (also see Chapter 15). Like the MMSE, the MoCA is a 30-point scale, with items that include 6 for orientation, 5 for memory, 6 for language, 6 for mental control/attention, 3 for visuospatial, and 4 for executive abilities (including clock hands). This broad range of coverage allows for increased sensitivity to mild cognitive impairments, making the MoCA a much better instrument for detecting early cognitive changes in broad range of disorders. In fact, examiners can use the MoCA as a brief MSX screening of most cognitive domains. There has been disagreement about the initial cutoff score of 26 being overly strict for detecting dementia. A recommended alternative cutoff score that minimizes false positives for dementia is less than 23. A salient difference between the MoCA and the MMSE is that the MoCA is a harder test. It also has floor effects with little variance among very impaired patients. Unfortunately, similar to the MMSE, education strongly affects MoCA scores.

There are other pros and cons to the MoCA. It has increasingly available psychometric support with normative data. There is also the availability of videoconferencing and telephone ("Blind MoCA) adminisitration. Less favorable for clinical access is that, since September of 2019, there have been restrictions on the use of the MoCA. The copyright owner requires certification (with a fee) for use. Perhaps more problematic is the requirement to enter patient data into an online database, where the forms are scored. Patients, or their proxies, would have to give informed consent, an added process that is a disincentive to use the MoCA in routine clinical settings. Finally, unfortunately, the MoCA has been widely circulated in public and on the internet, thus potentially compromising its use.

ROWLAND UNIVERSAL DEMENTIA ASSESSMENT SCALE (RUDAS)

The RUDAS aims to be a mental status scale relatively free of educational, linguistic, and sociocultural effects. The RUDAS has six items, including delayed recall memory, visuospatial construction (copy of a cube), and semantic word fluency. Its other items are unique. They are left-right disorientation on body parts, probing of judgment involved in crossing a street ("safety question"), and alternating hand movements with fist and palm. These items are aimed at avoiding a multicultural bias, and the RUDAS is more robust to the effects of years of education and variations in native language compared with comparable scales. Most of the discriminability of the RUDAS, however, appears to be from its practical "shopping list" delayed recall items with up to five registration repetitions and its word fluency composed of generating a list of animals. It is unclear how much left-right disorientation and the judgment question add to the cognitive assessment. Left-right

disorientation occurs from disturbance of a personal body map in the left parietal region (see Chapter 12) and is not a substitute for disorientation for time and place, which are disturbed from impairments in attention or memory. Paradoxically, the judgment question is one that may be extremely culturally dependent. The alternating motor movements are more a test of bradykinesia than of motor praxis and may be of value as an indicator of psychomotor slowing. The RUDAS has similar sensitivity for dementia but may be less sensitive for mild cognitive impairment than the MoCA, although more specific for both and much better overall than the MMSE.

SAINT LOUIS UNIVERSITY MENTAL STATUS EXAMINATION (SLUMS)

Like the MMSE, MoCA, and RUDAS, the SLUMS has a 30-point scale, which includes orientation, delayed recall memory, calculation, semantic word fluency, digit span backward, and clock drawing. It has two unique items: immediate story recall and visuospatial figure recognition-orientation. This instrument has the advantage of assessing most cognitive domains impacted by early dementia. The SLUMS is shorter than the MMSE, MoCA, or RUDAS, with a mean administration time of approximately 7 minutes. The cutoff scores for dementia are less than 20 if less than 12 years of education and less than 21 for high school graduates. Its most discriminative items appear to be the word fluency for animals, memory (delayed recall), digit span backward, and the immediate story recall. Preliminary data suggests that the SLUMS, at cutoffs of less than 20 for less than 12 years of education and less than 27 for high school graduates, may be one of the most sensitive mental status scales for mild cognitive impairment among scales of 15 minutes or less. The SLUMS, like the RUDAS, requires more research to validate its use and establish its value in screening for mild cognitive impairment.

ADDENBROOKE COGNITIVE EXAMINATION-III (ACE-III) AND ITS MINI-ACE DERIVATIVE

The ACE scales are comprehensive instruments that have shown great value in patient screening and assessment in studies throughout the world. They are noteworthy for their broad cognitive content and their applicability for assessing dementia syndromes beyond typical Alzheimer disease. Investigators have applied the ACE tests to distinguish typical Alzheimer disease (with decreased delayed recall memory and orientation) versus other disorders, such as fronto-temporal dementia (with decreased phonemic verbal fluency). The original 100-item ACE contains delayed recall memory, language and verbal fluency measures, and the clock drawing combined with the elements of the MMSE. A revised version (ACE-R) defines cognitive subscales, and a further revision (ACE-III) removes the elements of the MMSE. Administration time for the ACE-III ranges from 15 to 20 minutes. The ACE-R and ACE-III are highly correlated thanks to the incorporation of items that replace the cognitive constructs of the MMSE. The further introduction of an abbreviated version of the ACE-III, the 30-point Mini-ACE, provides a 5-minute mental status scale with items for orientation, delayed recall of an address, a semantic word list, and clock drawing. The Mini-ACE is excellent for detecting Alzheimer disease and dementia but, like the other scales of 5 minutes or less, it is not as sensitive for mild cognitive impairment as longer scales.

SURVEY OF GENERAL MENTAL STATUS SCALES

There are a great many mental status scales, and it is not possible to individually review all of them in detail. In addition to the instruments covered in the first part of this chapter, there are a number of other scales that are worth mentioning. The reader can refer to the literature for the remaining mental status scales outlined in Tables 16.3 and 16.4.

Some other mental status scales that take less than 15 minutes to administer are the Modified Mini-Mental State Exam (3MS), 7-Minute Screen (7MS), Abbreviated Mental Test (AMT), Short Orientation Memory Concentration Test (S-OMCT), and the Cognitive Capacity Screening Examination (CCSE). The 3MS is a revision of the MMSE that adds date and place of birth, animal naming, similarities, and another delayed recall task. It allows for assignment of partial credit on some items, broadening the range of scores from 0 to 100. The 7MS includes enhanced cued recall, temporal orientation, clock drawing, and word (semantic) fluency. This scale has been useful in screening for different types of dementia, as well as Alzheimer disease. The 10-item AMT asks patients their age and dates of birth, orientation questions, the identification of two persons, two information items, and finishes asking patients to count backward from 20 to 1. Rather than testing declarative episodic memory, the AMT tests orientation and

semantic memory. The S-OMCT, also known as the Six-Item Impairment Test (6-CIT), Blessed OMC, or Short Blessed Test, has three orientation items and asks the patient to remember a three-line address. The test includes two reversal tasks: months of the year backward, and counting backward from 20 to 1. The 30-item CCSE is a somewhat longer mental status scale, which incorporates attention, mental tracking, and arithmetic items along with testing orientation and memory (some with a Brown-Petersen distraction task). It is useful for identifying cognitive disturbances among medical patients, particularly if there is a delirium component.

Some other mental status scales that may take longer than 20 minutes to administer are the Alzheimer Disease Assessment Scale-Cog (ADAS-Cog), Cognitive Abilities Screening Instrument (CASI), Mattis Dementia Rating Scale (MDRS), Neurobehavioral Rating Scale (NBRS), and Neurobehavioral Cognitive Status Examination (NCSE or Cognistat). These instruments assess multiple domains often with separate subtests and are more sensitive to mild cognitive changes at the price of the brevity that is of value for screening in a clinical environment. The (ADAS-Cog), although rarely used in a routine clinical setting, is important to mention because of its prominence as a major outcome measure in research. This 70-item scale covers multiple cognitive domains with a good track record for longitudinal monitoring in Alzheimer disease clinical drug trials. The CASI is a longer composite that includes the basic elements of the MMSE, the 3MS, and the Hasegawa Dementia Screening Scale from Japan. Designed for cross-cultural studies, this test includes attention, concentration, orientation, memory, language, visuo-spatial construction, word-list generation, abstraction, and judgment. The MDRS starts with difficult items and proceeds with easier items only if the answers to the initial items were incorrect. It is composed of five subtests: attention, initiation and perseveration, construction, conceptual, and memory with initiation and perseveration and memory having the best correlation with functional level. The 28-item NBRS, which measures mood and behavior as well as cognition, is particularly applicable for the assessment of head-injured patients but may also be used for patients with dementia. Each item has a scale score of 0 to 6 based on patient observation, with the results yielding 6 factor scores. The NCSE or Cognistat (which

TABLE 16.3 General Mental Status Scales of ≤5 Minutes

Abbreviation	Name	Reference
3WR	Three-Word Recall	Kuslansky G, Buschke H, Katz M, et al. Screening for Alzheimer's disease: the memory impairment screen versus the conventional three-word memory test. *J Am Geriatr Soc.* 2002;50:1086–1091.
ABCS	AB Cognitive Screen	Molloy DW, Standish TI, Lewis DL. Screening for mild cognitive impairment: comparing the SMMSE and the ABCS. *Can J Psychiatry.* 2005;50:52–58.
AMT	Abbreviated Mental Test	Hodkinson HM. Evaluation of a mental test score for assessment of mental impairment in the elderly. *Age Ageing.* 1972;1:233–238.
BAS	Brief Alzheimer Screen	Mendiondo MS, Ashford JW, Kryscio RJ, et al. Designing a Brief Alzheimer Screen (BAS). *J Alzheimer Dis.* 2003;5:391–398.
BCS	Brief Cognitive Scale	Krishnan LR, Levy RM, Wagner HR, et al. Informant-rated cognitive symptoms in normal aging, mild cognitive impairment and dementia. Initial development of an informant-rated screen (Brief Cognitive Scale) for mild cognitive impairment and dementia. *Psychopharmacol Bull.* 2001;35:79–88.
CDT	Clock Drawing Test	Sunderland T, Hill JL, Mellow AM, et al. Clock drawing in Alzheimer's disease. A novel measure of dementia severity. *J Am Geriatr Soc.* 1989;37:725–729.
MAT	Mental Alteration Test	Salib E, McCarthy J. Menta Alteration Test (MAT): a rapid and valid screening tool for dementia in primary care. *Int J Geriatr Psychiatry.* 2002;17:1157–1161.
Mini-Cog	Mini-Cog	Borson S, Scanlan J, Brush M, et al. The Mini-Cog: a cognitive 'vital signs' measure for dementia screening in multi-lingual elderly. *Int J Geriatr Psychiatry.* 2000;15:1021–1027.
MIS	Memory Impairment Screen	Buschke H, Kuslansky G, Katz M, et al. Screening for dementia with the memory impairment screen. *Neurology.* 1999;52:231–238.
MOST	Memory Orientation Screening Test	Clionsky MI, Clionsky E. Development and validation of the Memory Orientation Screening Test (MOST): a better screening test for dementia. *Am J Alzheimer Dis Other Demen.* 2010;25:650–656.
RDST	Rapid Dementia Screening Test	Kalbe E, Kessler J, Calabrese P. Validity of the DemTect and the RDST for the earlier detection of dementia. Abstract at Annual Meeting Int College Geriatric Psychoneuropharmacology, Barcelona, Oct. 10–12 2002.
SDS	Symptoms of Dementia Screener	Mundt JC, Freed DM, Greist JH. Lay person-based screening for early detection of Alzheimer's disease: development and validation of an instrument. *J Gerontol B Psychol Sci Soc Sci.* 2000;55:163–170.
SIS	Six-Item Screener	Callahan CM, Unverzagt FW, Hui SL, et al. Six-item screener to identify cognitive impairment among potential subjects for clinical research. *Med Care.* 2002;40:771–781.
SMQ	Short Memory Questionnaire	Koss E, Patterson MB, Ownby R, et al. Memory evaluation in Alzheimer's disease. Caregivers' appraisals and objective testing. *Arch Neurol.* 1993;50:92–97.
S-OMCT	Short Orientation Memory Concentration (6-CIT, Short Blessed)	Katzman R, Brown T, Fuld P, et al. Validation of a short Orientation-Memory-Concentration Test of cognitive impairment. *Am J Psychiatry.* 1983;140:734–739.
SPMSQ	Short Portable Mental Status Questionnaire	Pfeiffer E. A short portable mental status questionnaire for the assessment of organic brain deficit in elderly patients. *J Am Geriatr Soc.* 1975;23:433–441.
STMS	Short Test of Mental Status	Kokmen E, Naessens JM, Offord KP. A short test of mental status: description and preliminary results. *Mayo Clin Proc.* 1987;62:281–288.

(Continued)

TABLE 16.3	General Mental Status Scales of ≤5 Minutes *(Cont'd)*	
Abbreviation	**Name**	**Reference**
T&C	Time and Change	Froehlich TE, Robison JT, Inouye SK. Screening for dementia in the outpatient setting: the time and change test. *J Am Geriatr Soc*. 1998;46:1506–1511.
TE4D-Cog	Test for the Early Detection of Dementia from Depression	Mahoney R, Johnston K, Katona C, Maxmin K, Livingston G. The TE4D-Cog: a new test for detecting early dementia in English-speaking populations. *Int J Geriatr Psychiatry*. 2005;20(12):1172–1179.
VFC	Verbal Fluency–Categories	Isaacs B, Kennie AT. The Set test as an aid to the detection of dementia in old people. *Br J Psychiatry*. 1973;123:467–470.
WORLD	Modified WORLD Test	Leopold NA, Borson AJ. An alphabetical 'WORLD'. A new version of an old test. *Neurology*. 1997;49:1521–1524.

TABLE 16.4	General Mental Status Scales of >5 Minutes	
Abbreviation	**Name**	**Reference**
3MS	Modified Mini-Mental State Examination	Teng EL, Chui HC. The Modified Mini-Mental State (3MS) examination. *J Clin Psychiatry*. 1987;48:314–318.
7MS	7-Minute Screen	Solomon PR, Hirschoff A, Kelly B, et al. A 7 minute neurocognitive screening battery highly sensitive to Alzheimer's disease. *Arch Neurol*. 1998;55:349–355.
ACE-III; Mini-ACE	Addenbrooke's Cognitive Examination-III; Mini-ACE	Beishon LC, Batterham AP, Quinn TJ, et al. Addenbrooke's Cognitive Examination III (ACE-III) and Mini-ACE for the detection of dementia and mild cognitive impairment. *Cochrane Database Syst Rev*. 2019;12:CD013282.
ACE-R	Addenbrooke's Cognitive Examination-Revised	Mioshi E, Dawson K, Mitchell J, et al. The Addenbrooke's Cognitive Examination Revised: a brief cognitive test battery for dementia screening. *Int J Geriatr Psychiatry*. 2006;21:1078–1085.
ADAS-Cog	The Alzheimer's Disease Assessment Scale–Cognitive Subscale	Kueper JK, Speechley M, Montero-Odasso M. The Alzheimer's Disease Assessment Scale–Cognitive Subscale (ADAS-Cog): modifications and responsiveness in pre-dementia populations. A narrative review. *J Alzheimer Dis*. 2018;63(2):423–444.
BCRS/GDS	Brief Cognitive Rating Scale/Global Deterioration Scale	Reisberg B, Ferris SH. Brief Cognitive Rating Scale (BPRS). *Psychopharm Bul*. 1988;24:629-636. Reisberg B, Ferris SH, de Leon MJ, Crook T. Global Deterioration Scale (GDS). *Psychopharm Bul*. 1988;24:661–663.
CASI	Cognitive Abilities Screening Instrument	Teng EL, Hasegawa K, Homma A, et al. The Cognitive Abilities Screening Instrument (CASI): a practical test for cross-cultural epidemiological studies of dementia. *Int Psychogeriatr*. 1994;6:45–58.
CAST	Cognitive Assessment Screening Test	Drachman DA, Swearer JM, Kane K, et al. The Cognitive Assessment Screening Test (CAST) for dementia. *J Geriatr Psychiatry Neurol*. 1996;9:200–208.
CCSE	Cognitive Capacity Screening Examination	Kaufman DM, Weinberger M, Strain JJ, et al. Detection of cognitive deficits by a brief mental status examination: the Cognitive Capacity Screening Examination, a reappraisal and a review. *Gen Hosp Psychiatry*. 1979;1:247–255.
DECO	Deterioration Cognitive Observée	Ritchie K, Fuhrer R. The validation of an informant screening test for irreversible cognitive decline in the elderly: performance characteristics within a general population sample. *Int J Geriatr Psychiatry*. 1996;11:149–156.
DemTect	DemTect	Kalbe E, Kessler J, Calabrese P, et al. DemTect: a new, sensitive cognitive screening test to support the diagnosis of mild cognitive impairment and early dementia. *Int J Geriatr Psychiatry*. 2004;19:136–143.

(Continued)

Abbreviation	Name	Reference
DQ	Dementia Questionnaire	Silverman JM, Breitner JC, Mohs RC, et al. Reliability of the family history method in genetic studies of Alzheimer's disease and related dementias. *Am J Psychiatry*. 1986;143:1279–1282.
FCSRT	Free and Cued Selective Reminding Test	Grober E, Sanders AE, Hall C, Lipton RB. Free and cued selective reminding identifies very mild dementia in primary care. *Alzheimer Dis Assoc Dis*. 2010;24:284–290.
FOME	Fuld Object Memory Evaluation	Mast BT, Fitzgerald J, Steinberg J, MacNeill SE, Lichtenberg PA. Effective screening for Alzheimer's disease among older African Americans. *Clin Neuropsychol*. 2001;15:196–202.
HVLT	Hopkins Verbal Learning Test	Brandt J. The Hopkins Verbal Learning Test: development of a new memory test with six equivalent forms. *Clin Neuropsychol*. 1991;5:125–142.
MDRS	Mattis Dementia Rating Scale-2	Matteau E, Dupré N, Langlois M, et al. Mattis Dementia Rating Scale 2: screening for MCI and dementia. *Am J Alzheimers Dis Other Demen*. 2011;26(5):389–398.
MCAS	Minnesota Cognitive Acuity Screen	Knopman DS, Knudson D, Yoes ME, et al. Development and standardization of a new telephonic cognitive screening test: the Minnesota Cognitive Acuity Screen (MCAS). *Neuropsychiatry Neuropsychol Behav Neurol*. 2000;13:286–296.
MMSE	Mini-Mental State Examination	Folstein MF, Folstein SE, McHugh PR. "Mini-mental state". A practical method for grading the cognitive state of patients for the clinician. *J Psychiatr Res*. 1975;12:189–198.
MoCA	Montreal Cognitive Assessment	Nasreddine ZS, Phillips NA, Bédirian V, et al. The Montreal Cognitive Assessment, MoCA: a brief screening tool for mild cognitive impairment. *J Am Geriatr Soc*. 2005;53(4):695–699.
Mont	Montpellier Screen	Artero S, Ritchie K. The detection of mild cognitive impairment in the general practice setting. *Aging Ment Health*. 2003;7:251–258.
NBRS-R	Neurobehavioral Rating Scale-Revised	Levin HS, High WM, Goethe KE, et al. The neurobehavioural rating scale: assessment of the behavioural sequelae of head injury by the clinician. *J Neurol Neurosurg Psychiatry*. 1987;50:183–193.
NCSE & Cognistat	Neurobehavioral Cognitive Status Examination (also known as Cognistat)	Kiernan RJ, Mueller J, Langston JW, et al. The Neurobehavioral Cognitive Status Examination: a brief but quantitative approach to cognitive assessment. *Ann Intern Med*. 1987;107:481–485.
R-CAMCOG	Rotterdam Version of the Cambridge Cognitive Examination	De Koning I, Dippel DW, van Kooten F, et al. A short screening instrument for poststroke dementia: the R-CAMCOG. *Stroke*. 2000;31:1502–1508.
RUDAS	Rowland Universal Dementia Assessment Scale	Basic D, Rowland JT, Conforti DA, et al. The validity of the Rowland Universal Dementia Assessment Scale (RUDAS) in a multicultural cohort of community-dwelling older persons with early dementia. *Alzheimer Dis Assoc Disord*. 2009;23(2):124–129.
SASSI	Short and Sweet Screening Instrument	Belle SH, Mendelsohn AB, Seaberg EC, et al. A brief cognitive screening battery for dementia in the community. *Neuroepidemiology*. 2000;19:43–50.
SLUMS	Saint Louis Mental Status Examination	Tariq SH, Tumosa N, Chibnall JT, Perry MH 3rd, Morley JE. Comparison of the Saint Louis University Mental Status Examination and the Mini-Mental State Examination for detecting dementia and mild neurocognitive disorder–a pilot study. *Am J Geriatr Psychiatry*. 2006;14(11):900–910.
TICS-M	Telephone Interview of Cognitive Status-Modified	Breitner JC, Welsh KA, Brandt J, et al. Telephone screening for dementia—a practical method for population-based twin studies of Alzheimer's disease and related disorders. *Gerontologist*. 1991;31:333.
TYM	Test Your Memory	Hancock P, Larner AJ. Test Your Memory test: diagnostic utility in a memory clinic population. *Int J Geriatr Psychiatry*. 2011;26:976–980.

has computerized versions) includes a graded series of questions in five areas: language (fluency, comprehension, repetition, naming); visuospatial constructions; memory (recall of 4 words at 10 minutes with category prompts, followed by multiple choices); calculation; and verbal reasoning (similarities, comprehension). Like the MDRS, each section begins with a difficult item, and if the patient gets that item correct, no other questions in the section are given.

Information and Informant-Based Rating Instruments

There are a number of scales or inventories that gather information for the purpose of arriving at a rating, usually of severity of impairment (Table 16.5). These instruments include, at least in part, an incorporation of noncognitive, functional information. Some of these consist of the examiner's impression of the patient's status or change based on acquired information on the patient's performance. Others are more in the nature of informant-based questionnaires used for rating the patient, rather than direct patient

assessments. Several of these instruments do combine mental status testing with functional ratings, and there is much overlap.

BLESSED DEMENTIA SCALE (BDS)

This is a two-part scale consisting of a rating scale assessing the functional status as reported by informants (the Blessed Dementia Rating Scale) and a mental status examination (The Information-Memory-Concentration Test). The rating scale asks a series of questions probing the patient's self-care capabilities and activities of daily living. In the absence of an informant, medical records and alternate sources can supply information for this scale. The Information-Memory-Concentration Test has led to a brief six-item mental status screening test, the S-OMCT described earlier.

CLINICAL DEMENTIA RATING SCALE (CDR)

The CDR is a global rating scale for staging patients diagnosed with dementia (Table 16.6). The CDR evaluates cognitive, behavioral, and functional aspects of Alzheimer disease and other dementias. Rather than a

TABLE 16.5	Information-Based Ratings	
Abbreviation	**Name**	**Reference**
AD8	Eight-Item Informant Interview for the detection of Dementia	Galvin JE Roe CM, Powlishta KK, et al, The AD8, a brief informant interview to detect dementia. *Neurology*. 2005:65:559–564.
BRS	Blessed Dementia Scale	Blessed G, Tomlinson BE, Roth M. The association between quantitative measures of dementia and of senile changes in the cerebral gray matter of elderly subjects. *Br J Psychiatry*. 1968;114(512):797–811.
CDR	Clinical Dementia Rating Scale	Morris J. Clinical Dementia Rating: a reliable and valid diagnostic and staging measure for dementia of the Alzheimer type. *Int Psychogeriatr*. 1997;8:173–176.
CIBIC Plus	Clinician Interview-Based Impression of Change, Plus Carer Interview	Olin JT, Schneider LS, Doody RS, et al. Clinical evaluation of global change in Alzheimer's disease: identifying consensus. *J Geriatr Psychiatry Neurol*. 1996;9:176–180.
GPCOG	General Practitioner Assessment of Cognition	Brodaty H, Pond D, Kemp NM, et al. The GPCOG: a new screening test for dementia designed for general practice. *J Am Geriatr Soc*. 2002;50:530–534.
IQCODE	Informant Questionnaire on Cognitive Decline in the Elderly	Jorm AF, Jacomb PA. The Informant Questionnaire on Cognitive Decline in the Elderly (IQCODE): socio-demographic correlates, reliability, validity and some norms. *Psychol Med*. 1989;19:1015–1022.
IQCODE-SF	Informant Questionnaire on Cognitive Decline in the Elderly-Short Form	Jorm AF. A short form of the Informant Questionnaire on Cognitive Decline in the Elderly (IQCODE): development and cross-validation. *Psychol Med*. 1994;24:145–153.

TABLE 16.6   Clinical Dementia Rating Scale

	Healthy CDR 0	Questionable Dementia CDR 0.5	Mild Dementia CDR 1.0	Moderate Dementia CDR 2.0	Severe Dementia CDR 3.0
Memory	No memory loss or slight inconstant forgetfulness	Mild consistent forgetfulness; partial recollection of events; "benign" forgetfulness	Moderate memory loss, more marked for recent events; defect interferes with everyday activities	Severe memory loss only highly learned material retained; new material rapidly lost	Severe memory loss; only fragments remain
Orientation	Fully oriented		Some difficulty with time relationships; oriented for place to place and person and examination but may have geographical disorientation	Usually oriented in time, often	Oriented to person only
Judgment + Problem Solving	Solves everyday problems well; judgment good in relation to past performance	Only doubtful impairment in solving problems similarities, differences	Moderate difficulty in handling complex problems; social judgement usually maintained	Severely impaired in handling problems, similarities, differences; social judgment usually impaired	Unable to make judgements or solve problems
Community Affairs	Independent function at usual level in job, shopping business and financial affairs, volunteer and social groups	Only doubtful or mild impairment, if any, in these activities	Unable to function independently at these activities though may still be engaged in some; may still appear normal to casual inspection	No pretense of independent function outside of home	
Home + hobbies	Life at home, hobbies, intellectual interests well maintained	Life at home, hobbies, intellectual interests well maintained or only slightly impaired	Mild but definite impairment of function at home; more difficult chores abandoned; more complicated hobbies and interests abandoned	Only simple chores preserved; very restricted interests, poorly sustained	No significant function at home outside of own room
Personal Care	Fully capable self-care		Needs occasional prompting	Requires assistance in dressing, hygiene, keeping of personal effects	Requires much help with personal care; often incontinent

CDR, Clinical Dementia Rating.
From Morris JC. The Clinical Dementia Rating (CDR): Current version and scoring rules. *Neurology* 43(11):2412–2414.

mental status examination or inventory, the rater simply makes a judgment on six categories based on all the information available. The scoring system for the CDR is somewhat complicated and heavily dependent on the memory scores, but the CDR has good interrater reliability in staging dementia. This instrument is a widely used scale in both Alzheimer disease centers and dementia research.

GENERAL PRACTITIONER ASSESSMENT OF COGNITION

The General Practitioner Assessment of Cognition (GPCOG) is a screening test that combines a cognitive test of the patient and an informant interview into a brief instrument (approximately 5 minutes) applicable for primary care. The cognitive test includes orientation, clock drawing, awareness of a current news event, and recall of a name and an address. The examiner asks the informant to compare the patient's current function with the patient's function a few years prior. The informant interview inquires about memory, word-finding difficulties, trouble managing finances, difficulties managing medication, and independence in transportation. For detecting cognitive impairment in the elderly, the GPCOG is at least as sensitive and specific as the MMSE and more robust to education and cultural differences.

INFORMANT QUESTIONNAIRE ON COGNITIVE DECLINE IN THE ELDERLY (IQCODE) AND SHORT FORM (SHORT IQCODE)

The 26-item Informant Questionnaire on Cognitive Decline in the Elderly (IQCODE) and its 16-item short form are informant-based questionnaires for evaluating cognitive and functional changes. Both versions ask informants to rate changes on a 5-point Likert scale of the patient's performance on items of memory, orientation, judgment, and instrumental activities of daily living. These instruments aim to establish the presence of cognitive decline from a premorbid level by focusing on common functional tasks. Using different cutoff scores, both the full and short versions of the IQCODE have good sensitivity and specificity for dementia.

Survey of Behavior Inventories Useful in Neurobehavior

Mental status examiners often need to evaluate behavior and mood, areas that are less amenable to actual tests or tasks. Consequently, some familiarity with behavioral and mood inventories is helpful. Although not comprehensive, this brief survey of these inventories, along with Tables 16.7 and 16.8, provide a background for thinking about and using these inventories. The tables include inventories that an examiner could easily apply but not structured interviews requiring significant skill and training to administer. The tables also include inventories that an informant or the patient could complete. Similar to prior sections, this section evaluates in greater depth a select group of eight widely used inventories: four assessing general behavior and four assessing for anxiety and depression.

GENERAL BEHAVIOR INVENTORIES

Brief Psychiatric Rating Scale (BPRS). The BPRS is a 16-item instrument that documents and quantifies the results of an open-ended interview. The examiner rates behavioral symptoms, such as anxiety, hostility, affect, guilt, orientation on a 7-point Likert scale from absent to extremely severe. The subscales are less reliable and valid than the total score. Although the BPRS provides little information on specific behaviors, it does reveal five factors in the elderly: withdrawn depression, agitation, cognitive dysfunction, hostile-suspiciousness, and psychotic distortion. In summary, the BPRS is brief, provides a quantitative score of global psychopathology, and can be useful in monitoring patients and their responses to treatment.

Cohen-Mansfield Agitation Scale (CMAI). This instrument is one of the best scales to measure agitation in dementia. The CMAI is a 15-minute, informant-based instrument that measures agitation as defined by inappropriate, abusive, or aggressive verbal or motor activity that is not explained by needs or confusion. The CMAI consists of 29 agitated behaviors rated on a 7-point frequency scale, with 7 representing a behavior that is exhibited several times in a day. It yields three factors: verbal and physical aggressive behavior, physically nonaggressive behavior such as pacing and

TABLE 16.7	**Behavior Scales—General**	
Abbreviation	**Name**	**Reference**
AES-C	Apathy Evaluation Scale, Clinician Version	Marin RS, Biedrzycki RC, Firinciogullari S. Reliability and validity of the Apathy Evaluation Scale. *Psychiatry Res.* 1991;38(2):143–162.
BPAQ	Buss Perry Aggression Questionnaire	Buss AH, Perry M. The aggression questionnaire. *J Pers Soc Psychol.* 1992;63(3):452–459.
BPRS	Brief Psychiatric Rating Scale	Overall JE, Gorham DR. The brief psychiatric rating scale. *Psychological Reports.* 1962;10(3):799–812.
BSI	Brief Symptom Inventory	Derogatis LR, Melisaratos N. The Brief Symptom Inventory: an introductory report. *Psychol Med.* 1983;13(3):595–605.
CBI	Cambridge Behavioural Inventory	Wedderburn C, Wear H, Brown J, et al. The utility of the Cambridge Behavioural Inventory in neurodegenerative disease. *J Neurol Neurosurg Psychiatr.* 2008;79:500–503.
CPRS-R	Revised Conners' Parent Rating Scale	Conners CK, Sitarenios G, Parker JD, Epstein JN. The revised Conners' Parent Rating Scale (CPRS-R): factor structure, reliability, and criterion validity. *J Abnorm Child Psychol.* 1998;26(4):257–268.
DAIR	Dementia Apathy Interview and Rating	Strauss ME, Sperry SD. An informant-based assessment of apathy in Alzheimer disease. *Cogn Behav Neurol.* 2002;15(3):176–183.
E-BEHAV-AD	Empirical Behavioral Rating Scale	Auer SR, Monteiro IM, Reisberg B. The empirical behavioral pathology in Alzheimer's disease (E-BEHAVE-AD) rating scale. *Int Psychogeriatrics.* 1996;8(2):247–266.
GAF	Global Assessment of Functioning	Hall RC. Global assessment of functioning: a modified scale. *Psychosomatics.* 1995;36(3):267–275.
GHQ	General Health Questionnaire	Goldberg DP, Hillier VF. A scaled version of the General Health Questionnaire. *Psychol Med.* 1979;9(1):139–145.
IA	Apathy Inventory	Robert PH, Clairet S, Benoit M, et al. The Apathy Inventory: assessment of apathy and awareness in Alzheimer's disease Parkinson's disease and mild cognitive impairment. *Int J Geriatr Psychiatry.* 2002;17(12):1099–1105.
NBRS	Neurobehavioral Rating Scale	Levin HS, High WM, Goethe KE, et al. The Neurobehavioural Rating Scale: assessment of the behavioural sequelae of head injury by the clinician. *J Neurol Neurosurg Psychiatry.* 1987;50(2):183–193.
NPI	Neuropsychiatric Inventory	Cummings JL, Mega M, Gray K, Rosenberg-Thompson S, Carusi DA, Gornbein J. The Neuropsychiatric Inventory: comprehensive assessment of psychopathology in dementia. *Neurology.* 1994;44(12):2308–2314.
OASS	Overt Agitation Severity Scale	Yudofsky SC, Kopecky HJ, Kunik M, Silver JM, Endicott J. The Overt Agitation Severity Scale for the objective rating of agitation. *J Neuropsychiatry Clin Neurosci.* 1997;9(4):541–548.
PCL-R	Psychopathy Checklist-Revised	Hare RD, Neumann CS. Structural models of psychopathy. *Curr Psychiatry Rep.* 2005;7(1):57–64.
SAS	Starkstein Apathy Scale	Starkstein SE, Mayberg HS, Preziosi T, Andrezejewski P, Leiguarda R, Robinson RG. Reliability validity and clinical correlates of apathy in Parkinson's disease. *J Neuropsychiatry Clin Neurosci.* 1992;4(2):134–139.

TABLE 16.8	Behavior Inventories—Anxiety and Depression	
Abbreviation	**Name**	**Reference**
BDI	Beck Depression Inventory	Beck AT, Steer RA, Carbin MG. Psychometric properties of the Beck Depression Inventory: twenty-five years of evaluation. *Clin Psychol Rev*. 1988;8(1):77–100.
BAI	Beck Anxiety Inventory	Beck AT, Epstein N, Brown G, Steer RA. An inventory for measuring clinical anxiety: psychometric properties. *J Consult Clin Psychol*. 1988;56(6):893–897.
BDC and BAI	Burns Depression Checklist and Burns Anxiety Inventory	Burns DD. The Burns Depression Checklist (BDC) and the Burns Anxiety Inventory (BAI). The feeling good handbook. New York, NY: William Morrow and Co. Revised and updated; 1999.
CES-D	Center for Epidemiological Studies Depression Scale	Radloff LS, Teri L. Use of the Center for Epidemiological Studies-Depression Scale with older adults. *Clin Gerontologist*. 1986;5(1–2):119–136.
CMAI	Cohen-Mansfield Agitation Inventory	Cohen-Mansfield J. Conceptualization of agitation: results based on the Cohen-Mansfield Agitation Inventory and the Agitation Behavior Mapping Instrument. *Int Psychogeriatr*. 1996;8(Suppl 3):309–315.
CSDD	Cornell Scale for Depression in Dementia	Alexopoulos GS, Abrams RC, Young RC, Shamoian CA. Cornell Scale for Depression in Dementia. *Biol Psychiatry*. 1988;23(3):271–284.
DMAS	Dementia Mood Assessment Scale	Sunderland T, Minichiello M. Dementia Mood Assessment Scale. *Int Psychogeriatrics*. 1997;8:329–331.
GAD-7	Generalized Anxiety Disorder 7-Item Scale	Spitzer RL, Kroenke K, Williams JB, Löwe B. A brief measure for assessing generalized anxiety disorder: the GAD-7. *Arch Int Med*. 2006;166(10):1092–1097.
GDS	Geriatric Depression Scale	Yesavage JA, Brink TL, Rose TL, et al. Development and validation of a geriatric depression screening scale: a preliminary report. *J Psychiatric Res*. 1982;17(1):37–49.
HAM-A	Hamilton Anxiety Rating Scale	Hamilton MAX. The assessment of anxiety states by rating. *Br J Med Psychol*. 1959;32(1):50–55.
HAM-D	Hamilton Depression Rating Scale	Williams JB. A structured interview guide for the Hamilton Depression Rating Scale. *Arch Gen Psychiatry*. 1988;45(8):742–747.
MDI	Major Depression Index	Bech P, Rasmussen NA, Olsen LR, Noerholm V, Abildgaard W. The sensitivity and specificity of the Major Depression Inventory using the Present State Examination as the index of diagnostic validity. *J Affect Disord*. 2001;66 (2–3):159–164.
MADRS	Montgomery-Asberg Depression Rating Scale	Montgomery SA, Åsberg M. A new depression scale designed to be sensitive to change. *Br J Psychiatry*. 1979;134(4):382–389.
STAI	State Trait Anxiety Inventory	Elliott T, Shewchuk R, Richards JS. Family caregiver problem solving abilities and adjustment during the initial year of the caregiving role. *J Counsel Psychol*. 2001;48:223–232.
Y-BOCS	Yale-Brown Obsessive-Compulsive Scale	Goodman WK, Price LH, Rasmussen SA, et al. The Yale-Brown Obsessive Compulsive Scale: I. Development use and reliability. *Arch Gen Psychiatry*. 1989;46(11):1006–1011.
SAS	Zung Self-Rating Anxiety Scale	Zung WWK. A rating instrument for anxiety disorders. *Psychosomatics*. 1971;12(6):371–379.
SDS	Zung Self-Rating Depression Scale	Zung WWK. A self-rating depression scale. *Arch Gen Psychiatry*. 1965;12:63–70.

restlessness, and verbally agitated behaviors such as screaming or repetitive requests for attention.

NeuropsychiatricInventory-Questionnaire(NPI-Q). The NPI-Q is another excellent instrument for assessing neuropsychiatric disturbances among dementia patients. The examiner obtains information, usually from a caregiver, on frequency and severity of symptoms in 12 areas: delusions, hallucinations, agitation or aggression, depression or dysphoria, anxiety, elation or euphoria, apathy or indifference, disinhibition, irritability or lability, motor disturbance, nighttime behaviors, and appetite and eating changes (Table 16.9). This instrument has validity and reliability in identifying the neuropsychiatric features of Alzheimer disease. The NPI-Q has the added feature of obtaining separate measures of symptom severity and the degree of distress that they cause.

Overt Aggression Scale (OAS). Clinicians use the OAS to document aggressive behaviors based on observable criteria. The OAS categorizes observed aggression as verbal aggression, physical aggression against objects, physical aggression against self, and physical aggression against others. The OAS further categorizes the aggressive behaviors into four levels of severity and records the therapeutic interventions for each aggressive episode. The instrument is particularly useful for assessing aggression in institutionalized patients and documenting episodes and their responses to interventions.

TABLE 16.9   Behavioral Assessment—Neuropsychiatric Inventory Questionnaire (NPI-Q) (to be completed by clinician per informant report)

Informant: ? Spouse ? Child ? Other: _____

Please ask the following questions based on <u>changes</u>. Indicate "yes" only if the symptom has been present in the <u>past month</u>; otherwise, indicate "no."

<table>
<tr><td colspan="2" align="center">For each item marked "yes":</td></tr>
<tr>
<td>Rate the SEVERITY of the symptom (how it affects the patient):</td>
<td>Rate the DISTRESS you experience because of the symptom (how it affects you):</td>
</tr>
<tr>
<td>1 = Mild (noticeable, but not a significant change)

2 = Moderate (significant, but not a dramatic change)

3 = Severe (very marked or prominent; a dramatic change)</td>
<td>0 = Not distressing at all
1 = Minimal (slightly distressing, not a problem to cope with)
2 = Mild (not very distressing, generally easy to cope with)
3 = Moderate (fairly distressing, not always easy to cope with)
4 = Severe (very distressing, difficult to cope with)
5 = Extreme or very severe (extremely distressing, unable to cope with)</td>
</tr>
</table>

Please answer each question honestly and carefully.

Ask for assistance if you are not sure how to answer any question.

	Yes	No	Severity			Distress					
			1	2	3	0	1	2	3	4	5
DELUSIONS: Does the patient believe that others are stealing from him or her, or planning to harm him or her in some way?											
HALLUCINATIONS: Does the patient act as if he or she hears voices? Does he or she talk to people who are not there?											
AGITATION OR AGGRESSION: Is the patient stubborn and resistive to help from others?											
DEPRESSION OR DYSPHORIA: Does the patient act as if he or she is sad or in low spirits? Does he or she cry?											

(Continued)

TABLE 16.9   Behavioral Assessment—Neuropsychiatric Inventory Questionnaire (NPI-Q) (to be completed by clinician per informant report) (Cont'd)

ANXIETY: Does the patient become upset when separated from you? Does he or she have any other signs of nervousness, such as shortness of breath, sighing, being unable to relax, or feeling excessively tense?												
ELATION OR EUPHORIA: Does the patient appear to feel too good or act excessively happy?												
APATHY OR INDIFFERENCE: Does the patient seem less interested in his or her usual activities and in the activities and plans of others?												
DISINHIBITION: Does the patient seem to act impulsively? For example, does the patient talk to strangers as if he or she knows them, or does the patient say things that may hurt people's feelings?												
IRRITABILITY OR LABILITY: Is the patient impatient or cranky? Does he or she have difficulty coping with delays or waiting for planned activities?												
MOTOR DISTURBANCE: Does the patient engage in repetitive activities, such as pacing around the house, handling buttons, wrapping string, or doing other things repeatedly?												
NIGHTTIME BEHAVIORS: Does the patient awaken you during the night, rise too early in the morning, or take excessive naps during the day?												
APPETITE AND EATING: Has the patient lost or gained weight, or had a change in the food he or she likes?												

MOOD INVENTORIES

Beck Anxiety Inventory (BAI). The BAI is a self-report anxiety inventory consisting of 21 questions. The BAI assesses frequency of anxiety symptoms over a 1 week period while minimizing their relationship with depression. Fourteen items ask about somatic symptoms and 7 ask about cognitive symptoms associated with anxiety. Patients rate the severity of each of these items on a 4-point Likert scale. The BAI is a valid and reliable instrument for detecting anxiety, including among elderly patients.

Beck Depression Inventory (BDI). This is a widely used self-report inventory for current depression. The BDI includes both cognitive and physical symptoms of depression. The patient answers the 21 items of the BDI on a continuum of severity from 0, "I don't feel sad," to 3, "I am so sad or unhappy that I can't stand it." This instrument has adequate criterion validity and test-retest reliability and is useful for the general screening for depression in the elderly.

Cornell Scale for Depression in Dementia (CSDD). This scale is useful for depression among impaired dementia patients. There are 18 items that can be answered by informants rather than by the patients. It is included here because, among patients with dementia, the CSDD may be the best instrument for quantifying their depression.

Geriatric Depression Scale (GDS), Short Version. There have been a number of versions of the GDS. The 15-item version has proven to be a good instrument for rating depression in the elderly. The GDS uses items with ecological validity for older people and generally avoids the emphasis on physical symptoms present in other instruments (Table 16.10). It is a self-report

TABLE 16.10   *Geriatric Depression Scale (Short Version)*
1. Are you basically satisfied with your life?
ª2. Have you dropped many of your activities and interests?
ª3. Do you feel that your life is empty?
ª4. Do you often get bored?
5. Are you in good spirits most of the time?
ª6. Are you afraid that something bad is going to happen to you?
7. Do you feel happy most of the time?
ª8. Do you often feel helpless?
ª9. Do you prefer to stay home, rather than going out and doing new things?
ª10. Do you feel you have more problems with memory than most?
11. Do you think it is wonderful to be alive now?
ª12. Do you feel pretty worthless the way you are now?
13. Do you feel full of energy?
ª14. Do you feel that your situation is hopeless?
ª15. Do you think that most people are better off than you are?

ª"Yes" answers indicating depression, otherwise "no" answers indicate depression. The Geriatric Depression Scale can be a self-rating or observer-rated inventory.

From Yesavage JA. Geriatric depression scale. *Psychopharmacol Bull*. 1988;24:709.

inventory, but the examiner can also complete the GDS-15. This instrument may be best for older patients who are cognitively normal or have only mild dementia, using the CSDD for more impaired patients.

Conclusions

The choice of the appropriate mental status scale, rating instrument, or behavior scale depends on the clinical need and context. Regardless of choice, most of these tools can screen and identify patientsneeding further diagnostic assessment. For shorter cognitive assessments (≤5 minutes) for dementia screening in a busy clinical practice, the CDT, MIS, Mini-Cog, SIS, SPMSQ, and STMS are appropriate instruments. In this group, the Mini-Cog, STMS, and Mini-ACE particularly stand out because of their content. The use of longer cognitive assessments (≥5 minutes), such as the MMSE, MoCA, RUDAS, SLUMS, and ACE-III, allow for a broader assessment for cognitive impairment. The MoCA and SLUMS may prove to be the most sensitive for mild cognitive impairment, but the RUDAS and ACE-III are good choices as well. Mental status screening is greatly improved with the addition of information-based instruments that assess functional status and with behavior inventories when there are behavioral or mood symptoms. Finally, mental status examiners need some familiarity with the role of neuropsychological testing, a topic that is discussed in Chapter 17.

Overview of Neuropsychological Testing

The neuropsychological examination is the ultimate extension of the mental status examination (MSX). Neuropsychological testing involves the administration of standardized, validated, and reliable instruments to patients, usually under the supervision of a professional neuropsychologist. Referral for this testing is necessary in some patients who have undergone prior levels of MSX and require even more investigation. The mental status examiner must know when to refer for neuropsychological testing, the nature of the tests administered, and how to interpret the results. When this testing is obtained, the referring clinician must integrate and incorporate the results into the complete neurocognitive profile of the patient. This chapter addresses these points. Rather than a compendium of neuropsychological instruments, it is an overview of the neuropsychological process including common test batteries and the neuropsychologist's report.

General Concepts of Neuropsychological Assessment

INDICATIONS AND ADVANTAGES

Neuropsychological assessment is a more "formal" process than mental status testing in the clinic or at the bedside. A neuropsychological assessment requires referral to a testing service, where trained neuropsychologists or psychometricians administer the tests in a standardized manner, minimizing environmental confounding variables. This referral should take place only after the clinician has taken a neurobehavioral history, made behavioral observations, and performed an MSX in the context of the clinical assessment. This clinical examination helps guide the choice of neuropsychological tests and procedures. Compared with most mental status tasks, neuropsychological tests have strong psychometric properties and have undergone both validation, often in different populations, and various forms of reliability testing. These instruments also have age- and education-based normative data, and, depending on the test, there may even be normative data for different sociocultural, linguistic, or ethnic groups.

There are a number of indications for referral for neuropsychological testing. In general, neuropsychological assessment is useful in distinguishing cognitive changes from normal and in characterizing the cognitive profile. Extensive and in-depth neuropsychological testing is best for the evaluation of mild or subtle impairments not detected on the clinic or bedside MSX, including mental status scales and inventories. This is possible because neuropsychological instruments allow for comparing the patient's performance with others of his or her age and education. A score that is normal for one older or less educated individual may be very abnormal for a younger or more educated person who might have scored at ceiling on mental status screening. Consequently, patients who continue to complain of memory or other cognitive impairment, particularly those of high intellectual background, may need a referral for neuropsychological testing.

There are several other indications for a neuropsychological referral. One is when it is difficult to differentiate the cognitive manifestations of depression, psychosis, or other psychiatric syndromes from an underlying neurodegenerative or other brain disorder. Neuropsychological testing is of further value in quantifying the actual cognitive profile, including the patient's strengths and weakness and degree of impairment. This information can be useful in addressing recovery, functional interventions, or rehabilitation programs. A comprehensive neuropsychological assessment can help in differential diagnosis when it provides the referring clinician with an analysis of the patient's cognitive profile and its compatibility with different disorders. Without other clinical information, however, neuropsychological testing by itself cannot diagnose causative diseases or etiology. Finally, there is a role in neuropsychological assessment for capacity and competence assessments and in forensic and legal situations.

LIMITATIONS AND CONCERNS

There are often concerns about the time that it takes to complete and report the results of neuropsychological testing. First, a full assessment cannot be done when the patient is first seen by the referring clinician. Neuropsychological testing requires scheduling an extended period of time in a controlled setting. This testing may require 2 to 7 hours and more than one session, hence it is not practical for screening for mental status impairments. Testing for a prolonged period can be quite challenging for cognitively impaired patients, and there are "state" effects with increasing fatigue and waning cooperation. If the session is too long, this can result in worse performance on later tests. Another drawback to neuropsychological assessment is the delay in generating a report. They require a period of time for scoring and interpretation, which delays the availability of the report and makes it less useful when urgent clinical decision-making is needed. The neuropsychologist must assure the timely availability of the neuropsychological report for patient care and its integration with the referring clinician's diagnosis and management.

Another area of concern in neuropsychological testing is the effects of demographic variables. The patient's age, education, sociocultural or ethnic background, and sex can affect test performance. Very old age and very high or low educational levels have highly significant effects on these instruments. There are age-related changes in psychomotor speed, sustained and complex attention, retrieval of information, and other aspects of cognition (see Chapter 6, Box 6.3). Neuropsychological tests have shown decreased performance on timed scores and "fluid" intelligence with aging, but relative preservation of verbal scores, narrative language, and established skills. After age, education has immense effects on how patients perform on these tests. Differences in test performance between those with grade school versus higher education can be profound, not only from differences in knowledge and familiarity

with the content, but also because of differences in comfort in taking paper and pencil (and increasingly computerized) tests. Although normative data adjusted for age and education are a strength of neuropsychological assessment, age and education may still impact on the clinical significance of the testing results. Other variables, such as sex differences, appear negligible for most tests, but sociocultural, linguistic, and ethnic differences can be substantive. Neuropsychologists have attempted to construct "culture-fair" tests as much as possible and, for the most part, are aware of these variables in interpreting the test results.

A final concern is establishing the presence of change from a prior level of cognitive functioning. The interpretation of the results of these tests depends on an estimation of the patient's estimated premorbid capabilities. Most often there are no prior or premorbid tests of cognition for comparison. The neuropsychologist must then estimate premorbid levels of functioning using patient characteristics, demographic formulas, or performance on select measures such as the North American Adult Reading Test (NAART). Most commonly, an estimate of premorbid status is derived from the patient's prior educational and occupational attainment. Other measures of premorbid cognition include demographic formulas, such as the Barona Index, or formulas that combine demographic information with vocabulary or word pronunciation tests, such as the Vanderploeg equation. These formulas can generate a wide range of potential premorbid estimates, and a preferred method to assess premorbid cognitive level is the ability to read aloud and pronounce irregular words. The NAART consists of 50 irregular words of decreasing frequency, for example, "island" or "cellist," whose pronunciation cannot be read aloud correctly using common phonemic rules and require familiarity and past educational exposure. The NAART, however, is based on language, a cognitive domain that is sensitive to brain injury, and estimates of premorbid cognitive ability from word reading ability may be unreliable in patients with dementia or other brain disorders.

Neuropsychological Batteries and Testing

There are many neuropsychological tests that are available (see Lezak et al, 2012), some of which are clearly similar or the source of mental status tasks described in prior chapters. The neuropsychological assessment usually groups tests into a battery that targets the major domains of cognition. Multiple cognitive functions can affect performance on each test, which increases the value of a battery approach with neuropsychological interpretation of the entire profile. There is no single, best neuropsychological battery of tests, but all batteries should aim to cover mental control/attention, language, memory, visuospatial skills, executive abilities, and other major cognitive domains (Table 17.1). Batteries can be predominantly "fixed" or predetermined, or they may be "flexible," with the neuropsychologist choosing the appropriate tests

based on the clinical question and the features of the patient. Often, the battery has a fixed core of tests with additional flexible choices as deemed indicated.

Historically, the two best-known fixed batteries for brain disease are the Halstead-Reitan Neuropsychological Battery (HRNB) and the Luria-Nebraska Neuropsychological Battery (LNNB). In addition to the trademark category test (discerning the principle embedded in arrangements of figures and shapes), the HRNB includes many "neurophysiological" tests that are not traditional paper and pencil tests. Among these are the tactual performance test (placing different shaped blocks without vision),

TABLE 17.1 Example of Neuropsychological Test Battery	
Domain	**Neuropsychological Test**
Attention and Fundamental Functions	WAIS subtests—Digit Span within Working Memory Index
	Trail Making-A and the Processing Speed Index (also executive)
	(Continuous Performance Test, Digit Vigilance Test, Paced Auditory Serval Attention Test, others)
Language and Speech	Boston Naming Test
	Controlled Oral Word Association Test ("F-A-S"); semantic verbal fluency
	Aphasia Test (e.g., Boston Diagnostic Aphasia Examination, Multilingual Aphasia Examination, Wechsler Test of Adult Reading, others)
Memory and Semantic Knowledge	Wechsler Memory Scale versions
	California Verbal Learning Test (and other supraspan word learning tests such as the Rey Auditory Verbal Learning Test, Hopkins Verbal Learning Test
	Rey-Osterrieth Complex Figure Test Delayed Recall
	(Rivermead Behavioral Memory Test, Test of Memory Malingering, others)
Constructional, Perceptual, and Spatial Abilities	Rey-Osterrieth Complex Figure Test Copy
	WAIS subtests—Block Design within Perceptual Reasoning Index
	(Hooper Visual Organization Test, Bender Visual Motor Gestalt Test, others)
Praxis and Related Cortical Movement Abnormalities	Halstead-Reitan Neuropsychological Battery (HRNB) subtests (e.g., such as finger oscillation (tapping), grooved pegboard, tactile performance)
Calculations and Related Functions	WAIS subtests—Arithmetic within Working Memory Index
Executive Operations and Attributes	Wisconsin Card Sort Test
	Trail Making-B
	Controlled Oral Word Association Test (i.e., "F-A-S")
	(Range of other available tests include the Stroop Test discussed in Chapter 13, Delis-Kaplan Executive Functions System, HRNB Category Subtest, Tower of London, Figural Fluency Tests, others)
Behavior (emotion/personality/psychopathology)	Minnesota Multiphasic Personality Inventory-2
	(Milton Clinical Multiaxial Inventory, Thematic Apperception Test, others)
General	(Wide Range Achievement Test, Shipley Institute of Living Scale)

Parentheses indicate optional tests

seashore rhythm test (judging the similarity of auditory rhythmic pattern), speech sound perception test (identifying spoken nonsense syllables), finger oscillation (tapping) test (tapping a mechanic counter as fast as possible with index finger), sensory perceptual and lateral dominance examinations, and the frequent addition of the grooved pegboard test and hand grip strength on a dynamometer. The entire HRNB is not based on current knowledge of the organization of behavior in the brain and is not a sensitive battery for the detection of mild cognitive deficits or for brain-behavior localization. Nevertheless, some of these HRNB subtests have proven useful and may be incorporated in flexible batteries. The 2- to 3-hour LNNB was a product of brain-behavior observations made by Alexander Luria and consists of 269 brief items that assess motor, rhythm, tactile, visual, oral language, writing, reading, arithmetic, memory, and intellectual functions. An additional scale consists of the items drawn from the other scales found to be maximally sensitive to brain dysfunction, and there are right and left hemisphere scales. The LNNB is open to errors of omission, issues of reliability and validity, and lack of normative data, and is only used by a small group of neuropsychologists.

Most commonly used batteries have a core base on the Wechsler Adult Intelligence Scale (WAIS) plus a number of other popular tests that cover the major cognitive domains, including some subtests of the HRNB. The current version of the WAIS (WAIS-IV; WAIS 5 pending) has 10 core subtests, which yield the Full Scale IQ, and five supplemental subtests. The WAIS-IV has four indices: verbal comprehension (information, similarities, vocabulary), working memory (arithmetic, digit span), perceptual reasoning (block design, matrix reasoning, visual puzzles), and processing speed (digit-symbol coding, symbol search). Although the WAIS was not original designed for the assessment of cognitive disorders, the extensive experience and large normative data with the WAIS provides a basis for interpreting the subtests in relation to cognitive changes. The pattern of performance on subtest scores can be informative as to the type of disturbance. Furthermore, the verbal comprehension and perceptual reasoning indices yield a General Ability Index, which is a measure of cognitive abilities that is less vulnerable to impairments of processing speed and working memory.

To the WAIS core, neuropsychologists can complete the battery from a large array of available neuropsychological tests (Table 17.2). Although there are likely regional variations, by and large, there is some consistency in the choice of additional tests. For coverage of the cognitive domains of memory and language, among the most popular are the Wechsler Memory Scale-III (WMS-III), California Verbal Learning Test (CVLT), Boston Naming Test (BNT), and Controlled Oral Word Association Test (COWAT). The WMS-III includes 18 subtests, such as paired-associate learning and logical memory, and yields information about various kinds of memory and learning processes. The WMS-III provides a comprehensive assessment of memory with subtest scores and summary memory index, but it may take an hour to administer. The CVLT is a supraspan auditory learning test that measures recent verbal memory and new learning (see another supraspan test, Chapter 9, Tables 9.1 and 9.2). A list of 16 or 9 words (depending on CVLT version) that are repeatedly rehearsed by the patient is followed by an interference task. After a 20-minute delay, the patient must recall the words freely and through multiple choice. The BNT is a sensitive confrontational naming test, which presents a series of 60 line drawings of increasing naming difficulty. Because patients may misname the line drawings due to visuospatial patterns, the BNT test includes conceptual and phonemic cueing trials. The COWAT asks the patient to say as many words as they can think of in 1 minute that begin with a given letter of the alphabet (usually "F", "A", and "S" in English), excluding proper nouns, numbers, and the same word with a different suffix, for example, shout, shouted, shouting. The score is the total number of words generated in all categories and stratified by age and years of education (Table 17.3). Related category fluency asks the patient to say as many words as they can think of in 1 minute for a given category, for example, animals, vegetables, or tools.

For the cognitive domains of perception and executive functions, among the most popular tests are the Rey-Osterrieth Complex Figure Test (CFT), Trail Making Tests (TMK), and Wisconsin Card Sort Test (WCST). The CFT is a test of construction, planning, and visual memory. The patient must copy a complex design containing 36 scorable elements and must reproduce it after a delay (Fig 17.1 and Chapter 10,

TABLE 17.2	**Example of Common Neuropsychological Tests**
Test Name	**Description**
Bender Visual Motor Gestalt Test	Classic test of visual-perceptual and visual-motor functioning
Boston Diagnostic Aphasia Examination	Extensive assessment of language functions
Boston Naming Test	60-item confrontational naming test ("mini" version has 15 items)
California Verbal Learning Test	Supraspan auditory learning test described in text
Continuous Performance Test	Test of sustained attention
Controlled Oral Word Association Test	Verbal fluency based on number of words that start with a certain letter ("F-A-S")
Delis-Kaplan Executive Function System	Series of tests that assess a number of executive functions, such as abstraction and deductive reasoning
Digit Vigilance Test	Attention measured by visual tracking
Figural Fluency Tests	Generation of as many figures as possible within time and spatial constraints
Finger Oscillation Test	HRNB finger tapping test for motor speed and agility
Grooved Pegboard	This test involves putting grooved pins in pegboard for fine motor ability
HRNB Category Test	Executive task that involves discerning the principle embedded in arrangements of figures and shapes
Halstead-Reitan Neuropsychological Battery (HRNB)	Original neuropsychological battery for brain disease, described in text
Hooper Visual Organization Test	Visual integration of "cut up" pictures, like a visual puzzle
Luria-Nebraska Neuropsychological Battery (LNNB)	Alternate neuropsychological battery for brain disease, described in text
Minnesota Multiphasic Personality Inventory-2 (MMPI-2)	Assesses personality and psychopathology with validity scales for effort and malingering
Millon Clinical Multiaxial Inventory	Alternative to MMPI-2
Multilingual Aphasia Examination	Alternative to Boston Diagnostic Aphasia Examination
North American Reading Test (NAART)	Irregular word reading test, described in text
Paced Auditory Serial Attention Test	Difficult serial addition tasks for testing attention and concentration
Repeated Battery for the Assessment of Neuropsychological Status (RBANS)	Brief screening and monitoring battery composed of five domains and multiple subtests, described in text
Rey Auditory Verbal Learning Test	Original supraspan verbal learning task and an alternative to the California Verbal Learning Test
Rey-Osterrieth Complex Figure Test	Complex figure copy and delayed recall, described in text
Rivermead Behavioral Memory Test	Excellent memory test for everyday real-life memory
Shipley Institute of Living Scale	General abilities tested by vocabulary knowledge and abstract sequential patterns
Stroop Test	Word, color, and color-word reading for response interference
Tactual Performance	Tests tactile perception, spatial memory, and speed of motor performance
Test of Memory Malingering	Visual recognition test to detect malingering in memory
Thematic Apperception Test	Projective test for assessing personality and emotions
Tower of London	Assesses strategy in alternate ring placements on pegs, an executive task
Trail Making Tests A and B	Visual sequencing tests, described in text
Semantic (Word) Fluency Test	Verbal fluency for categories, such as animals, vegetables, or tools
Wechsler Adult Intelligence Scale-III	The WAIS-III is a common core test for most neuropsychiatric batteries. The subtests are very informative. The WAIS-III is described in text

(Continued)

Test Name	Description
Wechsler Memory Scale-III	Comprehensive memory test with highly informative subtests, described in text
Wechsler Test of Adult Reading	Reading test estimates of premorbid cognitive ability, alternative to NAART
Wide Range Achievement Test	General assessment in multiple areas reflective of premorbid achievement, also an alternative to NAART
Wisconsin Card Sort Test	Executive set shifting test, described in text

TABLE 17.3 FAS and Animal Fluency Normative Data

Controlled Oral Word Association Test (COWAT). The patient must generate as many words as possible in 1 minute that begin with a given letter of the alphabet (usually F, then A, then S in English, total 3 minutes). These word lists exclude proper nouns, numbers, and the same word with a different suffix. The score is the total number of words generated in all categories.

Education (years)	Age 16–59 Years			Age 60–79 Years			Age 80–95 Years		
	0–8	9–12	13–21	0–8	9–12	13–21	0–8	9–12	13–21
Percentile Score									
90	48	56	61	39	54	59	33	42	56
80	45	50	55	36	47	53	29	38	47
70	42	47	51	31	43	49	26	34	43
60	39	43	49	27	39	45	24	31	39
50	36	40	45	25	35	41	22	29	36
40	35	38	42	22	32	38	21	27	33
30	34	35	38	20	28	36	19	24	30
20	30	32	35	17	24	34	17	22	28
10	27	28	30	13	21	27	13	18	23
Mean	38.5	40.5	44.7	25.3	35.6	42.0	22.4	29.8	37.0
SD	12.0	10.7	11.2	11.1	12.5	12.1	8.2	11.4	11.2

Semantic Word Fluency. The patient must generate as many words as possible in 1 minute that are within a given category, in this case animals. The score is the total number of animals generated.

Education (years)	Age 16–59 Years			Age 60–79 Years			Age 80–95 Years		
	0–8	9–12	13–21	0–8	9–12	13–21	0–8	9–12	13–21
Percentile Score									
90		26	30	20	22	25	18	19	24
75		23	25	17	19	22	16	17	20
50		20	23	14	17	19	13	14	16
25		17	18	12	14	16	11	12	14
10		15	16	11	12	13	9	11	12
Mean		19.8	21.9	14.4	16.4	18.2	13.1	13.9	16.3
(SD)		4.2	5.4	3.4	4.3	4.2	3.8	3.4	4.3

SD, Standard deviation.
From: Tombaugh TN, Kozak J, Rees L. Normative data stratified by age and education for two measures of verbal fluency: FAS and animal naming. *Arch Clin Neuropsychol.* 1999;14(2):167–177.

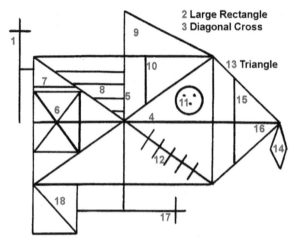

2 Large Rectangle
3 Diagonal Cross

13 Triangle

Fig. 17.1 Rey-Osterrieth Complex Figure scoring key.

SCORING:
Correct, properly placed: 2 points
Correct, improperly placed: 1 point
Distorted, improperly placed: ½ point

	Direct Copy	0-min. Delay	30-min Delay
1. Cross (upper left)			
2. Large Rectangle			
3. Diagonal Lines in Rectangle			
4. Horizontal Midline in Rectangle			
5. Vertical Midline in Rectangle			
6. Small Rectangle within Large Rectangle			
7. Small Line Segment Above Small Rectangle			
8. Horizontal Parallel Lines within upper left section of Large Rectangle			
9. Triangle above right section of Large Rectangle			
10. Short Vertical Line within upper right section of Large Rectangle			
11. Circle with Three Dots			
12. Diagonal Parallel Lines within lower right section of Large Rectangle			

	Direct Copy	0-min. Delay	30-min Delay
13. Sides of Triangle on right side of Large Rectangle			
14. Diamond attached to Triangle on right			
15. Vertical Line within Triangle on right			
16. Horizontal Line within Triangle on right			
17. Cross below Large Rectangle			
18. Square below lower left section of Large Rectangle			

Fig. 10.3). The TMK Tests, TMK-A and TMK-B, and their variants are also discussed in Chapter 7 (Fig. 7.6) and Chapter 13 (Fig. 13.3). TMK-B is a test of visual scanning and task switching, or cognitive flexibility. There are 25 targets on the page, which the subject needs to connect, alternating between numbers (1–13) and letters (A–L). The examiner records the time taken to complete the task, as well as the number of errors (corrected by the examiner while taking the test). The WCST is an executive functions test that assesses the ability to discern a strategy and shift responses accordingly. The patient must sort 64 cards on the basis of 4 stimulus cards containing geometric forms of different numbers, colors, and shapes. The patient must deduce the sorting principle from the examiner's "right" or "wrong" response to each placement. After 10 consecutive cards have been correctly sorted, the examiner shifts the principle of sorting, and the patient must shift to this new strategy.

The neuropsychological assessment often concludes with a "personality" or behavior inventory. Perhaps the most well-known is the Minnesota Multiphasic Personality Inventory-2 (MMPI-2). The MMPI-2 is a questionnaire originally developed to measure clinical personality disorders and psychopathology. The MMPI-2 has 10 clinical scales, which assess 10 major categories of abnormal human behavior (hypochondriasis, depression, hysteria, psychopathic deviate, femininity/masculinity, paranoia, psychasthenia, schizophrenia, mania, and social introversion). The MMPI-2 also contains validity scales, which assess the patient's general test-taking attitude and whether items were answered in a truthful and accurate manner. The MMPI-2 validity scales are useful in assessing for malingering or embellishment. There is a "Restructured Form" of the MMPI-2, which contains 338 items and 9 validity and 42 homogeneous substantive scales.

To these traditional batteries and tests, there is the addition of a brief neuropsychological battery, the Repeated Battery for the Assessment of Neuropsychological Status (RBANS). This instrument contains five domains made up of subtests: immediate memory (list learning, story memory), visuospatial/constructional (figure copy, line orientation), language (picture naming, semantic fluency), attention (digit span, coding), and delayed memory (list learning, list recognition, story memory, figure recall). The subtests are brief, and the entire battery takes approximately 30 minutes. Studies indicate that the RBANS has value as a screening instrument and cannot take the place of the usual and more extensive neuropsychological assessment.

The RBANS has been particularly useful in repeat evaluations and measuring change over time.

The Report and Interpretation

Timeliness, format, and organization are initial considerations in the neuropsychological report (Table 17.4). Timeliness of the report, as well as the availability of the neuropsychologist to discuss it, are essential in clinical decision-making. The format is a consideration because some neuropsychological reports may be relatively unstructured and narrative with limited outline of the findings and their interpretation. Most reports, however, are professionally organized into an initial extensive interview followed by a description of the tests, the summary of the results, and a discussion with conclusions. Sometimes these reports are quite long, of 10 to 20 pages in length, and may lack practicality in a busy clinical setting. Referring clinicians may be tempted to go straight to the discussion and conclusions and miss the valuable history obtained by

TABLE 17.4 Structure of the Neuropsychological Assessment and Report	
Indication for Referral	Mild or subtle deficits
	Cognitive severity for intervention, rehabilitation
	Distinguish psychiatric conditions
	Pattern of cognitive profile
	Capacity, legal
Battery and Tests	Cognitive domains assessed
	Fixed or flexible battery
	Individual tests chosen
Test Administration	Length, requiring more than one session
	Administration by psychometrist or neuropsychologist
	Fatigue, waning effort, cooperation
	Emotional or psychiatric factors
Context of Results	Clinical assessment and testing
	Demographic variables such as age, education, sociocultural, and linguistic
	Premorbid estimation and method used
	Normative data used to compare patient
Content of Report	Timelines and availability
	Organization of report, including the history and interview
	Table with actual scores, numerical data, and applicable norms
	Process interpretation and qualitative description of cognitive performance
	Pattern of cognitive deficit and presence of scatter
	Conclusions

an interviewer who spent time listening to the patient and informant. It is important for the report to contain or make available the numerical data, for example, the actual patient scores, percentiles, and normative comparisons. Just as they look at their own lab, x-rays, and brain scans, referring clinicians should get used to reviewing the actual neuropsychological data.

Once the report is received, the referring clinician needs to consider other information in interpreting the results. The test results are not meaningful in and of themselves. The neuropsychological report occurs in the context of the history and behavioral observations, clinical information, and the clinician's MSX. The neuropsychological assessment should be highly complementary to the clinician's MSX, whether it was a brief examination, scales and inventories, or an extended neurobehavioral status examination. The referring clinician must place the patient's performance on these tests within the context of the patient's personal characteristics, such as the patient's age, education, sociocultural background, primary language, and other factors. The referring clinician must also consider the results in the context of the patient's estimated premorbid status and how it was determined. Some knowledge of the normative data used for comparison can be useful in understanding whether the patient was impaired. In addition, consider the patient's emotional and psychiatric status (anxiety, depression, motivation) and whether it was a factor in test performance.

Two other aspects of interpretation of a neuropsychological report are whether all major cognitive domains were covered and whether there was discrepant performance across these different domains. Quickly assess whether the batteries were too long or short and whether there were appropriate tests for the clinical problem and referral question. Most normal patients show a relative homogeneous performance across cognitive domains, but patients often do better on some tests versus others. Some areas are sensitive to brain disorders such as mental control/attention or psychomotor speed, whereas other areas are more resilient to brain disease such as breadth of word knowledge or fund of general information. The presence of variability of performance across different tests can provide diagnostic clues in terms of etiology and underlying mechanisms. The pattern of this "scatter" on neuropsychological measures, with some low scores and other normal ones, suggests the cognitive areas that are particularly affected by disease or specific disorders.

The patient's performance on neuropsychological tests benefits from a qualitative as well as a quantitative interpretation. The clinician can scrutinize the neuropsychological report for any "process" interpretation of how and what strategies were used to perform the tasks. In addition to the presence of errors and absolute results, this "process approach" observes and analyzes the steps and strategy used in actual performance on the cognitive tasks. A process interpretation may be more likely if a skilled neuropsychologist was present during the administration of the tests, as opposed to a psychometric technician. In this regard, the availability of the neuropsychologist to discuss the results can be extremely valuable.

Conclusions

The neuropsychological assessment plays an important role in mental status assessment. The mental status examiner must be knowledgeable on when to refer for neuropsychological testing, on the nature of the administered tests, and on the interpretation of the results. Neuropsychological testing is particularly valuable in assessing for mild or subtle cognitive deficits, determining severity of cognitive impairment for management, differentiating from psychiatric conditions, evaluating the cognitive profile patterns, and processing legal or capacity issues. The referring clinician should understand something of the content of the battery and the major or more common neuropsychological tests used in assessing the patient. Finally, in interpreting the neuropsychological report, referring clinicians must place the results in the context of the patient's clinical evaluation, personal characteristics, and his or her own mental status evaluation

Chapter 18

Tele-Neurobehavior and Computerized Cognitive Tests

The application of telemedicine extends to the administration of the mental status examination via telephone or videoconferencing and the use of computers for cognitive testing. "Tele-neurobehavior" is defined here as the use of telecommunications to evaluate neurocognition and related behavior in patients who are at different sites than the examiner. The COVID-19 pandemic has accelerated the need for tele-neurobehavior, which was already developing at a rapid pace. Similarly, the increasing role of computers in neuropsychology has spawned the field of dedicated computerized cognitive tests. These two areas are interrelated, not only in the interface with computer technology, but also in the automatization of cognitive testing. The future clearly signals greater application of mental status testing remotely, via tele-neurobehavior, often with the help of computerized stimuli and responses.

Tele-Neurobehavior

Telemedicine allows access to health care at a distance, including for people who live in remote places or who cannot easily travel to medical centers. Clinical visits via telephone or computer-based videoconferencing allow greater availability not only to routine medical care but also to neurological, psychiatric, neuropsychological, and other specialty evaluations. Patients need not travel to clinics only to linger in waiting rooms for brief in-person encounters with specialists or other clinicians. Moreover, with COVID-19 and other similar situations, telemedicine facilitates the maintenance of social distancing and, when necessary, isolation from others. In addition to direct communication via telephone, e-mail, or real-time "synchronous" videoconferencing, telemedicine includes "asynchronous" (store-and-forward) transmission of the patient's prior medical information,

laboratory findings, and neuroimaging. This section focuses on telephone and synchronous videoconferencing for mental status assessment before going on to discuss computerized cognitive testing.

Tele-neurobehavior involves the telephone or videoconferencing administration of the mental status tasks and mental status scales described in prior chapters. Some aspects of the mental status examination are more amenable to testing via telecommunications than others. Using telephone or videoconferencing, the mental status examiner can easily test mental control/attention, orientation, spoken language and speech, verbal memory and semantic knowledge, and visual stimuli recognition. The examination of constructional and spatial abilities, written calculations and related functions, and some executive operations require more planning and effort. Tele-neurobehavior also relies heavily on verbal responses from the patient, whereas, assessing visual, motor, or behavioral responses requires some modification of test administration. In summary, with some training and preparation, the examiner can perform a complete mental status examination via videoconferencing and much of it via telephone.

Despite its benefits, clinicians must first consider whether tele-neurobehavior for mental status assessment is appropriate for each patient. Most patients are comfortable with telephone encounters, and this continues to be an important choice, particularly for those who have visual or physical limitations that preclude videoconferencing. In addition, the elderly and those from lower educational and socioeconomic backgrounds may prefer telephone encounters because of a lack of familiarity, experience, comfort, or access to computers. Patients who are too cognitively impaired or disturbed may not be able to participate in either telephone encounters or videoconferencing.

After concluding a patient's eligibility for tele-neurobehavior there are several preliminary recommendations before testing. The examiner should have an initial routine that includes an introduction of himself/herself (identity, credentials, institution) and a request for verification of the patient's identity and location. The examiner needs to verify the patient's telephone number, should they get disconnected or it is needed during either a videoconferencing or a telephone session. Explain the purpose of the encounter and that it is private, confidential, and not being recorded without permission. The examiner then obtains informed consent from the patient or the caregiver if the patient is unable to give proper consent. The consent can be electronic but should be included in the clinical note. Determine who else, if anyone, will be participating in the session, either on the examiner's side, for example, other clinicians, trainees, therapists, or on the patient's side, for example, caregivers, facilitators. The examiner must assure that the patient is comfortable with this. If caregivers participate, determine if speakerphone, conference call, or, if video, a linked-in participation is indicated. The examiner then administers the mental status tests and tasks simulating, as much as possible, a traditional in-person session. Beyond the application of mental status tasks and the neurobehavioral status examination, there are specific considerations involved in the use of individual mental status scales by telephone or videoconferencing.

MENTAL STATUS SCALES BY TELEPHONE ENCOUNTERS

Examiners have introduced a number of modifications of the Mini-Mental State Examination (MMSE) for administration over the telephone. A 22-item version of the MMSE administered as part of the Adult Lifestyles and Function Interview (ALFI) omits eight items of the original MMSE that require visual cues or assessment. The ALFI-MMSE specifically omits the three-step command, reading and written samples, the intersecting pentagons, the floor orientation, and one of the two naming items (changing the other to asking for the name of the object they are speaking into). A 26-item version, the Telephone MMSE (TMMSE), modifies the ALFI-MMSE, adding back a three-step command and including recall of the patient's telephone number (Fig. 18.1). The TMMSE, which takes 5 to 10 minutes to administer, appears valid and comparable to the traditional MMSE with a cut-off score for dementia of ≤20. Another widely used MMSE-based scale is the Telephone Interview for Cognitive Status (TICS), an 11-item screening test (maximum score of 41 points) developed for assessing cognitive function in patients with Alzheimer disease. The TICS is longer than the MMSE as it includes a 10 word list learning task, responsive naming, and other items, yet it only takes approximately 10 minutes to administer on the telephone. The TICS has several variants itself (TICS-M, TICS-30, TICS-40), which include delayed word recall or other changes (Table 18.1). Two additional telephone scales derived from the MMSE are the 34-item Telephone Modified Mini-Mental Status Exam (T3MS), and the 4-item Telephone Assessed Mental State (TAMS).

Telephone-administered mental status scales that are not derived from the MMSE similarly omit visual items and other comparable modifications to traditional scales. These scales include the Structured Telephone Interview for Dementia Assessment (STIDA), Six-Item Screener, Telephone Screening Protocol (TELE), Telephone Cognitive Assessment Battery (TCAB), Hopkins Verbal Learning Test (HVLT), Memory Impairment Screen by Telephone (MIS-T), Category Fluency Test (CF-T), Blessed Telephone Information-Memory-Concentration Test (Blessed TIMC), Cognitive Assessment for Later Life Status (CALLS) instrument, and others (Table 18.2). Of particular interest is the Telephone Montreal Cognitive Assessment (MoCA), or the "MoCA-Blind," which is the MoCA stripped of its visual elements (Fig. 18.2). This version has 22 items with a cutoff for cognitive impairment of 19.

Advantages and Disadvantages. Telephone screening tools appear to have sufficient sensitivity and specificity to screen for dementia. These tools, particularly those that are derived from the MMSE, have adequate validity and reliability when compared with the in-person MMSE, but must be further validated with the NBSE or with neuropsychological testing. Telephone mental status scales are of particular value for follow-up assessments and monitoring the course of patients with dementia, but, like most mental status scales, they cannot accurately detect mild cognitive impairments. Contributing to this is that they are limited to verbal responses and are not good for assessing visuospatial or sensorimotor impairments. Their administration can be very difficult for patients with severe dementia and for those who are hearing impaired. In addition, the examiner must assure that patients do not take notes, write words down, consult external aids such as calendars, or ask for help during testing.

PATIENT NAME: _____ ID#:_____ PATIENT LOCATION: _____

Exam Date: _____ Date of Admit: _____ Examiner: _____

Patient Data: Age: _____ Years of Education: _____ Handed: RT/LT Sex: _____ Race: _____

Orientation:
1. Date _____
2. Year _____
3. Month _____
4. Day _____
5. Season _____
6. Phone number where you can usually be reached _____
7. Hospital _____
8. City _____
9. County _____
10. State _____

Registration:
11. Cook _____
12. Blue _____
13. Horse _____

Recall: (after ~3 min)
19. Cook _____
20. Blue _____
21. Horse _____

Language:
22. What is the name of the object through which we are speaking?_____
23. No, ifs, ands, or buts _____
24. Say hello, _____
25. tap the mouthpiece of the phone 3 times, _____
26. then say "I'm back". _____

TOTAL SCORE: _____/26

Attention: (only score highest one)
14. 93____ D____ _____
15. 86____ L____ _____
16. 79____ R____ _____
17. 72____ O____ _____
18. 65____ W____ _____

Fig. 18.1 26-Item Telephone Mini-Mental State Examination. (Modified from: Newkirk LA, Kim JM, Thompson JM, Tinklenberg JR, Yesavage JA, Taylor JL. Validation of a 26-point telephone version of the Mini-Mental State Examination. *J Geriatr Psychiatry Neurol.* 2004;17(2):81–87.)

MENTAL STATUS SCALES BY VIDEOCONFERENCING

The videoconferencing presentation of mental status scales is an improvement on telephone encounters, although the scales or testing must still be modified for administration. For example, examiners have used the MMSE as a 28-item version without the written sentence or copy of the intersecting pentagons, and this video-conferencing version has shown similar results as the

TABLE 18.1   The Telephone Interview for Cognitive Status (TICS) and Versions: Standard TICS, 41 items; TICS-M, 50 items; TICS-30, 30 items; TICS-40, 40 items
Instructions for Standard TICS [brackets indicate scoring]
To Proctor: In a couple of minutes, I am going to be asking [patient] a number of different questions to test his/her thinking and memory. Before we start, I need to ask you whether the address I have for your current location is correct. Please don't repeat it out loud if [patient] is in the room with you since I will be asking him/her the same question in a few minutes. Is your current address [patient's address]? Please be sure that all papers, pencils, books, calendars, newspapers, and everything else that might provide distraction or visual cues are removed from [patient's] sight. Also, please be sure that the room is quiet; there should be no television, radio, or music playing. Some of the questions may be difficult for [patient] to answer. He/She may ask you for help. If he/she does, just encourage him/her to do as well as he/she can. He/She should guess if necessary. Please do not give him/her any answers or hints. O.K.? If you are [patient] ready, please put him/her on the phone.
To Patient: I am going to ask you some questions to test your memory. Some of these are likely to be easy for you, but some may be difficult. Please bear with me and try to answer all the questions as best you can. If you can't answer a question, don't worry. Just try your best. Are you ready?
1. Please tell me your full name. [2] (Not in TICS-30 or TICS-40 [0])
2. What is today's date? What day of the week is it? or What season is it? [5]
3. Where are you right now? What number is that? What is your zip code? [5] (TICS-M has age and phone number [2]; TICS-30 and TICS-40 has address [3])
4. Please count backward from 20 to 1. [2]
5. I am going to read you a list of words. Please listen carefully and try to remember them. When I am done, tell me as many of the words as you can, in any order. Ready? The words are… cabin, pipe, elephant, chest, silk, theater, watch, whip, pillow, giant…. Now tell me all the words you can remember. [10]
6. I would like you to take the number 100 and subtract 7…. Now keep subtracting 7 from the answer until I tell you to stop. [5]
7. What do people usually use to cut paper? How many things are in a dozen? What do you call the prickly green plant that lives in the desert? What animal does wool come from? [4] (TICS-30 and TICS-40 only have two [2])
8. Please repeat after me: "No ifs, ands, or buts." Now, please repeat this after me: "Methodist Episcopal." [2] (TICS-30 and TICS-40 only have one [1])
9. Who is the president of the United States right now? Who is the vice-president? [2] (TICS-M includes first and last names [4])
10. With your finger, tap five times on the part of the phone you speak into. [2] (Not in TICS-30 or TICS-40 [0])
11. I am going to say a word and I want you to give me its opposite. For example, if I said "hot," you would say "cold." What is the opposite of "west"? What is the opposite of "generous"? [2] (Not in TICS-30 or TICS-40 [0])
12. Delay Word Recall—(Not in TICS [0]; Present in TICS-M and TICS-40 [10])
For Standard TICS: Total Possible Score 41
Suggested qualitative interpretive ranges 33–41 nonimpaired, 26–32 ambiguous, 21–25 mildly impaired; ≤20 moderately to severely impaired

Brandt J, Spencer M, Folstein M. The telephone interview for cognitive status. *Neuropsychiatry Neuropsychol Behav Neurol.* 1988;1:111–117.

Fong TG, Fearing MA, Jones RN, et al. Telephone interview for cognitive status: creating a crosswalk with the Mini-Mental State Examination. *Alzheimers Dement.* 2009;5(6):492–497.

in-person 30-item version in the same patients. For videoconferencing, clinicians have administered the other in-person scales with similar modifications that primarily eliminate written responses or visuospatial constructions. Alternatively, it is preferable to still use the entire in-person scales by videoconferencing but with modification of administration. For example, for the full MoCA, instruct the patient to get a white sheet of paper and a pencil or pen, and then show the patient only the visual section (first eight points) of the MoCA via computer

TABLE 18.2 Mental Status Scales for Telephone Administration

Based Primarily or Originally Derived from MMSE
1. Telephone version of the MMSE (ALFI-MMSE)
2. The 26-point telephone version of the Mini-Mental Status Examination (TMMSE)
3. Telephone Interview for Cognitive Status (TICS)
4. Modified Telephone Interview for Cognitive Status (TICS-M) (also not TICS-30 and TICS-40 versions)
5. Telephone adaptation of the Modified Mini-Mental State Exam (T3MS)
6. Telephone Assessed Mental State (TAMS)
Not Based Primarily or Originally Derived from MMSE
7. Blessed Telephone Information—memory—concentration test (TIMC)
8. Brief Screen for Cognitive Impairment (BSCI)
9. Brief Test of Adult Cognition by Telephone (BTACT)
10. Cognitive Assessment for Later Life Status (CALLS)
11. Cognitive Telephone Screening Instrument (COGTEL)
12. Hopkins Verbal Learning Test (HVLT)
13. Memory and Aging Telephone Screen (MATS)
14. Memory Impairment Screen Telephone (MIS-T)
15. Minnesota Cognitive Acuity Screen (MCAS)
16. Short Portable Mental Status Questionnaire (SPMSQ-T)
17. Six-Item Screener (SIS)
18. Structured Telephone Interview for Dementia Assessment (STIDA)
19. Telephone Cognitive Assessment Battery (TCAB)
20. Telephone Montreal Cognitive Assessent (T-MoCA or MoCA-BLIND) and Short version of Telephone Montreal Cognitive Assessment (T-MoCA-Short)
21. Telephone Screening Protocol (TELE)

Castanho TC, Amorim L, Zihl J, Palha JA, Sousa N, Santos NC. Telephone-based screening tools for mild cognitive impairment and dementia in aging studies: a review of validated instruments. *Front Aging Neurosci.* 2014;6:16.

share screen (Fig. 18.3). After the patient completes this section, the examiner tells the patient to: "Please fold the paper in half and set it and your pencil off to the side (or place in a folder)." The rest of the MoCA remains the same except for vigilance (read a sequence of letters and have the patient tap every time he or she hears the letter "A") and orientation for place (ask the patient to give the name of the clinic or institution and city where you are at). These altered presentations need much more study, but the videoconferencing versions tend to be comparable to their paper-and-pencil versions at least for moderately impaired patients. In general, patients with severe or advanced dementia tend to do worse with videoconference assessments compared with in-person assessments.

There are a number of procedures that are particularly important for mental status scale presentations by videoconferencing. First, the examiner needs to attend to the environment. In addition to quiet, private places absent of distractions or interruptions, the environment needs good lighting without glare from windows, uncomplicated backgrounds without personal or controversial objects, and good sound acoustics. Second, the examiner should attend to the internet connectivity. On both the examiner's and patient's end, the connection should not be public or unsecured Wi-Fi, and the internet connection should be encrypted. There also needs to be sufficient broadband so that the video and audio do not freeze, fade, or break. Third, the examiner evaluates the equipment, including its readiness, video and audio quality, and the potential for technological problems as previously noted, (have the patient's telephone number ready if video fails). A large display size and widescreen may help in making behavioral observations and in projecting

MONTREAL COGNITIVE ASSESSMENT / MoCA-BLIND
Version 7.1 Original Version

Name:
Education:
Sex:
Date of birth:
Date:

MEMORY		FACE	VELVET	CHURCH	DAISY	RED	POINTS
Read list of words, subject must repeat them. Do 2 trials even if 1st trial is successful. Do a recall after 5 minutes.	1st trial						No points
	2nd trial						

ATTENTION

Read list of digits (1 digit/sec.) Subject has to repeat them in the forward order   [ ] 2 1 8 5 4
Subject has to repeat them in the backward order   [ ] 7 4 2   __ / 2

Read list of letters. The subject must tap with his hand at each letter A.   No point if ≥ 2 errors

[ ]   F B A C M N A A J K L B A F A K D E A A A J A M O F A A B   __ / 1

Serial 7 subtraction starting at 100

[ ] 93   [ ] 86   [ ] 79   [ ] 72   [ ] 65

4 or 5 correct subtractions: **3 pts**, 2 or 3 correct: **2 pts**, 1 correct: **1 pt**, 0 correct: **0 pt**   __ / 3

LANGUAGE

Repeat: I only know that John is the one to help today. [ ]
The cat always hid under the couch when dogs were in the room. [ ]   __ / 2

Fluency / Name maximum number of words in one minute that begin with the letter F.
[ ] _____ (N ≥ 11 words)   __ / 1

ABSTRACTION   [ ] train - bicycle
Similarity between e.g. banana - orange = fruit   [ ] watch - ruler   __ / 2

DELAYED RECALL	Has to recall words	FACE	VELVET	CHURCH	DAISY	RED		
	With no cue	[ ]	[ ]	[ ]	[ ]	[ ]	Points for UNCUED recall only	__ / 5
Optional	Category cue							
	Multiple choice cue							

ORIENTATION	[ ] Date [ ] Month [ ] Year [ ] Day [ ] Place [ ] City	__ / 6

© Z. Nasreddine MD   **www.mocatest.org**   Normal ≥ 18 / 22

TOTAL	__ / 22

Add 1 point if ≤ 12 yr edu

Administered by:_____

Fig. 18.2 Montreal Cognitive Assessment/MoCA-BLIND. (© Z. Nasreddine MD, Reprinted from www.mocatest.org.)

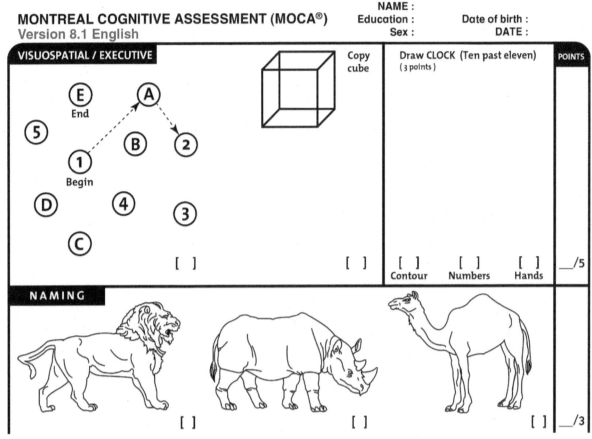

Fig. 18.3 Montreal Cognitive Assessment (MOCA©)-Visual Items. (Reprinted from www.mocatest.org.)

computerized stimuli with the screen-sharing option (rather than holding stimulus materials up to the camera). Fourth, the examiner, and facilitator if available, need to consider the patient's setup and whether he or she has all materials needed for the session. The examiner should ask the patient to hide the self-view window and help the patient arrange the camera for best visual transmission, including refocusing it on the patient performing a task as on a table. Finally, the role of a caregiver or facilitator during videoconferencing needs definition before or at onset of the session. A caregiver or facilitator can help with instructions and can discontinue the assessment if they observe significant patient distress or difficulties, but they should know the boundaries between facilitating the examination and trying to help the patient do better.

Advantages and Disadvantages. Tele-neurobehavior through videoconferencing greatly facilitates the examination of patients at remote sites and in

underserved areas. Patients are more likely to keep a tele-neurobehavior videoconferencing appointment than to present for an in-person assessment, and most patients and families seem to be satisfied with the telemedicine experience. Concerns with tele-neurobehavior via videoconferencing include the potential distancing effect on the clinician's relationship with the patient. There is less access to social feedback from eye contact (somewhat mitigated by the patient looking at the camera instead of at the examiner's image), facial microexpressions, and body language. There are also limitations on the ability to observe performance and behavioral responses during the administration of cognitive screening. Yet behavioral observations of the way the patient actually performs the tests can be as important as the endpoint scores. There are other aspects of mental status examination by videoconferencing that cannot be tested as well as in the in-person setting unless the examiner makes changes to the presentation, for example, screen sharing a computerized visuospatial stimulus, focusing the camera on the patient as he/she copies it, and then having them share screen or hold up their copy for a screen shot.

Computerized Cognitive Testing

Computers have opened up new ways to administer, record, score, and even interpret cognitive testing without relying on human examiners. Computerized cognitive tests are available for administration on smartphones, tablets, laptops, and desktop computers. Examiners can perform cognitive tests through downloaded software with computer-administered versions, or they can use web-based versions of cognitive tests. There are two types of computerized cognitive tests, those that are adaptations or conversions of traditional paper-and-pencil tests to computerized formats, and those that are primary computerized cognitive tests developed to take advantage of the speed and accuracy of computers.

Computerized testing has unique aspects that distinguish them from traditional mental status testing. They mostly relate to the exceptional ability to process multiple information at great speeds. Computers are very good for processing speed and reaction times, continuous performance and other attention tests, N-back and other working memory tasks. They are less helpful for traditional verbal delayed recall memory, language, visuospatial constructional ability, praxis, and written calculations. Another advantage of computerized cognitive tests is that they improve on the standardization of test administration and stimulus presentation. They can automate the recording of responses, report on many aspects of performance, calculate scores, and even modify test difficulty during testing (computer adaptive testing). Computers can quickly analyze scores in comparison to normative data and generate numerical results and interpretations based on statistical comparisons. Some computerized tests have an interpretive expert algorithm whose routines generate a clinical interpretation.

Computerized cognitive tests are not directly comparable to examiner-administered tests. Even when a traditional examiner-administered test is only slightly modified for computer administration, it still becomes a new and different test. This is because computerized and in-person administration differ in degree of examiner supervision, stimulus presentation, response methods, and a number of procedures during testing. For example, the patient may respond with keyboard strokes, use of a mouse, a response pad, a touch screen, or even voice recognition. For these reasons, even minimally modified computer adaptations of traditional tests are new instruments that need full psychometric determinations. Their reliabilities have been generally comparable to traditional testing, but their validities may not be fully established.

PART A: ADAPTATION OF CURRENT TRADITIONAL TESTS

Clinicians and investigators have adapted the current mental status examination, mental status scales and inventories, and neuropsychological tests for computerized administration. There is no standard way to modify most traditional tests for computerized presentation, with most modifications trying to simulate the in-person test as much as possible. Computerized mental status scales range from the clock drawing to the Alzheimer Disease Assessment Scale-Cog (ADAS-Cog) and the Informant Questionnaire on Cognitive Decline in the Elderly (IQCODE). Computerized neuropsychological tests include versions for Digit Span Forward and Backward, Controlled Oral Word Association Test and verbal fluency measures, Boston Naming Test, supraspan verbal learning tests such as the Hopkins Verbal Learning Test-Revised, Repeatable Battery for the Assessment of Neuropsychological Status, Wisconsin Card Sort Test, Stroop Test, and many others. Variations of administration of these tests range from computer facilitation, observation during testing on a computer or tablet, to total self-administration. Because of the differences from their traditional format, computerized versions need normative and other psychometric data. The normative data from traditional tests does not automatically apply to a computerized version of the same test. The examiner's report should include the main modifications and adaptation of the standardized in-person tests, whether traditional norms were used, and any consequent limitations in the interpretation.

PART B: PRIMARY COGNITIVE TESTS DEVELOPED FOR COMPUTERIZED PRESENTATION

There has been increasing development of automated cognitive batteries designed specifically to take advantage of computer technology and speed in processing (Table 18.3). These computerized tests may be intended for clinicians, neuropsychologists, and others, and they are sometimes linked to commercial cognitive rehabilitation

TABLE 18.3   **Primary Computerized Cognitive Tests**
1. Amsterdam Cognition Scan
2. Automated Neuropsychological Assessment Metrics (ANAM)
3. Brain on Track (BoT) test
4. BrainCheck
5. Cambridge Brain Sciences: Online Cognitive Assessment
6. Cambridge Cognitive Examination CAT Battery (computerized adaptive testing)
7. Cambridge Neuropsychological Test Automated Battery (CANTAB)
8. CANS-MCI (Computer administered neuropsychological screen)
9. CANTAB Mobile and CANTAB insight
10. Clinical Dementia Rating (CDR) Computerized Assessment System
11. CNS Vital Signs
12. CogniFit
13. COGNIGRAM Digital Cognitive Assessment System
14. Cognistat Assessment System (CAS-II) and Cognistat Five
15. Cognitive Assessment Screening Instrument (CASI)—computerized
16. Cognitive Function Scanner (CFS)
17. Cognitive Skills Index (CSI)
18. Cognitive Symptom Checklists
19. Cognivue
20. CogScreen: Aeromedical Edition
21. COGselftest and Cogselftest-Medinteract
22. CogSport
23. Cogstate tests
24. Computer Assessment of Mild Cognitive Impairment (CAMCI)
25. Computerized Neuropsychological Test Battery (CNTB)
26. Computerized Neuropsychological Testing System (WebCNP)
27. Digital Montreal Cognitive Assessment (MoCA)
28. Food for the Brain Cognitive Function Test
29. Headminder Concussion Resolution Index (CRI)
30. Immediate Post-Concussion Assessment and Cognitive Testing (ImPACT)
31. Lumosity NeuroCognitiv Performance Test
32. MemTrax Test
33. MicroCog
34. Mindstreams tests
35. Neurobehavioral Evaluation System-3 (NES-3)
36. NeuroTrax–BrainCare testing
37. NIH Toolkit and NIH EXAMINER
38. Philips' IntelliSpace Cognition
39. Specialty Automated Systems Online Cognitive Tests
40. Tablet-Based Cognitive Assessment Tool (TabCat)
41. TestMyBrain (TMB) Digital Neuropsychological Toolkit
42. Touch Panel-Type Dementia Assessment Scale

See: Zygouris S, Tsolaki M. Computerized cognitive testing for older adults: a review. *Am J Alzheimers Dis Other Demen.* 2015;30(1):13–28.

programs. Moreover, there are primary computerized tests designed for specific evaluations, such as for concussions, sports-related monitoring, mood disorders, epilepsy, cardiovascular surgery, military- or deployment-related monitoring, and age-related neurocognitive disorders. They can range from a computer-assisted battery, in which an examiner presents the stimuli and records the responses, all the way to fully self-administered tests, with the immediate availability of reports detailing and interpreting performance. Most commonly they depend on an examiner who provides instruction and helps initiate the testing. The National Institutes of Health (NIH) Toolbox Cognitive Battery, although meant for research,

is worth reviewing because the individual descriptions of the computerized cognitive tasks give an overall picture of the nature and content of primary computerized cognitive tasks and their brevity (Table 18.4).

Advantages. There are a number of advantages of computerized testing. They are fast (<2 hours) tests that can accurately measure performance on time sensitive tasks, such as information processing speed and response times. They are automated in their administration and scoring, with interpretive algorithms and the ability to tailor the testing to the patient's abilities through computerized adaptive testing. Overall, they are more cost-effective than

TABLE 18.4 National Institutes of Health (NIH) Toolbox Cognitive Battery		
Episodic Memory	Picture Sequence Memory Test; 7 minutes	Participants are asked to reproduce a sequence of pictures that are shown on the screen. Different practice sequences and test items for participants of different ages.
Executive Function and Attention	Flanker Inhibitory Control and Attention; 3 minutes	Measures attention and inhibitory control. Participant focuses on a given stimulus while inhibiting attention to stimuli flanking it.
Working Memory	List Sorting Working Memory Test; 7 minutes	Measures working memory. Participant recalls and sequences different visually and orally presented stimuli.
Language	Picture Vocabulary Test; 4 minutes	Measures receptive vocabulary administered in a computer adaptive test (CAT) format. Respondents select the picture that most closely matches the meaning of the word.
Language	Oral Reading Recognition; 3 minutes	Measures reading decoding skill and crystallized abilities. Participant is asked to read and pronounce letters and words as accurately as possible.
Executive Functions	Dimensional Change Card Sort Test; 4 minutes	Measures cognitive flexibility and attention. Pictures are presented varying along two dimensions (e.g., shape and color). The dimension for sorting is indicated by a cue word on the screen.
Processing Speed	Pattern Comparison Processing Speed Test; 3 minutes	Measures speed of processing. Participants discern whether two side-by-side pictures are the same or not, with 85 seconds to respond to as many items as possible. Items are simple so as to purely measure processing speed.
Immediate Recall (supplemental)	Auditory Verbal Learning Test; 3 minutes	Measures immediate recall. Unrelated words presented via audio recording and participant recalls as many as possible. Supplements Picture Sequence Memory Test or an alternative if participant's visual limitations preclude administering Picture Sequence Memory Test. Version differs from some other available versions.
Processing Speed (supplemental)	Oral Symbol Digit Test; 3 minutes	Measures speed of processing. Symbols on the screen are associated with a number, then presented with symbols without numbers. Participant says each number that goes with that symbol. Supplements Pattern Comparison Processing Speed Test or as an alternative when a participant's motoric limitations preclude administering the Pattern Comparison Processing Speed Test.

in-person tests and more accessible to patients in remote and underserved areas. Testing can occur in a variety of environments from hospital inpatients to sports teams on the field.

Disadvantages. There are a number of potential challenges to the adoption of primary computerized cognitive tests. First, most of the currently available computerized cognitive tests lack sufficient validation and reliability determinations and normative data across different populations. Reliability can vary significantly with different computer and screen variables and with environmental factors, such as sitting on a couch or are a table, good versus poor lighting, the presence of distractions and interruptions, and the motivation and effort expended by the patient in performing the tests. Second, for software installed programs, there are issues with their interaction with the user's operating system and hardware (central processing unit speed, memory, clock, screen resolution, and refresh rate). Although the web-based versions mitigate some of these issues, they raise additional concerns about the privacy and security of patient data transmitted over the internet. Third, there are issues with the use and dissemination of these computerized cognitive tests. Many are targeted to end-users or to others without training in the field, and general marketing can result in errors in the interpretation and application of the results of these tests. Ultimately, the examiner needs information on the test's psychometrics and administration variables, technical specifications, security measures for patient data, and the qualifications for those who can administer and interpret these tests.

Conclusions

Tele-neurobehavior is an increasing part of the future of clinical mental status testing. Neurobehavioral status examination tasks and mental status scales can be effectively administered by telephone and, especially, by videoconference, often with slight modifications. They are most effective for established dementia rather than for detecting milder cognitive difficulties or evaluating severe dementia. Tele-neurobehavior can be particularly useful and efficient in the patient's cognitive follow-up.

Computerized cognitive tests are also an increasing part of the future. Computerized versions of standard neuropsychological tests can increase efficiency provided that they have been validated and have reliability and other psychometric determinations as for a new test. Primary computerized cognitive tests are particularly suited for rapid, efficient, and cost-effective screening for specific cognitive disorders, such as concussions, or for monitoring, such as in clinical drug trials. These tests also need more psychometric evaluations and normative data from large and diverse populations. This technology may keep growing in importance, in areas such as greater automated speech assessment, virtual reality evaluations for visuospatial and other abilities, and sensorimotor tracking.

Index of Mental Status Tasks

Arousal, Attention, and Other Fundamental Functions

AROUSAL

1. **Verbal and Physical Stimulation.** If a patient is not awake or responding to the environment, the examiner loudly calls the patient's name while tapping him/her and, if still unresponsive, the clinicians applies pressure to the sternum or a fingernail or pinches the Achilles tendon.

2. **Responsiveness to Stimulation.** The examiner notes the type of responsiveness to stimulation. Note eye, verbal, and motor responses. Note whether the patient maintains eyes open and visually fixates, tracks stimuli, or attains eye contact. Note the presence of any verbal responses and their content. Finally, note any reactive movements to stimulation, reflex actions, or posturing. In addition, observe the patient's overall behavior for hypoactivity, hyperactivity, or movement abnormalities, such as myoclonus or tremors. The examiner can semiquantify the eye, verbal, and motor responses with various scales, such as the Glasgow Coma Scale (Chapter 7, Table 7.2).

ATTENTION

1. **Verbal Digit (or Letter) Span.** The examiner explains, "I am going to repeat a series of numbers. Please immediately repeat the same numbers after I give them to you." Random digits are given, one per second, starting with three, at a regular rhythm of presentation (Chapter 5, Fig. 5.1). The patient must repeat the entire sequence in the same order immediately after presentation. If the patient can correctly repeat three digits, the examiner presents four digits, and then five digits, and so forth at increasing series. If the patient incorrectly repeats a string of digits, then another string

of digits at the same series level is repeated. The examiner stops when the patient incorrectly repeats two strings of digits at the same series level. His/her digit span is the level just before missing both trials. A normal performance is correct recitation of seven (±2) digits. A patient attaining fewer than five digits may have a significant attentional problem.

2. **Visual Sequence Span.** An equivalent of the Digit Span Test may be performed as a nonverbal sequence span test using visual stimuli. The examiner asks the patient to serially tap four squares or blocks in the same sequence as tapped by the examiner (Chapter 7, Fig. 7.3). The test can be done with or without verbal input from the examiner or verbal responses from the patient. The procedures are otherwise the same as for the Digit Span Test.

3. **Digits (or Letters) Backward.** In the backward digit span, the patient repeats digits beginning with the last number and in reverse order to the first number. The instructions and methodology are the same as for the forward Digit Span Test with the examiner continuing until the patient incorrectly repeats two strings of digits backward at the same series level. A normal performance is correct backward recitation of five (±2) digits. A patient failing at three or fewer digits may have a significant attentional problem.

4. **Serial Subtraction Tests.** Two common serial subtraction tests are counting backward from 100 by 7s and counting backward from 20 by 3s. In the first, the examiner asks the patient to subtract by 7 beginning with the number 100, for example, 93, 86, 79, 72, 65, et cetera. The number of errors are the number of incorrect subtractions; if the patient makes

an incorrect subtraction at one level, the examiner corrects the patient and instructs the patient to continue subtracting from the corrected number. Alternatively, the subsequent "correct" subtractions are determined from the incorrect number, that is, if the patient subtracts 7 from 100 as 94, then the subsequent correct subtraction is 87 and not 86. An alert patient should be able to get three or more subtractions in a row. Counting backward from 20 by 3s is a similar, but easier, version of serial subtractions.

5. **Spelling "World" Backward.** The examiner gives the patient a word, often the word "world," and asks the patient to spell it backward beginning with the last letter and finishing with the first letter. In contrast to the serial subtraction tasks, the scoring of word backward is by "error of place," that is, a correct performance would require a "d" in the first place, an "l" in the second, et cetera. For example, the score for a response of "d-r-l-o-w" is 3 as the "r" and "l" are absent or in the wrong place, and the score for a response of "d-o-w" is 1.

6. **Calendar in Reverse Order.** Additional reversal tasks include the months of the year in reverse order beginning with December and finishing with January. An easier version is to have the patient recite the days of the week backward from Saturday to Sunday. The item is missed if it is absent or if it is in the wrong sequence.

7. **"A" Cross-Out Test.** The examiner recites a list of 30 or more letters, one per second, and instructs the patient to tap on a table only when they hear the letter "A." An abnormal performance includes any errors of omission in which the patient fails to tap for an "A," or errors of commission in which the patient taps for a letter other than "A." This test can also be done visually by asking the patient to cross out the letter "A" in a written paragraph or on a piece of paper with random letters scattered on the page (Chapter 7, Fig. 7.4). Alternatively, the patient can cross out every instance of a particular letter in a magazine or newspaper paragraph. More than a single omission in 60 seconds suggests a disturbance in sustained attention. Harder versions of this continuous performance measure involve indicating a target letter whenever it appears in a specific sequence, for example, "A" only when followed by "B," or crossing out whole words that have a certain letter.

8. **Visual Search Cancellation Task.** Visual search tasks, which overlap with visuospatial processing, may be administered timed or untimed and involve searching for a target letter or figure on a piece of paper with scattered nontarget, random letters or figures (Chapter 7, Fig. 7.5; Chapter 10, Fig. 10.10). The patient indicates the target letter or figure wherever it appears by marking it or circling it. A good format has at least 60 stimuli and 10% targets, and the patient should be able to locate all of them.

9. **Serial Ordering of Digits.** The examiner can ask the patient to serially order digits by asking the patient to reorder a forward digit span in an ascending order from smallest to largest. For example, if given the series "2-1-3," the correct answer would be "1-2-3." This task has a working memory component but can also indicate difficulties with attention. Most people can serially order four or more digits.

10. **Modified Clinical "N-Back."** In the classical test, the participant hears a series of digits or letters and is asked to indicate if a letter was previously presented a set number of places back, for example, for N-3, the participant would indicate the ones shown in capital letters: n t s j o a **J** p q s t u **S**. In a simpler clinical variation, the examiner recites a long series of digits and, once the examiner stops, asks the patient to repeat the next to last digit in the sequence ("N-1") or, for more challenging testing, two or three back from the last digit in the sequence ("N-2" and "N-3"). Most people have difficulty beyond the N-3 level.

11. **Paced Auditory Serial Addition Test (PASAT).** There are clinical variants of the PASAT, which is a relatively challenging attentional test. It requires the addition of the last numbers in a sequence of numbers, and it can be administered as cumulative addition (adding the last number to the prior sum). Alternatively, ask the patient to add the successive overlapping pairs as rapidly as possible: 5, 2, 7, 3, 4, et cetera (adds last to next to last for 7, 9, 10, 7). This test overlaps with calculations ability and is often difficult for people who are unimpaired.

12. **Trail making A ("Trail Making A") Test** (Chapter 7, Fig. 7.6). The patient must draw a line connecting 25 randomly arrayed numbered circles in ascending numerical order (1-2-3, etc.). After a practice sample, the examiner tells the patient to go as fast as possible without lifting the pencil or pen, points out errors as they occur so that the patient can correct them, and times the overall performance. On the standard timed version, which also reflects psychomotor speed, an average completion time is <30 seconds, and an impaired completion time is greater than approximately 78 seconds. The examiner can give a version of the Trail making A Test in an untimed version to assess strictly for errors (as is done in the Montreal Cognitive Assessment).

13. **Simultaneous Divided Attention Task.** Evaluate the ability to divide attention by simultaneous tasks, such as having the patient do a forward digit span while manually tracking the examiner's moving finger with their index finger. The examiner compares the results of this divided attention task to the results from the single task forward digit span.

14. **Face-Hands Test.** In this divided attention test, the examiner touches the patient on the hands and cheek simultaneously in 10 trials (4 contralateral, 4 ipsilateral, 2 symmetric). Any error in recognizing where the patient was touched suggests impairment, most often from dementia or frontal lobe disease.

PSYCHOMOTOR SPEED AND ACTIVITY

1. **Finger Tapping Test.** This is a test of psychomotor speed and should be tested with both the left and right index finger for approximately 10 seconds each. The patient must keep tapping an index finger on a table until the examiner instructs the patient to stop. A modification of this requires the patient to perform a repetitive movement with the opposite hand, such as supination and pronation, while having them finger tap with the other hand. The examiner records the rapidity of tapping.

2. **Counting Speed.** There are several timed speed tasks available in a routine clinical encounter. First, the examiner has the patient count from one as fast as possible and records the number reached in 10 seconds. Second, the examiner asks the patient to recite the alphabet, or write it in uppercase letters, as fast as possible. The written alphabet should take the patient 30 seconds or less to accomplish. Third, the examiner asks the patient to draw lines between a series of three and five dots as rapidly as possible.

3. **Pole Grasp Test.** Patients grasp a measuring pole at the bottom, let it go, and then grasp it as fast as possible before it falls. The distance between the original and final grasp reflects reaction time.

ORIENTATION

1. **Orientation to Date and Time.** The examiner asks the patient to state the current date and place. Orientation in the clinical setting is a sensitive general measure of awareness, attention, and memory. In the absence of a watch or other obvious display of the time, the patient's knowledge of the exact time of day can be a further extension of the assessment for temporal orientation. Ask the patient to tell you what time it is at the present moment. Normal subjects are orientated to within 4 hours of the time, 3 days of the date, and 2 days of the week, but they should know the month and year.

2. **Orientation to Place.** The next most common disorientation occurs to place, that is, home, clinic or hospital, city, county, state or province, and specific floor or localization in a building. In addition to inquiring whether the patient knows where they are, the examiner can ask what kind of place it is and under what circumstances they are there. Asking for the patient's telephone number is another "place" orientation item. Patients should not be disoriented to place, but they may be off on the floor or ward if they are hospitalized or the city/location if they were taken there without their full awareness.

Language and Speech

SPOKEN LANGUAGE AND SPEECH

1. **Conversational Fluency.** Language fluency is the ability to produce words, phrases, and sentences proficiently and smoothly. The language examination starts with listening to the patient's fluency during spontaneous discourse (with permission, an

auditory recording can be made for later analysis). The examiner may elicit conversation with questions or by asking the patient to describe an activity or a picture, such as the "Cookie Theft" picture from the Boston Diagnostic Aphasia Examination (Chapter 8, Fig. 8.2). The examiner should have a checklist of items to consider for conversational fluency, including approximate words/minute, flow (interruptions from word-finding pauses, hesitancy, or effort), phrase length (four or more words/phrase), presence of agrammatism or telegraphic output (loss of prepositions, conjunctions, and other "functor" words), and presence of dysprosody (Chapter 8, Tables 8.1 and 8.2). Phonemic distortions and substitutions and increased inter-syllabic pauses due to "apraxia of speech" may accompany nonfluent aphasia. During the course of conversational speech, also listen for the information content, for the presence of paraphasic errors (word or phonemic substitutions), and for dysarthric speech.

2. **Controlled Word Association Test.** The examiner instructs the patient to name as many English words that begin with the letter "F" (or "A" or "S") as they can in 1 minute and as quickly as possible. These letters reflect word frequencies in English and vary with the language tested (e.g., in Spanish the corresponding letters would be "P," "M," and "R"). Tell the patient: "I will say a letter of the alphabet. Then I want you to give me as many English words that begin with that letter as quickly as possible. I do not want you to use words that are proper names. Also do not use the same word again with a different ending, such as 'eat' and 'eating' or 'sixty' and 'sixty-one.' Begin when I say the letter." Do not count close word variations of the same word, such as "six," "sixth," "sixtieth," but do count word variations with a different meaning, for example, "sixteen." Normal subjects can list 15 + 5 words/minute for each letter.

3. **Category Word-List Generation (verbal fluency).** Ask the patient to generate a list of as many animals as possible (or other category of items such as grocery items, articles of clothing, cities, colors) in 1 minute. "I am going to ask you to name as many animals as you can in 1 minute. An animal is any living thing that is not a plant. Please wait until we are ready to begin." Do not count proper nouns, plurals, and repetitions in the total correct, but do count word variations or subcategory items (e.g., include both dogs and beagles). Do not suggest subcategories (e.g., "zoo animals"). Normal subjects can list 18 + 6 animals/minute without cueing.

4. **Naming.** The examiner tests word production primarily with confrontational naming, that is, asking the patient to name common items pointed out in the room or a series of pictures, such as the 15-item version of the mini–Boston Naming Test. In confrontational naming, the examiner should test a range of common and uncommon words across different word frequencies. Six readily accessible high-frequency items for naming include key, ring, button, collar, nose, chin; and six additional lower-frequency items include earlobe, eye lashes, lapel, shoelaces, sole or heel of shoe, and watch band or crystal. The examiner may increase the difficulty of word production tasks by asking the patient to "name-by-definition," that is, the examiner provides a definition of an object or action, and the patient provides the appropriate name. A guide to normal performance on all these tasks involves correctly naming all high-frequency items and at least four of six low-frequency ones.

5. **Sentence Comprehension Screening.** The examination of sentence comprehension involves a series of tasks of increasing difficulty. First, there are simple axial and one-step commands such as "close your eyes" and "point to the floor." This can be followed with yes-or-no questions such as "Are you sitting down?" and "Does March come before April?" Then do sequential commands such as "Touch your nose and then your chin" and "first point to the ceiling and then to the door." Finally, evaluate complex grammatical sentence comprehension, for example, "If the lion was killed by the tiger, which animal is dead?" "If we were in a crowd of people and I said, 'there's my wife's brother,' would I be pointing to a man or a woman?"

6. **The Token Test.** A good way of testing comprehension is the token test. This involves presenting 20 tokens of 5 colors each having 2 shapes and 2 sizes and giving commands such as "put

the red circle on the green rectangle" or "before touching the yellow circle, pick up the red rectangle." The examiner can substitute commonly available objects for the tokens, such as pen, pencil, and different coins (Chapter 8, Table 8.3). The sequence of commands include "put the pencil on the coin" and "touch the coin with the pen."

7. **Word Comprehension.** The examiner needs to test the ability to comprehend words and sentences. Problems with word comprehension may be initially evident on confrontational naming tasks. When this occurs, testing should be followed up with word recognition tests. The simplest procedure is to return to misnamed items from the prior naming testing. Give the patient the name and ask him/her to identify it. They can do this by either pointing to the object or picture or by identifying (defining or describing) the item. This "two-way" naming deficit, in which the patient can neither name an item nor point to it on command (despite being able to repeat the name), represents abnormal word comprehension.

8. **Repetition.** The examiner asks the patient to repeat digits, multisyllabic words, phrases, and sentences. Note that tests of repetition do not include "serial speech," which are overlearned sequences (such as counting 1, 2, 3, etc., or the reciting the alphabet) as serial speech is relatively preserved in most aphasics. Begin with single word or short phrase repetitions, for example, "constitutional," "Mississippi River," "hopping hippopotamus," or "Methodist Episcopal," then proceed to longer utterances and sentences. "I'm going to read some sentences to you. Please repeat them back to me exactly the way I say it." Examples include "No ifs, ands, or buts," "they heard him speak on the radio last night," "the truck rolled over the stone bridge," and "the quick brown fox jumped over the lazy dog." The examiner may allow one reattempt at repetition of the sentence if the patient requests it. If the patient succeeds, the examiner may ask for repetition of more complex sentences, for example, "if he comes soon, we will all go away with him."

9. **Prosody.** There may be changes in prosody or intonation at the sentence level and in the stressed or accented syllable in a word (lexical stress). In addition to listening for changes in pitch (rising or falling) and stress (often increased loudness), further screening for prosody can be done with repetition of sentences in different tones and asking the patient to interpret them and then to repeat them with a certain meaning. For example, for prosodic comprehension, emphasize bolded and italicized word in the sentence: ____ I *AM* going to the other movies. ____ I am going to the *OTHER* movies. ____ *I* am going to the other movies. ____ I am going to the other *MOVIES*. ____ I am *GOING* to the other movies. For prosodic fluency, ask the patient to say the sentence with determination, sadness, anticipation, emphasis on himself/herself, and type of place or action.

10. **Speech Examination.** The examiner independently evaluates for apraxia of speech and for dysarthrias during the speech examination. Testing for apraxia of speech, or disturbed speech programming, involves testing for repetition of polysyllabic phrases. The examiner asks the patient to repeat each of the syllables, /pa/, /ta/, and /ka/, individually over and over again as quickly as possible (alternating motor rates), and then to repeat the three together in the sequence /pa-ta-ka/ over and over as quickly as possible (sequencing motor rates). An alternative approach is to ask the patient to repeat the words "catastrophe," "artillery," or "articulatory" as many times as possible in 5 or 10 seconds. The evaluation for dysarthrias involves listening to the patient's speech for loudness, vocal cord function (strained if too apposed, breathy if too open), resonance or nasality from escape of air, articulatory disturbances from labial or lingual mispronunciation, and evidence of slurring from cerebellar system dysfunction. In addition, the examiner may ask the patient to maintain an "aah" sound loudly and for as long as possible to assess respiratory and vocal power.

WRITTEN LANGUAGE AND READING

1. **Reading Test.** The examiner starts by asking the patient to read aloud a short standard paragraph (or, for expediency, a paragraph from a newspaper

or magazine). This reading material should be at the eighth-grade level. Then the examiner tells the patient: "I am going to present a list of words to you, one at a time. Please read each word out loud to the best of your ability." The examiner then asks the patient to read regular words (usual grapheme-phoneme pronunciation), irregular words (irregular grapheme-phoneme pronunciation), and pseudowords (pronounceable nonsense words) aloud, e.g., "mint, blitor, colonel, shout, yacht, flarmic, bouquet, chrome, strotinale, quick, thartrist, pint." When the patient reads aloud, the examiner looks for differential difficulties in the ability to read 1) regularly spelled words (e.g., mint, shout, chrome, quick); 2) irregularly spelled words (e.g., colonel, yacht, bouquet, pint); or 3) pronounceable pseudowords (blitor, flarmic, strotinale, thartrist).

2. **Reading Comprehension.** For reading comprehension, the examiner first presents a list of written names of objects in the room, such as door, sink, table, window, telephone, and then asks the patient to read them and point to the object. If this is successful, then the examiner presents two or more sentences with commands instructing the patient to do something, for example, "Fold this paper in half and put it on the table," and "point to the source of illumination in this room." Reading comprehension may also be tested with written word-picture matching tests and by asking the patient to comprehend words spelled orally.

3. **Writing Test.** First, the examiner asks the patient to copy single letters and a few printed words. Those with apraxic agraphia or spatial agraphia may have abnormal copying. Second, the examiner asks the patient to write a series of words dictated by the examiner. These words can be similar to the ones noted earlier for reading and should include regular words, irregular words, and nonsense pseudowords. Third, the examiner requests the patient to write at least two sentences, one sentence to dictation complete with punctuation, and a second sentence composed by the patient. Examples of sentences to dictation are: "The children are the heirs of the earth"; "it is hard to gauge the size of a sieve"; and "the bride was taken down the aisle by the colonel." Finally,

the examiner can elicit sentences for composition with a command, such as "describe what you did today in a full sentence."

Memory and Semantic Knowledge

DECLARATIVE EPISODIC MEMORY

1. **Three to Four Word Recall.** The examiner can screen declarative episodic memory through the patient's ability to recall a list of words. One easy test in the clinical setting is a three to four word-learning task. On initial presentation, the examiner repeats the words until the patient can repeat all three or four words in no specific order three times in a row, and the examiner records the number of trials necessary for correct repetitions. To avoid further continued rehearsal during the subsequent "interference" period, the patient must do other tasks, such as recalling three current events in the news or performing other cognitive testing. After a 1 or more minute delay, the patient is asked to spontaneously recall the three or four words. A normal recall performance is at least three words. Finally, for missed words, the examiner may ask them to identify the words in a multiple-choice recognition task.

2. **Verbal (Word) List Learning Tests.** For the more extended examination, it is preferable to administer a list of 8 or 10 words with multiple initial repetitions (Chapter 5, Table 5.4; Chapter 9, Table 9.1). Tell the patient that you are going to repeat a list of words; "Please remember them. I will ask you to repeat the word list immediately after I finish." The examiner reads the word list and asks the patient to immediately recall as many words as possible from the list. The examiner repeats this process four or five times. After an interference interval, which can range from 10 to 30 minutes, during which time the patient's attention is engaged in other tasks, the examiner tests the patient's spontaneous recall of the 8 or 10 words. Normal individuals learn most of the list after three or four repetitions and spontaneously recall two-thirds or more of the words on delayed recall. One valuable calculation is the "savings score." This score is the delayed recall score divided by the repetition score on the last registration trial. A savings score of less than 50%

is strongly suggestive of a memory problem not due to decreased registration. The examiner then checks recognition memory and retrieval by giving categorical and/or multiple-choice clues for the words that are not recalled. Normal elderly patients recognize most of the 8 to 10 words. A 2 or more Recognition Index (Total Recognition/2X Delayed Recall) suggests a predominant retrieval deficit, rather than a predominant encoding or storage deficit as seen in Alzheimer disease.

3. **Alternative Verbal Memory Tests.** There are other practical ways to evaluate episodic recent memory in the verbal domain. First, the examiner can give his or her name and that of at least one other in the room, and minutes later ask the patient to recall the names. Disturbed recent memory is suggested if the patient cannot retain any names after 5 minutes. Second, the examiner can ask the patient to recall a sentence, such as the Babcock sentence: "The one thing a nation needs to be rich and strong is a large, secure supply of wood." The patient must repeat it until it is learned and is then required to recall it after 5 minutes. Third, the examiner can ask the patient to recall a story (Chapter 9, Table 9.3). First instruct the patient: "I am going to read you a short story. Please listen carefully because afterward I want you to tell me the story as accurately as possible." Afterward, after an interference interval, say: "Tell me everything that you remember about the story." The examiner concludes by asking specific questions about the content of the short story.

4. **Paired Associate Learning.** Ask the patient to learn unrelated word pairs (e.g., stove-letter). Give a list of four word pairs (include easy pairs and hard pairs of less related items), one word pair at a time (2 seconds). After an interference interval, memory for those pairs is typically tested by having them either recall one of the words in response to the word it was paired with during encoding (e.g., recall the word that was paired with "stove"), or by asking them to distinguish between word pairs that were encoded together (e.g., stove-letter) and word pairs composed of two words that were studied, but were not paired during encoding (e.g., stove-dance), known as associative recognition).

5. **Visual Memory Tests.** One of the easiest visual memory tests involves asking the patient for delayed recall of three or four previously copied nonsense figures (Chapter 9, Fig. 9.4). Use geometric figures that elicit minimal verbalization or verbal associations. Patients may also reproduce from memory any other drawing copied earlier during visuospatial testing (e.g., intersecting pentagons, cube). Scoring is based not on visuospatial accuracy but on the general outline and semblance of the drawing to the copied model. An example of grading is 2 for accuracy, 1 for recognizable semblance, and 0 for incorrect. Subsequently, they may identify the drawings from pictures of other drawings in a multiple-choice recognition task of at least twice as many nonsense geometric figures. In addition, there is a visual-visual paired associate learning version that pairs three nonsense or geometric figures with colors and asks the patient to reproduce the figures later on presentation of the paired colors.

6. **Complex Figure Delayed Recall.** A further related visual memory task is the reproduction from memory of a previously copied complex figure. The examiner may use the Rey-Osterrieth Complex Figure or an alternative complex figure (Chapter 10, Fig. 10.3; Chapter 17, Fig. 17.1). Without prior notification, the patient is asked to reproduce the figure at 3 minutes and/or at 30 minutes after the initial copy.

7. **Visual Hidden Items.** There are several other visual memory tasks that can be easily done in a clinical encounter or at the bedside. One task involves asking the patient to recall item and location of four items previously hidden in the room. The examiner hides the items in the room while the patient observes, aware that this is a memory test. The examiner then asks the patient to identify the object and its location after a 5-minute delay. Grading should include 2 for both item and its correct location, 1 for correct item but incorrect location, and 1 for correct location but incorrect item.

8. **7/24 Non-Verbal Memory Test.** Another test is the "dot localization" test of memory using 7 tokens placed on a board of 24 empty squares (Chapter 9, Fig. 9.5). The examiner places the tokens in 7 of the squares, shows the patient, then

removes the board. After a delay of 5 minutes, the examiner reintroduces the tokens and the blank board and instructs the patient to place the tokens in the same prior squares.

9. **Remote Memory.** The examiner assesses retrieval of remote information by asking the patient to recall four or more current events or historical events that have occurred during the individual's lifetime. The examiner could facilitate this by asking the patient to name major historical events from the last two decades, probing for details (Chapter 9, Table 9.4). The chosen events should consider the patient's age and sociocultural background and should also be sufficiently salient such that it would be reasonable for the patient to have been exposed to information about the event. Alternatively, the examiner may also start by asking the patient to relate four major events, with some detail, in the past few months. Another alternative is to ask the examinee to name the prior four presidents or prime ministers in proper sequence beginning with the current leader.

10. **Autobiographical Memory.** The examiner asks questions concerning autobiographical history, such as the patient's family, residences, and jobs. Sample questions are: "Tell me about the home that you grew up in?" "Tell me about how you met your spouse?" The examiner can determine the patient's particular interests and query him/her on them, for example, specific television shows or sports events. A more formal assessment of autobiographical events asks questions similar to the Autobiographical Memory Interview. Examples of potential questions are descriptions of favorite grade school or middle school memories, first remembered birthday, description of secondary school graduation, earliest memory of grandparents, and others. Scores are calculated on the level of specificity of personal details of the experience, for example, 0 indicating no specificity and 3 indicating the ability to describe events of a discreet time and place.

DECLARATIVE SEMANTIC MEMORY

1. **Semantic Word Knowledge.** The examiner can test semantic knowledge of words by speaking word names and asking the patient to identify them, that is, ask the patient "What is a…" Present the words one at a time and give the patient sufficient time to think of an answer. The words should range from low frequency to high frequency and cover animate and inanimate categories. The patient may show word comprehension by providing definitions, descriptions of the use or function, or common associations for the words. For example, if the patient cannot define the word, ask the patient to describe its use or its associations, for example, "doctor" for stethoscope. If the patient is still unsuccessful, the examiner may ask the patient to demonstrate use, where possible, or to indicate an association from a multiple-choice array of four definitions to choose from.

2. **Semantic Naming.** On listening to the patient's conversation during the initial interview, look for the presence of noun omissions and compensatory circumlocutions or nonspecific pronouns or names. The examiner then performs a confrontational naming test (see Spoken Language and Speech, #4) and records the missed items. Later, the examiner gives the patient the missed names from the confrontational naming test and asks the patient to define or describe what the names mean. If the patient cannot recognize the meaning of a word that he would be expected to know, then this is consistent with semantic anomia.

3. **Multiple Category Word Lists.** During the language examination when evaluating category word-list generation, ask the patient to generate word lists from multiple categories, that is, animals, fruits and vegetables, and inanimate objects such as tools or makes of cars. The patient may also generate within-class lists (Thing Categories Test), such as "all things" predominantly red, blue, round, et cetera.

4. **Semantic-Word Picture Matching.** Semantic-word picture matching is an alternative way to test word comprehension. This procedure requires sets of semantically related pictures (e.g., haystack, barn, chickens, plow). The examiner speaks word names ("plow") and asks the patient to identify the word by choosing the picture that matches the word. The examiner can create at least four displays of four pictures each for the patient to choose from, and the patient should undergo multiple trials.

5. **Object-Action Semantic Associations.** The examiner may want to avoid language altogether and test semantics strictly through visual-visual matching tasks. The examiner presents 10 objects or pictures of objects, one at a time, and asks the patient to match them with one of an array of 10 action pictures, for example, a saw with a carpenter working and a pot with a chef cooking. The stimulus items should range from low frequency to high frequency and belong to different categories. Patients with semantic deficits may make errors in matching the correct object/picture and its semantically associated action picture. Subsequently, the examiner can reverse the order of the task. The examiner presents the action pictures and asks the patient to point to the corresponding object/picture.

6. **Picture Semantic Associations.** Another nonverbal test of semantic associations involves showing the patient arrays of objects or pictures and asking the patient to indicate which ones go together. There are multiple trials. Each trial consists of an array of two pairs of two vertically arranged objects/pictures (Chapter 9, Fig. 9.6). In one of the pairs, the target object (top picture) is semantically associated with the lower picture, whereas in the other pair, the same target object is not semantically associated with the lower picture. The patient must indicate which pair contains the semantically associated objects. For the different trials, the objects or pictures should range from low frequency to high frequency and belong to different categories.

7. **Category Sorting Task.** An alternative semantic task involves identifying the category or class of an item, either from words or objects/pictures. One way to do this is by sorting an array of written words or an array of objects/pictures by predefined categories (e.g., living vs. nonliving, fruits vs. vegetables, tools vs. nontools). The examiner can also ask the patient to group 10 or more familiar objects/pictures according to use, color, material, or situation in which they are normally found.

8. **"Draw an Animal" Test.** The patient must draw a picture of specific animals, such as a dog, giraffe, or camel. This exercise is particularly useful for distinguishing subordinate deficits from relatively retained superordinate groupings, such as the outline of a generic animal rather than one with specific identifying details (Chapter 9, Fig. 9.7).

Constructional, Perceptual, and Spatial Abilities

CONSTRUCTIONAL ABILITIES

1. **Simple Figure Copy.** Ask the patient to copy a simple two-dimensional figure such as a circle or a diamond, a complex two-dimensional figure such as a rectangle, or three-dimensional figures such as a box, cube, or napkin holder ("Benson figure") (Chapter 10, Fig. 10.2). For the best constructional task performance, have a pre-printed design for copy, separate, blank white sheets of paper (uncomplicated and unlined), and a black pen or a pencil without eraser. The introductory instructions include: "Please make a copy of the picture exactly as you see it." Those who make errors and wish to start over again should be allowed to do so. There are different methods for grading the drawings. First, they should be reviewed for abnormal or fragmented spatial relationships, absence of detail or impoverished essential features, stimulus-boundedness ("closing-in" or drawing over the master copy), loss of three-dimensional perspective, or neglect of one part of the drawing. Second, there are suggested grading systems for the copy of a circle (closed to within 1/8" = 1; circular = 1); of a diamond (4 sides = 1; 4 closed angles = 1; sides of equal length = 1); and of a rectangle (both figures 4 sided = 1; overlaps resembles original = 1). For the cube and Benson figure, a suggested grading system is included in Chapter 10, Fig. 10.2.

2. **Complex Figure Copy.** The Rey-Osterrieth Complex Figure is the original complex figure test (Chapter 10, Fig. 10.3), but there are other alternative ones. These constructional tasks have the advantage of having a formal scoring system and normative data for assessing the patient's performance. The examiner gives the patient a blank piece of paper and places the stimulus figure in front of them. The complex figure task requires

the patient to copy the entire figure as best as he/she can, and, although not given a time limit, the patient receives encouragement to complete it. To assess strategy, the examiner may change the patient's pencil or pen to different colored ones at different points in the drawing, thus indicating the sequence and strategy for copying the figure. The scoring system includes 18 specific items (Chapter 17, Fig. 17.1). As an additional visual memory task, they may reproduce the complex figure from memory (Chapter 9) and the strategy for completion can be analyzed as an executive task (Chapter 13).

3. **Freehand Drawing Tasks.** These tasks add the element of visual imagery and remove the guide of a prescribed drawing to copy. The examiner provides the patient with a blank sheet of paper and instructs the patient to draw a house, a dog, a flower (e.g., a "daisy in a flowerpot"), or even a person (the "draw-a-person" test). The patient instructions are: "I would like you to draw simple pictures. I know that you may not be an artist, but please draw the pictures as well as you can." Evaluate the drawings in terms of the features noted for simple figural constructions. In addition to perceptual and spatial disturbances, these drawings can also reflect semantic deficits (see Declarative Semantic Memory, #8).

4. **Clock Drawing Task.** The freehand drawing of a clock can be administered in a number of ways, but the simplest is the presentation of a blank paper with the instructions to "draw the face of a clock." The examiner then has the patient put in the numbers and the hands to read "10 after 11" or, alternatively, "5 past 4." There are many scoring systems for the clock, some of which attempt to distinguish the main cognitive factors that impact on clock drawing (Chapter 10, Table 10.2). The easiest is to evaluate for the contour of the circle, the order and quadrant placement of the numbers (whether within or outside of the circle), and the presence of two hands: a short hour hand, and a long minute hand meeting near the center of the clock face (Chapter 10, Fig. 10.4).

5. **Tasks With Constructional Tools.** The examiner, where indicated, may want to test constructional ability with additional tests, such as block assembly, tinker toys (or match sticks, toothpicks), or picture arrangement. Most of these tests, however, require special stimuli or procedures for testing and scoring performance and are highly dependent on visuomotor coordination and basic motor ability. For example, block construction can employ four Koh's blocks, which have sides that are red, white, or half red and half white. The examiner presents pictures of different four-block arrangements and asks the patient to take the blocks and make a design that looks like the pictures. The examiner can use other constructional tools, including readily available items such as match sticks or toothpicks, for freehand constructions.

6. **Paper Folding Tasks.** One additionally potentially useful constructional task, which does not require blocks or constructional tools, is paper folding. The examiner folds the paper in different ways, for example, exactly in half, quarters, two triangles, along the diagonal, et cetera, and asks the patient to fold their paper in an identical way.

PERCEPTUAL ABILITIES

1. **Visual Form Discrimination.** When viewing images, people must be able to recognize form at the basic, geometric level. The reconstruction and eventual recognition of basic forms and shapes is a process that underlies the ability to recognize objects, which are made up of basic forms and shapes. The easiest screen is to have the patient match two or three previous constructions with the correct choice out of a field of different geometric forms (Chapter 10, Fig. 10.5). The examiner should note any strategy that the patient uses in matching the figures and whether it is a serial, feature-by-feature analysis rather than a rapid global analysis of configuration.

2. **Unconventional Views.** Although requiring more stimulus materials, this evaluation can be done as a multiple-choice matching task using complex forms or shapes or objects in unconventional views. Each figure is presented with four other match figures varying in shape, rotation, or distortion of the figure, and the patient is asked to indicate which match figure corresponds to the

stimulus figure. Alternate views of objects can be easily created by taking pictures of objects from different points of view, for example, aerial, side, from below, and others.

3. **Cross-Hatched Figures.** A form of visual perceptual screening that overlaps with figure-ground discrimination tests involves asking the patient to identify figures obscured by cross-hatching (Chapter 10, Fig. 10.6A).

4. **Figure-Ground Discrimination.** When viewing images, people experience some figures as projecting into the foreground, whereas others recede into the background. The brain organizes the visual field into figures that stand out from their surroundings (ground). Figure-ground discrimination, which is evident at the V2 level, is a basic perceptual process that can be tested with hidden or embedded and overlapping figures (Chapter 10, Fig. 10.6B). The patients may also identify three or four overlapping figures made up of overlapping line drawings, originally popularized as the Poppelreuter figures test.

5. **Visual Perceptual Organization or Completion.** When viewing images, people automatically organize what they see into figures, objects, and scenes. This process of integration allows the apprehension of intact figures from dilapidated or incomplete ones. The inability to apprehend and integrate at the single form or object level is sometimes called "integrative agnosia." The examiner tests visual organization with incomplete or fragmented drawings, such as the Street Figures (part of the original Street Completion Test), cut-up or fragmented pictures as represented in the Hooper Visual Organization Test (Chapter 10, Fig. 10.6C). The fragmented or cut-up figures have to be reconstructed mentally and identified.

6. **Global-Local Processing.** Loss of the global precedence is easily tested with the "Navon" figures, which consist of letters or numbers made up of smaller letters or numbers (Chapter 10, Fig. 10.6D). With the stimuli held approximately 2 feet from the patient, ask him or her, "What do you see?" Patients may recognize the smaller numbers or letters and miss the global one without having to be redirected to the larger figures.

SPATIAL ABILITIES

1. **Visual Search of Scene.** It is important to present a complex drawing to the patient, generally representing a familiar scene, and assess whether the patient can identify the whole theme or situation, as well as the constituent parts (Chapter 10, Fig. 10.7; Chapter 8, Fig. 8.2). The complex picture should be oriented to the patient's body axis. Note if the patient is unable to put the entire scene together and if the patient misses seeing or describing a part or a side of the picture. The following are the specific items graded on the Cookie Theft Picture: girl, boy falling, cookie jar, mother washing, sink overflowing, and window.

2. **Dot Visual Search Task.** The examiner asks the patient to locate and circle dots on a page (Chapter 10, Fig. 10.8). To formally quantify this task, include 40 dots within an 11- $\times$ 17-inch field and score the maximum number of correctly circled dots: 15 = 1, 25 = 2, 32 = 3, 36 = 4, 39 = 5, 40 = 6.

3. **Timed Visual Search Task.** For more precise assessment of visual search abilities, the examiner can present a timed task consisting of a field of a specific letter, with an embedded odd letter. The patient's task is to find the odd letter as fast as possible. For example, the patient may search for the letter "Q" embedded among 29 "Os" and, conversely, the letter "O" embedded among 29 "Qs." Begin timing once the stimuli are displayed and record the time to recognition of the target letter in seconds.

4. **Line Bisection.** This task consists of a test sheet with a series of horizontal lines differentially placed on the paper (Chapter 10, Fig. 10.9). (A simple line bisection can be done with just one line, rather than a series of lines.) The examiner asks the patient to divide each line in half by placing a mark at the center of each line. "Using a pen or pencil, please draw an 'X' where you think the center of the line is. Do not use a ruler or any other measuring instrument; just use your best guess." On this line bisection, the degree of displacement is directly proportional to the length of the line used. Accepted range of scores will only include marks made within 20% of the stimulus midpoint

(±10% of midpoint). Incorrect responses are evaluated as to whether neglect is in left or right field.

5. **Visual Search Cancellation Task.** This task is basically the same as for visual attention and involves scanning for a specified figure or letter on a piece of paper with scattered nontarget, random figures or letters (Chapter 7, Fig. 7.5; Chapter 10, Fig. 10.10). The examiner can administer the test timed or untimed. The patient indicates the target figure or letter wherever it appears by marking it or circling it. The examiner may also give the patient with suspected hemispatial neglect an "attention" cancellation task (See Attention, #7). The patient is instructed to circle the letter "A" (the target) every time they see that letter in a written paragraph.

6. **Gap Test.** The patient must indicate (circle or cross out) all the circles with a gap (Chapter 10, Fig. 10.11). Failure to cross out all gaps facing in one direction, either left or right, indicates allosteric neglect, whereas failure to cross out all gaps on one side of the page indicates egocentric neglect.

7. **Double Simultaneous Stimulation.** Stimuli, such as fingers, are simultaneously presented or held up in each hemifield, and the examiner asks the patients to report the number of objects or fingers while maintaining their gaze fixed on the examiner. Unilateral extinction occurs when the patients fail to detect the stimuli on one side.

8. **Conceptual Neglect.** Conceptual neglect is an inability to visualize the left side of an imagined representation and can be considered a form of hemispatial neglect affecting visualization. Patients with conceptual neglect may fail to report structures on the left side of their visualization, which differs depending on which end of the corridor or street they imagine themselves to be. The examiner asks the patients to imagine themselves looking down from one end of a familiar corridor or street and to describe what is on each side of the corridor or street. The examiner then repeats the task by asking the patients to imagine themselves looking down from the other end of the same corridor or street.

9. **Dressing Disturbance or "Apraxia."** This task involves asking the patient to put on a coat four times. In the first condition, the examiner or a facilitator holds the coat in an open manner with the inside facing and subject. In the second condition, the patient must remove the hanging coat and put it on by themselves without orientation clues. In the third and fourth conditions, one or both sleeves are inside-out. The maximum score is 4. The examiner observes whether the patient gets muddled in attempting to put on the garment, inserting a limb into the wrong area and orienting the garment incorrectly (body-garment disorientation). Dressing problems can also be observed in correctly arranging the collar or finding the pockets.

10. **Environmental Disorientation.** Testing for environmental orientation includes orienting to a route and its landmarks. The examiner or facilitator can evaluate this by guiding the patient around his or her environment, pointing out at least 10 landmarks along the way. The examiner instructs the patient to remember the route and the indicated landmarks. Subsequently, after returning back to the starting point, the examiner asks the patient to guide the examiner along the same route, pointing out the previously indicated landmarks. The examiner notes the necessity for route cues and redirection and the recall of landmarks en route.

11. **Familiar Route Recall.** The examiner asks the patient to recall a familiar local route known to the examiner as well, for example, a common route to the clinic, hospital, familiar building, or monument. The patient must identify key intersections, roads, or buildings along the route and the correct direction from them. The examiner can also ask the patient to draw a schematic of a familiar route. The patient must trace one of the routes, including labeling of the landmarks, corridors, or street names on the drawing.

12. **Map Reading.** The examiner asks the patient to read a two-dimensional map. It can be a standard road map, or one created by the examiner of a local area. The examiner asks the patient to imagine walking a designated route and to trace it on the map. Alternatively, the examiner can ask the patient to place major cities or landmarks on a familiar map.

13. **Simultanagnosia Tasks.** In addition to evaluating the patient's ability to entirely "see" all parts of a complex scene or only isolated items or segment of items in the picture, the examiner presents the

patient with pairs of stimuli, such as two circles, and evaluates whether the patient only reports seeing one or has to look around with some effort to see both circles. The examiner then presents the two circles connected with a "linker" that makes them into glasses or a bicycle and evaluates whether the patient now reports seeing the whole drawing (Chapter 10, Fig. 10.12).

14. **Oculomotor Apraxia.** In the absence of primary visual field deficits, oculomotor apraxia is the inability to voluntarily direct one's gaze to a particular point. For testing, the patient focuses his or her gaze on the examiner's nose. First, the examiner asks the patient to move their gaze to moving targets in each quadrant while maintaining their head straight. Second, the examiner asks the patient to move their gaze to stationary targets in each quadrant, again without moving their heads. The patients must quickly move their gaze directly to the targets in the peripheral field without evidence of undershooting, overshooting, or searching, and the maximum score is 8. A delay in the onset of eye movement on command may be the most sensitive indicator of oculomotor apraxia.

15. **Optic Ataxia.** This is the inability to voluntarily direct one's hand movements toward visually presented targets. The examiner asks the patient to use the right hand to touch a moving target in each peripheral quadrant while maintaining their gaze on the examiner's nose. This is repeated with stationary targets and with the left hand. The patients must quickly reach out and touch the object without undershooting, overshooting, or searching movements. Scoring for the hand-eye coordination: 0 = total miss; 1 = near miss; 2 = accurate with a maximum score of 16.

VISUAL AGNOSIAS

1. **Object/Picture Comprehension.** The examiner presents 10 objects visually and asks the patient to name them and, if unsuccessful, describe their function or pantomime their use. In visual agnosia, it is best to start with 10 real objects and then to repeat the task with photographs or line drawings. The stimulus items are presented visually only, for example, the patient must not touch, manipulate, or induce sounds from the object. The stimulus items range from low frequency to high frequency and belong to different categories. Subsequently, the examiner reverses the order of the task. The examiner names items previously missed and asks the patient to point to the corresponding object in an array. The examiner must exclude semantic deficits by asking the patient to define the named item and its function ("What is a....?"), pantomime its use, and/or identify it by touch and manipulation (or hearing it if appropriate). Patients with visual agnosia should be able to perform these last tasks yet still not be able to recognize the object by sight.

2. **Visual Appearance and Matching.** The examiner then presents the patient with a matching task involving two visual arrays of objects. The two arrays contain similar items, although not necessarily identical in all aspects. The examiner instructs the patient to "put together the two things that are visually the same." The patient must match the items in the first array with the corresponding items in the second array. Once completed, the examiner further asks the patient to describe the visual appearance or visual attributes of the items, that is, the basic shape, color, size, et cetera. The patients can also sort the items by these attributes. Patients with apperceptive agnosia due poorly on this task; those with associative agnosia do well.

3. **Drawing Tasks.** One potentially useful test is to have the patient draw a copy of common visual items that the patient has not been able to identify, for example, flower, dog, whistle, or others. Patients with apperceptive agnosia do poorly in copying the item; those with associative agnosia are able to draw a recognizable copy but still do not recognize it.

4. **Atypical/Unusual Perceptual Tasks.** Patients with apperceptive visual agnosia may not be able to identify objects or pictures in atypical or unusual views but recognize them in typical and normal views. Atypical or unusual views include direction of view, lighting and shadow, size, color, or texture. The examiner may create his/her own stimuli or use established unusual views tests, such as the progressive silhouettes from the Visual Object and Space Perception battery.

5. **Examination for Prosopagnosia.** The examiner tests familiar face recognition with photographs

of famous, well-known, or familiar individuals (without any salient hairstyle, glasses, etc.). For example, the examiner can present eight black and white portraits of politicians or entertainers that are presumably well-known to the vast majority of people in their sociocultural and temporal cohort. The examiner asks the patient to name the person. If the patient cannot name the person, the patient should describe whether the person looks or feels familiar and the type of person, for example, politician, entertainer, or other associated aspects of the individual. Normal is presumed to be a perfect score but varies with prior exposure to these faces. To test for more general semantic deficits, the examiner must ask the patient for information about any familiar face that they fail to recognize in the face recognition task. After a delay, the patient is given the name of the missed famous person and asked to describe something about them. This can be salient facial characteristics or semantic characteristics such as general occupation, living or dead, specific accomplishments, and others.

6. **Face-Face Matching.** The examiner asks the patient to match photographs of unfamiliar faces with the same face among other photographs in an array. This task can include four stimuli faces, which are presented one at a time, and an array of eight other photographs laid out in front of the patient. The 8 photographs in the array include the 4 stimuli faces, in somewhat different poses or angles of view, and 4 foils who are similar in appearance to the stimuli faces. The patient is asked to indicate which face in the array is the same person as the stimuli face. The face matching task is patterned after the Benton Face Recognition (Benton, 1983), which matches faces in front-view with others in front-view, three-quarters view, or in different lighting. Normal is presumed to be a perfect score.

7. **Name-to-Face Matching.** To assess types of errors, the examiner shows the patient displays, each with 4 faces of people of the same sex. In each display, three of the four people are famous. One of the four faces is the index face, and the others are a semantically related famous face (e.g., same profession or fame), a semantically unrelated

famous face, and an unfamiliar but visually similar face (Chapter 10, Fig. 10.13). For each display, the examiner names the index person and asks the patient to point to that person's picture among the four choices. The examiner determines the numbers of errors and whether semantically related or visually related.

8. **Color Processing Tests.** The examiner presents the patient with at least six different color patches (or the Ishihara Color Plates) and asks the patient to 1) name the color; 2) indicate the named color; and 3) sort the items of the same color. In color anomia and color agnosia, patients cannot name colors on presentation, and they cannot point to named colors, but they can correctly sort them. To distinguish color anomia and color agnosia, the examiner should present the patient with a series of incorrectly colored line drawings, for example, a blue banana, a green dog, and others, and asks if the colors are correct. The examiner can also ask the patient to correctly color line drawings. In color agnosia, but not color anomia, the patient cannot judge the correct color for common objects and incorrectly colors them. Note, if a patient fails to name or point to named colors and cannot sort colors that go together, then they may have achromatopsia, or loss of color vision, in which case everything looks black and white or gray scale, either bilaterally or in one hemifield.

9. **Auditory Processing Tests.** The examination starts by assuring that the patient does not have a primary hearing impairment before proceeding to cortical auditory processing. One of the main tests involves the examination of responses to prerecorded environmental sounds. Four pictures are presented with each environmental sound. The four choices were either correct, acoustically related, semantically related, or totally unrelated. The patient must point to the corresponding picture. They can also be discriminated as same or different. If more in-depth testing is possible, discrimination can be extended to prerecorded pure tones of varying frequency, intensity, duration, phoneme pairs, and sequences varying only in a regular interstimulus interval (also consider the Seashore Rhythm Test). The ability to localize sounds in space may be evident or may require

special testing given the bilaterality of sound transmission. In the auditory modality, the examiner may give special consideration to evaluating patients for loss of prosody or for one of the amusias (music processing disorder).

10. **Olfactory Processing Tests.** Odor or olfactory agnosia can result from right anterior temporal disease and may present with altered dietary preferences or appreciation, considering that much of eating involves olfaction. These patients are able to detect smells, evident with simple screens such as recognizing the presence of coffee, vanilla, lemon, or tobacco, but cannot recognize what they are. Olfactory agnosia is further tested using the University of Pennsylvania Smell Identification Test (UPSIT) or similar tests. The UPSIT is a standardized set of 40 common odorants, which are embedded in "scratch and sniff" fragrance labels and administered in a multiple-choice format. Initially, the examiner evaluates the detection and intensity of the odors. Then the examiner evaluates whether they are familiar or unfamiliar.

Praxis and Related Cortical Movement Abnormalities

APRAXIA

1. **Limb Apraxia Examination: Pantomime-Imitation-Gesture Comprehension.** The examiner begins with both verbal "transitive" commands, that is, pretending to use an object in a task, and verbal "intransitive" commands, that is, performing symbolic gestures (Chapter 11, Table 11.3). Common transitive commands include pretending to comb their hair or brush their teeth, and common intransitive commands include waving good-bye and beckoning others to approach them. The examination usually focuses on testing both upper limbs, first the dominant hand and then the nondominant hand independently, avoiding going from one hand to the other so as to avoid self-cuing. If the patient fails to perform the movement on verbal command, then the examiner pantomimes the action and asks the patient to imitate it. Should the patient continue to have difficulty, ask him/her to explain what the action

signifies or represents, that is, gesture comprehension. The examiner can further ask the patient to identify random gestures and whether they felt that the examiner's gestures were performed correctly or poorly.

2. **Axial and Lower Extremity Apraxia.** Apraxia testing needs to include the central axis of the body and the lower extremities (Chapter 11, Table 11.2). Begin evaluating for orobuccal-facial apraxia by asking the patient to pretend to suck through a straw or pretend to blow out a match. Then evaluate responses to whole-body commands, such as asking the patient to stand up, bow, or assume a boxer's stance. Next check for gait apraxia or a "magnetic gait," reported with normal pressure hydrocephalus, vascular dementia, and other frontal lobe conditions. These patients have a hard time getting started, as if their feet are glued to the ground, with subsequent slow, shuffling gait. The examiner can videotape this whole maneuver and time it for quantification (e.g., Timed Walk or Timed Up and Go Tests). In addition to asking them to initiate a gait, evaluate for the presence of a "foot grasp," similar to a hand grasp reflex, with curling down of the toes on stroking the plantar aspect of the feet. Further evaluate for lower extremity apraxia with commands such as writing on the floor while sitting and making figure threes or eights with their legs while supine.

3. **Real Object Choice or Use.** The examination of real object use can clarify the apraxia diagnosis. If necessary, the clinician can supplement the neurobehavioral status examination with instruments such as the Apraxia Battery for Adults-2, the Florida Apraxia Battery, the Cologne Apraxia Screening, the Test of Upper Limb Apraxia, Short Screening Test for Ideomotor Apraxia, Diagnostic Instrument of Limb Apraxia, and others.

4. **Ideational Apraxia.** Unlike patients with ideomotor apraxia, these patients can pantomime, imitate, and identify individual gestures, but cannot order them to correctly complete a series of movements in a multistep action, for example, they can pantomime brushing one's teeth but cannot do the sequence of opening the toothpaste, putting it on the toothbrush, and so on. The

examiner tests for ideational apraxia by telling the patient to imagine that all the items needed for a sequential task are in front of them, and then asking them to pantomime the multistep tasks with the items. Other examples of tasks include making a sandwich and preparing and mailing a letter. Errors are evident as a failure to perform the tasks in the correct sequence.

5. **Conceptual Apraxia.** Patients with conceptual apraxia demonstrate the wrong action to command because they are mistaken about the concept ("action semantics") behind the movement, particularly choosing the wrong tool for an action or choosing the wrong action associated with the tool. They make errors in tool-selection and tool-object knowledge with inability to indicate a tool based on its function or action. These patients, who often have advanced dementia, tend to substitute the wrong action for the tool. The examiner may ask the patient to pretend to brush their teeth, and the patient may comb his/her hair instead, or, if provided a toothbrush, brush their teeth with the back and not the bristle.

6. **Limb-Kinetic Apraxia.** The examiner asks the patient to do repetitive finger tapping; pick up a small coin with a pincer grasp; and rapidly twirl a coin between their fingers (Chapter 11, Table 11.4). On finger taps, the patient taps thumb with index finger in rapid succession with widest amplitude possible, each hand separately. The coin must be picked up without sliding it. Twirling the coin must be done in continuous, smooth movements. Patients with limb-kinetic apraxia may have irregular tapping movements, struggle to pick up the coin without using many fingers, and drop the coin on twirling it. They may also have difficulty with meaningless gestures because of loss of dexterity. The examiner must distinguish limb-kinetic apraxia from primary motor disturbances.

7. **Callosal Apraxias.** This is ideomotor or dissociation apraxia limited to the nondominant upper extremity. This shows both ideomotor apraxia with spatiotemporal errors on imitation and dissociation apraxia with unrecognizable movements on pantomime command, but only in the nondominant (usually left) arm and hand.

8. **Examination of Meaningless Movements.** The examiner has the patient imitate at least four unfamiliar and meaningless movements, such as those illustrated in Chapter 11, Fig. 11.3 . The examiner evaluates the patient for the ability to complete the movements without confusion or spatiotemporal errors.

RELATED CORTICAL MOVEMENT ABNORMALITIES

1. **Motor Neglect Syndromes.** Primary motor neglect is evident when the patient fails to spontaneously move an extremity or side of the body ("akinesia") or initiates the movement only after a notable delay ("hypokinesia"). Unilateral directional akinesia or hypokinesia is present when the patient fails or delays initiation of movement of a limb into the contralateral hemispace or in the contralateral direction. For detection of unilateral directional hypokinesia, the examiner additionally asks the patient to move the arms into contralateral hemispace. The difference between primary motor neglect and unilateral directional akinesia or hypokinesia is that the former is limb or body centered and the latter is space or direction centered. These syndromes are particularly evident in spontaneous activities and in performing bimanual actions, and they may improve when prompted to use the neglected limb or initiate the neglected movement.

2. **Alien Limb Phenomenon.** The "alien limb" moves, raises, or "acts on its own." In other words, this condition is a sensation of an "alien limb" because there are limb movements that the patients feel were not initiated by them or that were moved by someone else. The most common movement is spontaneous levitation of the nondominant limb, but there may be a range of semi-purposeful movements.

3. **Diagonistic and Agonistic Apraxia.** Callosal lesions can partially disconnect the hemispheres and result in either "diagonistic apraxia" characterized by intermanual conflict between the actions of the two limbs acting in opposition to each other, or "agonistic apraxia" characterized by automatic execution of commands with the opposite hand.

4. **Frontal Lobe Movements.** Advanced frontal lobe disease can result in "release" signs such as

grasp reflexes or the more extreme grope reflexes in which the patient cannot keep from actively reaching out for items in the environment or drawing over a stimulus. Frontal release signs may be associated with manifestations of a more general "environmental dependency syndrome" (Chapter 13). Patients with this condition may automatically manipulate or use objects in front of them ("utilization behavior"), imitate or mimic other people's observed behavior ("imitation behavior"), and copy their motor movements ("echopraxia") or their speech ("echolalia"). Dorsolateral frontal lesions may also result in motor perseveration, which includes an inability to stop movements or an inability to keep from returning to them. Paradoxically, in some cases there is the opposite, a motor impersistence or failure to maintain a movement or posture. In some frontally impaired patients there is a tendency for a body part to be easily moved with light touch or pressure ("mitgehen") or to be easily placed in an unusual position with gradual return ("mitmachen") or with prolonged maintenance of the unusual position ("catalepsy" or waxy flexibility). Additional frontal origin behaviors include disinhibition and poor impulse control from orbitofrontal lesions and stereotypies and compulsive-like behaviors from frontolimbic involvement.

Calculations and Related Functions

ACALCULIAS

1. **Mental Acalculia Screen.** Examiners most frequently rely on serial subtraction tests, which are also of value for assessing attention (see Attention, #4). Patients must count backward from 100 by 7s or count backward from 20 by 3s. In the first, the examiner asks the patient to subtract by 7 beginning with the number 100, for example, 93, 86, 79, 72, 65, et cetera. The number of errors are the number of incorrect subtractions; if the patient makes an incorrect subtraction at one level, the examiner corrects the patient or restarts serial subtraction from the incorrect number. Normal patients should be able to get three or more subtractions in a row. Counting backward from 20 by 3s is a similar, but easier, version of serial subtractions.

2. **Oral Problem Screen.** Some clinicians briefly screen for calculation difficulty with an oral word problem. Three examples of increasing difficulty are: Ask the patient to calculate the number of books on two shelves, if there are 18 books with twice as many on one shelf as the other. Ask the patient to report the number of nickels in $1.35, or the number of quarters in $6.75. Tell the patient: "The girl went to the store with $5 to buy 2 sodas for $1.85 each. What was her change?"

3. **Written Acalculia Screen.** A written assessment allows for a greater process interpretation of any errors in attempting to solve the calculation problems, such as carryover and placement errors. The patient performs these screening problems using paper and pen. For routine screening, it is not necessary to test all four major arithmetic operations, and problems in addition and subtraction may be sufficient. The patient can perform two simple double-digit calculations such as $47 + 18 = $ ___ and $82 - 16 = $ ___. During these calculations, have the patient specifically read the arithmetic signs and describe their operation.

4. **Acalculia Battery** (Chapter 12, Table 12.3). The complete acalculia battery includes eight areas to screen: reading and transcoding, number writing, spatial alignment, mental calculations and estimates, arithmetic signs, analog and ordinal processing, and numeracy including arithmetic reasoning and knowledge. First, ask the patient to read and transpose verbal numbers to Arabic numerals and vice versa. Second, ask the patient to write numbers of one, two, or more digits. Third, ask them to write a dictated addition and subtraction problem with double or triple digits without performing the problem. Fourth, ask the patient to calculate $4 + 13$, $21 - 3$, 6×5, and $25 \div 5$ in their head. The examiner can also ask the patient to serially subtract from 100 by 7s or from 20 by 3s, as has previously been described. Fifth, follow this up with actual performance on written calculations. Sixth, have them read the arithmetic signs themselves, and seventh, place numbers on an analog line. Finally, ask the patient for items reflective of numeracy. Start by asking the number of days in a week and the number of weeks in a half a year.

5. **More Extensive Mathematical Testing.** Instruct the patient that you are going to do arithmetic problems that range from easy to hard and not to worry about missing a problem but to just to complete them. There should be a wide number of both single digit and double-digit problems, two or more each of addition, subtraction, and multiplication with division being optional (Chapter 12, Table 12.4). During this testing, the examiner evaluates several other areas in addition to the problem itself. Have the patient read the problems out loud prior to performing them. During the calculations, observe for errors in borrowing, carrying over, sequencing, and spatially aligning the written calculations.

6. **Numeracy and Cognitive Estimations.** Finish with numeracy, evaluating mathematical knowledge, arithmetic reasoning, and cognitive estimations (Chapter 12, Table 12.5). This involves assessing the ability to apply mathematics to the real world. For example, the examiner can ask the patient to estimate the distance between New York and Paris or the height of the tallest building in the world.

GERSTMANN SYNDROME

1. **Digit Agnosia.** The examiner asks the patient to point to named fingers or to report, with occluded vision, which finger is indicated by the examiner. First, the examiner asks the patient to name each of the fingers on their hands and on the examiner's hands (Chapter 12, Table 12.7). The tests for digit agnosia particularly focus on the index, middle, and third fingers and can be extended to the toes. Second, the examiner asks the patient to point to named fingers on their own hands and on the examiner's hands. Although these tests assess naming or pointing to individual fingers on oneself and on others, the examination is really about the absence of "gnosis," or knowing the digits, rather than the absence of naming, or anomia for digit names. Both of these tasks may be failed because of aphasia or anomia, rather than because of true agnosia for digits or fingers; therefore if they fail naming and pointing tasks, a nonverbal test is indicated. The examiner can ask the patient to state, with occluded vision, the number of fingers between two fingers touched by the examiner. Alternatively, the examiner moves one of the patient's fingers on a hand while held out of the patient's sight, usually above and behind their head, and asks the patient to indicate, on the contralateral hand, the correct finger moved.

2. **Hand Picture Test for Digit Agnosia.** There is another good test for digit agnosia using drawings of hands. The examiner presents a drawing of the left and right hands in front of the patient. The hand drawings are with the palms down and the fingers facing the patient. On the drawing, the examiner asks the patient to point to the corresponding fingers named by the examiner. For nonverbal recognition, the examiner touches the fingers on the drawings and asks the patients to move his or her corresponding fingers. Alternatively, the examiner simultaneously touches pairs of fingers on the dorsal side of the patient's hand, unseen by the patient, and asks the patient to point to the corresponding fingers on the drawings of the hands.

3. **Right-Left Orientation.** For right-left discrimination, the examiner asks the patient to follow uncrossed and crossed right-left body commands followed by "Double-Own" and "Double-Other" commands (Chapter 12, Table 12.8). First, the examiner asks the patient to show his or her right and left hands. If this is correctly performed, the examiner asks the patient to identify body parts on the left and right side of both the patient's body and the examiner's body. In a right-handed patient, uncrossed commands are "point to your right ear," and crossed commands are "point to my (the examiner's) right shoulder." Double-Own commands are "point with your left hand to your left ear," or "point with your right hand to your left shoulder." Double-Other commands are "point with your right hand to my (the examiner's) right shoulder," or "point with your left hand to my (the examiner's) right ear." The examiner needs to keep in mind that patients may fail these tests not because of right-left disorientation but because of hemineglect, apraxia, language comprehension, or executive disturbances.

4. **Autotopagnosia and Somatotopagnosia.** These are agnosias for localization and orientation on a

body map, which is related to digit agnosia and right-left disorientation. Autotopagnosia is difficulty localizing on one's own body, whereas somatotopagnosia also includes difficulty localizing on the body parts of others or on pictures, drawings, or dolls. For testing, the examiner asks the patient to point to individual parts of the body (neck, ankle, ear, and so forth) and to name parts of the body. The examiner names a body part while asking the patients to point to the corresponding body part first on themselves and then on the examiner. The examiner can also point to their own body parts (or the patient's) while asking the patient to point to the corresponding body part on themselves (or on the examiner). The examiner evaluates for errors of localization to the surrounding body parts rather than the correct one (contiguity error) or in localization to an incorrect but semantically related body part (semantic error), for example, pointing to an eye when asked to point to an ear.

5. **Transitional Agraphia.** In addition to primary agraphia (see Written Language and Reading, #3), the agraphia of Gerstmann syndrome may extend to the transition between lexical elements to motor elements. The transitional components of this alexia may affect graphemic motor (sets of motor programs for writing), including allographic (style, script, upper or lower case) elements and the actual graphic codes for their motor execution. These patients may have these problems without evidence of upper extremity limb apraxia. On obtaining a writing sample, patients make corresponding errors in the direction, relative size, and ordering of strokes and in correctly using script or case.

Executive Operations and Attributes

EXECUTIVE OPERATIONS

1. **Serial Reversal Tasks.** These aspects of executive operations overlap with attention tests as previously described. The first is the Backward Digit Span in which the patient must repeat digits in reverse order, beginning with the last number. The examiner continues to administer series of digits until the patient incorrectly repeats two strings of digits backward at the same series level. A normal performance is correct backward recitation of five (±2) digits, or two less than the maximum forward digit span. The ability to spell "World" backward is another commonly used serial reversal task. The patient must give the letters placed in the correct place, that is, "d-l-r-o-w." The serial recitation tasks include counting backward by threes from 20, or sevens from 100. As previously discussed, the examiner asks the patient to subtract by 7 beginning from 100, for example, 93, 86, 79, 72, 65, et cetera. The number of errors are the number of incorrect subtractions from the prior response. Finally, the examiner may ask the patient to recite the days of the week backward or the months of the year backward beginning with December. Patients should be able to obtain a normal score on these last two serial reversal tasks.

2. **Four Working Memory Tasks.** A simple working memory task (involving both maintenance and manipulation) is to have the patient rearrange digits in ascending order from smallest to largest. For example, if given the series "2-1-3," the correct answer would be "1-2-3." Most people can serially order up to five or more digits. A second tests is a clinical variation of the N-Back, in which the examiner recites a long series of digits and, once the examiner stops, asks the patient to repeat the next to last digit in the sequence ("N-1") or, for more challenging testing, two or three back from the last digit in the sequence ("N-2" and "N-3") (See Attention, #10). A third task is a variation of the Brown-Peterson procedure, which aims to test working memory divorced from the effects of rehearsal. The examiner spells aloud a random, three-letter consonant syllable ("trigram") that the patient must remember. Immediately afterward, the patient is asked to count backward by 3s from a random number. After 10 seconds, the examiner interrupts the counting backward and asks the patient to recall the consonant trigrams. The examiner repeats this procedure at least four times. Fourth are complex span paradigms that require remembering a set of items in order and combined with a concurrent secondary task. One version is the reading span task in which patients read 2 to 6 sentences and must remember the last word of each sentence, which they have to repeat back in order at the end of the task.

3. **Fluency Tasks—Verbal and Nonverbal.** There may be a decline in the Controlled Oral Word Association Test (e.g., "F" word/minute task) out-of-proportion to any decline in categorial word-list generation (see Spoken Language and Speech, #2 and #3). In addition, there may be a decline in design fluency, or the number of free form designs/minute. One easily administered version of design fluency is the Five-Point Test (Chapter 13, Fig. 13.1). The examiner presents the patient with squares (typically 40) containing five dots and asks the patient to make as many unique designs as possible in 1 minute by connecting the dots within each square with straight lines. The patient does not need to use all the dots in the designs. The lines must be straight ones that connect dots, and the designs should not be repeated. The examiner can start with two examples. There are several variations of this design fluency test. One counts the number of unique designs in 5 minutes. Another restricts the total number of lines/square to four. A third version restricts to continuously connected straight lines. The examiner scores the total number of correct designs, the number of rule violations, and the number of repeated designs.

4. **Trail making B ("Trail Making B") Test.** In Part B of the Trail making Test (see Chapter 7, Fig. 7.6 for Trail making A), the patient must draw a line connecting numbers and letters in alternating sequence, that is, 1 to A then 2 to B then 3 to C, et cetera. The Trail Making test measures the time required to draw a line between scattered circles, but variants of this test can be administered untimed for error assessment (as in the Montreal Cognitive Assessment). There are other variations of the Trail making B, which change letters into Roman numerals, days of the week, or months of the year (Chapter 13, Fig. 13.3). For the numbers-months variation, tell the patient: "On this page are both numbers and months of the year. Begin at number 1 and draw a line from 1 to January, then to 2, then to February, and so on. Remember, first you have a number, then a month, then a number, and so on. Draw the lines as fast as you can. Begin." If the patient makes a mistake on the practice sample, point to the error immediately and explain it. If the patient makes an error on the real test, point to the error and return the patient's pen to the last correct circle and continue from that point.

5. **Alternating Coin Test.** One easy to implement set-shifting task involves alternating a coin between the examiner's hands and having the patient guess the hand that has the coin. The examiner starts with hands held behind the back, then brings them forward and asks the patient to state which hand has the coin. Then the examiner uncovers his hands indicating the correct response. The examiner repeats this procedure, moving the location of the coin out-of-sight behind his or her back according to different strategies. The first strategy is a right hand–left hand alternation of the coin. Once the patient determines the correct alternating strategy for three coins in a row, the examiner then switches to a two right-hand, two left-hand strategy until the patient gets five in a row. This is followed by a three right-hand, three left-hand strategy until the patient gets seven in a row. The inability to get the set within a strategy trial constitutes an abnormal response.

6. **Four Alternating Tasks.** In the alternate tapping task, the examiner asks the patient to reproduce a simple rhythm that the examiner taps on the table (Chapter 5, Fig. 5.3; Chapter 13, Table 13.2). The examiner instructs the patient to "tap twice when I tap once" for three trials, then "tap once when I tap twice" for another three trials. Then the examiner has the patient respond correspondingly to the following tapping sequence: 1-1-2-1-2-2-2-1-1-2. Alternatively, to exclude visual input, the examiner may tap out-of-sight underneath table and patient responds by raising a finger. Second, the patient must copy alternating programs such as a series of shapes, continuing the pattern to the end of the page (Chapter 13, Fig. 13.4A). Disturbances include perseveration of one of the letters or impersistence. Third, the patient can alternate symbols on a piece of paper. Ask the patient to write "0" and "+" in an ascending numerical pattern, that is, 0+00++000+++, et cetera. Fourth, the examiner asks the patient to give as many names as possible in 1 minute, alternating between categories such as fruits versus vegetables, animals versus tools, colors versus countries. The examiner records the

number of correct alternations/minute. This alternate word-list generation task overlaps with verbal fluency measures but with the examiner focusing on the number of correct alternations/minute.

7. **Three Sequencing Tasks.** The first task asks the patient to couple the first letters of the alphabet with the last letters and to continue as far as possible, for example, AZ-BY-CX-DW, et cetera. The last correct coupling is the patient's score. The second, or "Alphanumeric Sequencing Test," asks the patient to verbally count from 1 and recite the alphabet, but switching between numbers and letters, that is, "1-A-2-B-3-C-4-D-5-E-6-F-7-G-8-H-9-I-10-J-11-K." The number or errors is the number of mistakes in alternations. The third task, or Letter-Number Sequencing Test, asks the patient to repeat a mixed sequence of numbers and letters, for example, J-7-F-6-P-4, and then repeat the numbers in ascending order followed by the letters in alphabetical order. This is a more difficult test; many patients struggle attaining more than three numbers–three letters.

8. **Luria Three-Step Hand Sequence Test.** This test requires that the patient imitate three hand motions performed by the examiner. On a table, the examiner places his or her hand with a fist with the knuckles down, then the edge of the hand in a cutting motion, and then palm down with fingers extended (Chapter 13, Fig. 13.5, Table 13.2). The examiner demonstrates this hand sequence three times. Then the patient must perform the sequence three times in a row along with the examiner. Finally, the patient must perform the hand sequence six times in a row without error, without cues, and without verbalization. A normal untimed performance is a perfect score of six correct hand sequences in a row.

9. **Alternating Hand Open-Fist.** A simpler motor set-change task than the Luria Three-Step Hand Sequence Test is to have the patient do alternate hand movements such as alternate between one hand fisted and the other open palm down on the table, alternating simultaneously at a moderate pace.

10. **Spiral Loops Task.** The patient must copy a pattern of a set number of spiral loops without adding additional number of spirals (Chapter 13, Fig. 13.4B). The instructions are to copy the spirals exactly as they are to the end of the page.

11. **The Crossed Hands Test.** The examiner asks the patient to close their eyes and place their hands, palm down, in front of them. The examiner then instructs the patient to lift the hand opposite to the one touched by the examiner. There are 20 trials, and errors involve initially moving the touched extremity rather than the opposite one.

12. **The Antisaccades Test.** The examiner holds up index fingers in each of the patient's two visual fields and randomly moves one of them. Ask the patient to look to and from the examiner's moving index fingers and nose. When the patient is comfortable, the examiner asks the patient to look at the index finger that is NOT moving. After practice, the patient is asked to perform 20 serial antisaccades. An error occurs if the patient looks toward the moving finger. The Antisaccade score is as follows: ≤3 errors = 4; 4 errors = 3; 5 errors = 2; 6 errors = 1; >6 errors = 0.

13. **The Go-No-Go Test** (Chapter 5, Fig. 5.3; Chapter 13, Table 13.2). The examiner instructs the patient to "tap once when I tap once." The examiner runs three trials (1-1-1) then instructs the patient "do not tap when I tap twice." The examiner runs three trials (2-2-2) then instruct the patient to "tap once with I tap once but do not tap when I tap twice." Finally, the examiner runs 10 trials of mixed tapping (1-1-2-1-2-2-2-1-1-2) and records the errors of commission or omission.

14. **Color-Word Interference Test.** The patient must first read a list of color names in black and white and then name an array of colors. After this, the patient must rename the colors, but this time the colors are presented as contradictory color names. The patients must inhibit responses to the word names of colors and just name the colors that they are printed in. It is possible to administrator variations of this color-word interference test with simple stimuli, such as color words printed in different colors (Chapter 13, Fig. 13.6), and noting the patient's errors, delays, or struggles in naming the colors.

15. **Big-Little-Big Test.** Patients have to report whether the words "big" or "little" are printed in uppercase or in lowercase (Chapter 13, Fig. 13.7). "Say which SIZE each of these words are, one by one, as quickly as you can. Ignore what the word

says: say "big" for capitalized words and "little" for lowercase." The examiner records errors in correctly categorizing the case of the words.

16. **Hayling Sentence Completion Paradigm.** This asks patients to complete sentences with totally unrelated words or endings so that the sentence does not make sense. For example, if given the phrase "Mary had a little…."; "She laughed out…."; "The dog dug a…."; Jack and Jill went up the….", the patient must give entirely different responses than "lamb," "loud," "hole," and "hill," respectively. A series of these sentences can be constructed from common sayings and used to evaluate the patient's response inhibition.

17. **Contradictory Commands.** A related procedure is to instruct the patient to respond to your verbal commands but not to your contradictory gestures. For example, put out an outstretched hand and say "don't shake my hand"; throw a soft object and say "don't catch it"; show your open palms and say "don't show me your hands"; beckon to stand up and say, "please remain seated."

18. **Environmental Dependency Tasks.** The patient may manifest observable stimulus-bound behavior such as the compulsion to imitate the examiner's movements or to utilize ambient objects. "Stimulus-bound" behavior is evident when patients tend to touch items in the environment or approach other people beyond what the context or situation requires. Imitation behavior reflects environmental dependency and manifests as the tendency for patients to imitate the examiner's (or others') movements ("echopraxia") or speech output ("echolalia"). The examiner can test imitation by making deliberate, unusual movements or postures of the hand or face, or by saying nonsense words. Utilization behavior reflects environmental dependency and manifests as the tendency for patients to touch, take, and/or use whatever is in front of them. Finally, the presence of frontal grasp reflexes are part of the general spectrum of environmental dependency.

EXECUTIVE ATTRIBUTES

1. **Similarities and Differences.** Ask how two objects or concepts are similar or different or how they converge or diverge. "Please tell me in your own words what these words have in common (for similarities) or how they are different." Examples of similarities are apple-pear, coat-shirt, talking-listening, and others (Chapter 13, Table 13.3). For differences, the examiner can ask the difference between a lie and a mistake or between a poem and a statute.

2. **Interpretation of Idioms and Proverbs.** The examiner should start with simple idioms and progress to proverbs that are sufficiently hard to challenge the patient. Instruct the patient as follows: "I am going to give you some sayings. Some of them you may not have ever heard before. Please tell me in your own words what these words are trying to say." Common idioms include the meaning of "level-headed," "narrow-minded," and "warm-hearted" (Chapter 13, Table 13.3). Testing for proverb interpretation should include both familiar, common proverbs, whose interpretation may be recalled by memory or may reflect semantic difficulty, and unfamiliar proverbs that require the patient to actively abstract the underlying connotative meaning of the words (Chapter 13, Table 13.4). Ask the patient to explain the more general meaning of the proverb. If the patient gives a concrete response or is unable to interpret, give the patient the correct answer and explain that this is the expected type of response. Then continue with different proverbs until the patient fails two successive proverbs. Considering the patient's educational level and prior familiarity with proverbs, the examiner otherwise grades responses as accurate, correct but concrete (mere repetition or rephrasing of the statement given by the examiner), correct but irrelevant or bizarre, or incorrect.

3. **Judgment and Reasoning.** Additional tests of situational judgment can assess cognitive flexibility, cognitive estimations, and logical reasoning. Cognitive flexibility is exemplified by questions such as the "brick test": "Tell me all the things that you could you use a brick for?" Instead of a brick, the examiner could ask about other common objects with the aim of assessing the patients flexibility in coming up with multiple common and novel uses for objects. Cognitive estimations are exemplified by questions such as "How far is Paris from Los

Angeles?" or "How high is the tallest building in the world?" Clearly, these questions are knowledge dependent, but they can stretch the patient's judgment. Logical reasoning is exemplified by questions such as "Why are light-colored clothes cooler in summer than dark-colored clothes?" "John, Robert, and Michael are running a race. Michael is not behind Robert. John is the slowest. Who is ahead in the race?"

4. **Insight** (Chapter 13, Table 13.5). After completion of a full examination, a simple question to the patient—"And how concerned are you about your trouble?"—may demonstrate a lack of realization or a serious misinterpretation of the problem. The examiner compares the patient's responses with those of the caregiver, family, or other objective sources: 1) "Do you have a disease or disorder?"; 2) "Has your behavior changed over the last few years?"; 3) "Are you concerned about having an illness/problem?"; 4) "Have you had a behavior or personality change that has affected your life?"; 5) "Are you concerned about having an illness/problem that might be upsetting your family/friends?"; and 6) "Are you concerned that others may be seeing/perceiving you differently?"

5. **The Towers Tests.** This includes the Tower of Hanoi or the Tower of London and are particularly challenging complex problem-solving tasks. These tests require the patient to solve the arrangement of colored pegs or discs in an iterative process, often in a particular order of size. For the Tower of Hanoi, there are three rods and discs of different sizes arranged from the smallest on top to the largest below. The patient must move the discs to another rod, one at a time, by taking the upper disc and placing it on another rod without ever placing a larger disc on top of a smaller one. For 3 discs, a minimum number of moves is 7, and for 4 discs it is 15. Although the towers tests require special stimulus materials, a simpler clinical modification is to do the Towers of Hanoi procedure using three places on the table and three or four stacked coins of different sizes on one of the places. Have patients rearrange three stacks of coins by decreasing size. The main rule is that no coin can be placed on top of a smaller one.

The Neurologic Behavioral Examination (includes Social Cognition)

1. **Apathy.** The examiner probes for the patient's degree of motivation for initiating behavior, from productive activities or routine activities of daily living. One of the most widely used measurement scales for apathy is the Apathy Evaluation Scale and its variations, which takes approximately 10 to 20 minutes to complete (Chapter 14, Table 14.2).

2. **Emotion.** The examiner may assess emotion by evaluating the following features of mood and affect: the current mood state and its intensity, the present of emotional hyporesponsivity and indifference, episodes of emotional lability or dyscontrol, the presence of an impaired range of emotion, and the congruence of mood and affect with each other and with the context or situation (Chapter 14, Table 14.3).

3. **Social Behavior Checklist.** The examiner asks specific questions on a social cognitive questionnaire and observes for comparable behavior (Chapter 14, Table 14.4). Key questions include: Has there been a change in personality or behavior? If there is a change: Detached, unmotivated or apathetic? Is there socially inappropriate or disinhibited behavior? Has he/she violated social norms or rules? Does he/she fail to respond to social cues? Is there poor impulse control? Is there loss of sympathy or empathy? An easy to use Social Observation Inventory is included in Chapter 14, Table 14.5.

4. **Classic Theory of Mind (Mentalizing) Tasks.** Theory of Mind tests evaluate the ability to disregard one's own knowledge about the world and consider that someone else might have a different belief. A classic Theory of Mind false belief task is the Sally–Anne story: "Sally has a stroller and Anne has a toy box. Sally puts her doll in her stroller and goes out for a short time. While Sally is away, Anne moves the doll to the toy box. Sally comes back to get her doll. Where will Sally look for her doll?" (Does the patient understand that Sally has an erroneous belief of where her doll is?). This is a first-order false belief task; it can be escalated to second-order in which the

patient must understand that someone else has an erroneous belief about another character's belief. Additional examples of first-order and second-order false belief Theory of Mind tasks are depicted in scenarios 1 and 2 of Chapter 14, Figs. 14.2 and 14.3.

5. **Faux Pas Scenarios.** Non-false belief tasks of Theory of Mind assess social inference, such as faux pas tasks, that interpret the hidden meanings in scenarios. For example, in one example of a faux pas scenario Adam, John's boss, unexpectedly visits John at his office. John has a client with him and says, "Let me introduce Mr. Baker, one of our most important clients." The client interjects, "my name is not Baker, my name is Brown." In another faux pas scenario, Katie gives her in-laws a framed picture of her wedding. On a later visit, she discovers the picture stored in a drawer. Her mother-in-law, not recalling that it was a gift, comments, "that was my least favorite of your wedding pictures."

6. **Additional Theory of Mind Tasks.** Another test of Theory of Mind is the Reading the Mind in the Eye's test in which patients must infer the mental state of someone based on photographs of just their eyes. Second, the examiner can assess the patient's response to cartoons of humorous situations. The examiner can obtain cartoons from magazines or newspapers. A third, less commonly used test is the Awareness of Social Inference Test, which presents videos that focus on the ability to detect sarcasm. Fourth is the Strange Stories Test with stories that depend on knowing someone's mental state. Finally, there is the Hinting Test, which consists of brief vignettes that depend on understanding that a character dropped a hint.

7. **Facial Emotional Recognition.** The easiest way to screen for facial emotional recognition is to present the Ekman 60 Faces (Chapter 14, Fig. 14.4) and ask the patient to identify one of six basic emotions: happiness, sadness, surprise, fear, disgust, and anger.

8. **Sexual Behavior Checklist.** Crucial information for evaluating sexuality also include key questions such as the following: increased sexual frequency, the presence of public sexual behavior, an increase in actively seeking sexual experiences, a widened of sexual interests to previously unarousing stimuli, and evidence of sexual disinhibition.

9. **Oral/Dietary Behavior Checklist.** Crucial items for evaluating eating behavior are the following: the presence of hyperphagia or increased overall ingestion of food, altered food preferences, increased food preoccupation, absence of satiety, and hyperorality with ingestion, or orality of non-food or inedible items. Hyperorality may include gum chewing, oral tobacco, smoking, and other oral activities.

10. **Aggressive Behavior Checklist.** Crucial items for evaluating aggressive behavior are the following: the presence of verbal or physical aggressive episodes, reactive aggression with emotional reactions, instrumental aggression that was organized and planned, the presence of precipitants such as situational factors, and personality traits consistent with psychopathy. These personality traits include lack of guilt or remorse, lack of fear for punishment, risk-taking behavior, superficial charm and glibness, grandiosity, and the tendency to manipulate others.

11. **Thought, Speech, and Behavioral Content.** Disturbed content may underlie thoughts, speech, and behavior. By observing speech processes, the examiner can make deductions about patients' thought processes. The examiner is interested in evidence of delusions, hallucinations, or special preoccupations. In addition to the patient's reports, disturbed content may be evident in the patient's speech and motor behavior. For example, speech may be unusual in rate, quantity, loudness, and manifest blocking, clanging, or repetitions. There may be poor coherence, clarity, logicality, and overall intelligibility of language discourse. Look for circumstantiality (circuitous answers with overinclusion of unnecessary information), tangentiality (side-tracked answers with irrelevant and digressive information), or derailment (off-topic answers that are totally unrelated to the original conversation).

12. **Altered Perceptions.** Examiners are usually unable to elicit hallucinations in a clinical encounter; however, in some situations hallucinations can be brought out by holding a white piece of paper or an imaginary string between the fingers and asking the patient to describe what he or she sees. Illusions, however, can be precipitated with exposure to an image or sensory phenomena that is experienced as altered or distorted. The examiner should be particularly alert to any reports of misperceptions of the body or self.

Mental Status Scales

10 Select Mental Status Scales	Pages
SHORT (≤5 minutes)	
Clock Drawing Test	
Mini-Cog	
Six-Item Screener	
Short Portable Mental Status Questionnaire	
Short Test of Mental Status	
MODERATE (5–15 minutes)	
Mini-Mental State Examination	
Montreal Cognitive Assessment	
Rowland Universal Dementia Assessment Scale	
Saint Louis University Mental Status Examination	
LONG (15–30 minutes). Full scales not included here	
Addenbrooke's Cognitive Examination-III (ACE-III) is available from The University of Sydney—Diagnostic Dementia Tests; as a representative of the ACE-III, the Mini-Addenbrooke's Cognitive Examination (M-ACE) is included here.	

The Clock Drawing Test

INSTRUCTIONS

General setup: Equipment required includes a blank sheet of paper, a sheet of paper, a second paper with the drawing of a clock, a pen, and a chair/table for ease of drawing.

Patient Instructions (Rouleau et al., 1992):

PART A, Clock Drawing: The following instructions are given:

"I would like you to draw a clock, put in all the numbers, and set the hands for 10 after 11."

PART B, Clock Copy: Following the drawing, the patients should be instructed to copy, as accurately as possible, a clock from a model. The model should contain all the numbers on the clock, be 3 inches in diameter, and located on the upper part of an 8.5 × 11-inch sheet of paper. The hands on the model should be set for 10 after 11. The patient is then instructed to copy the model on the lower part of the same sheet of paper.

- Instructions can be repeated if necessary.
- Patients may use their nondominant hand for drawing the clock.

Name: _____
Date: _____

DRAW A CLOCK WITH ALL THE NUMBERS AND SET THE HANDS FOR 10 AFTER 11.

Name: _____

Date: _____

COPY THIS CLOCK BELOW.

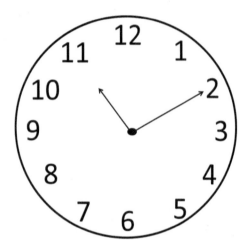

REFERENCES (multiple references reflect different scoring methods)

1. Hazan E, Frankenburg F, Brenkel M, Shulman K. The test of time: a history of clock drawing. *Int J Geriatr Psychiatry*. 2018;33:e22.
2. Mainland BJ, Amodeo S, Shulman KI. Multiple clock drawing scoring systems: simpler is better. *Int J Geriatr Psychiatry*. 2014;29:127.
3. Mendez MF, Ala T, Underwood KL, Zander BA. Development of scoring criteria for the clock drawing task in Alzheimer's disease. *J Am Geriatr Soc*. 1992;40:1095–1099.
4. Rouleau I, Salmon DP, Butters N, Kennedy C, McGuire K. Quantitative and qualitative analyses of clock drawings in Alzheimer's and Huntington's disease. *Brain Cogn*. 1992;18(1):70–87.
5. Sunderland T, Hill JL, Mellow AM, et al. Clock drawing in Alzheimer research. A novel measure of dementia severity. *J Am Geratr Soc*. 1989;37:725–729.

Mini-Cog

Name: _____

Date: _____

Step 1: Three Word Registration

Look directly at person and say, "Please listen carefully. I am going to say three words that I want you to repeat back to me now and try to remember. The words are [select a list of words from the versions below]. Please say them for me now." If the person is unable to repeat the words after three attempts, move on to Step 2 (clock drawing).

The following and other word lists have been used in one or more clinical studies. For repeated administrations, use of an alternative word list is recommended.

Version 1	Version 2	Version 3	Version 4	Version 5	Version 6
Banana	Leader	Village	River	Captain	Daughter
Sunrise	Season	Kitchen	Nation	Garden	Heaven
Chair	Table	Baby	Finger	Picture	Mountain

Step 2: Clock Drawing

Say: "Next, I want you to draw a clock for me. First, put in all of the numbers where they go." When that is completed, say: "Now, set the hands to 10 past 11."

Use preprinted circle (see next page) for this exercise. Repeat instructions as needed, as this is not a memory test. Move to Step 3 if the clock is not complete within 3 minutes.

Step 3: Three Word Recall

Ask the person to recall the three words you stated in Step 1. Say: "What were the three words I asked you to remember?" Record the word list version number and the person's answers below.

Word List Version: _____

Person's Answers: _____

TOTAL SCORE _____

Word Recall: (0–3 points)	1 point for each word spontaneously recalled without cueing.
Clock Draw: (0 or 2 points)	Normal clock = 2 points. A normal clock has all numbers placed in the correct sequence and approximately correct position (e.g., 12, 3, 6, and 9 are in anchor positions) with no missing or duplicate numbers. Hands are pointing to the 11 and 2 (11:10). Hand length is not scored. Inability or refusal to draw a clock (abnormal) = 0 points.
Total Score: (0–5 points)	Total score = Word Recall score + Clock Draw score. A cut point of <3 on the Mini-Cog has been validated for dementia screening, but many individuals with clinically meaningful cognitive impairment will score higher. When greater sensitivity is desired, a cut point of <4 is recommended as it may indicate a need for further evaluation of cognitive status.

Clock Drawing for Mini-Cog

Name: _____

Date: _____

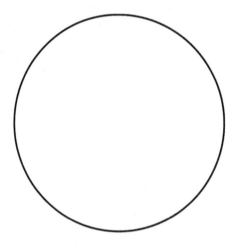

REFERENCES

1. Borson S, Scanlan JM, Chen PJ, et al. The Mini-Cog as a screen for dementia: validation in a population based sample. *J Am Geriatr Soc.* 2003;51:1451–1454.
2. Borson S, Scanlan JM, Watanabe J, et al. Improving identification of cognitive impairment in primary care. *Int J Geriatr Psychiatry.* 2006;21:349–355.
3. Lessig MC, Scanlan JM, Nazemi H, Borson S. Time that tells: critical clock-drawing errors for dementia screening. *Int Psychogeriatr.* 2008;20:459–470.
4. Tsoi KK, Chan JY, Hirai HW, Wong SY, Kwok TC. Cognitive tests to detect dementia: a systematic review and meta-analysis. *JAMA Intern Med.* 2015;175(9):1450–1458.
5. McCarten JR, Anderson P, Kuskowski MA, McPherson SE, Borson S. Screening for cognitive impairment in an elderly veteran population: acceptability and results using different versions of the Mini-Cog. *J Am Geriatr Soc.* 2011;59:309–313.
6. McCarten JR, Anderson P, Kuskowski MA, McPherson SE, Borson S, Dysken MW. Finding dementia in primary care: the results of a clinical demonstration project. *J Am Geriatr Soc.* 2012;60:210–217.
7. Scanlan J, Borson S. The Mini-Cog: receiver operating characteristics with the expert and naive raters. *Int J Geriatr Psychiatry.* 2001;16:216–222.

Six-Item Cognitive Screener

"I would like to ask you some questions that ask you to use your memory. I am going to name three objects. Please wait until I say all three words, then repeat them. Remember what they are because I am going to ask you to name them again in a few minutes. Please repeat these words for me: APPLE—TABLE—PENNY." (Interviewer may repeat names three times if necessary but repetition not scored.)

Care Partners: To be eligible for this project, a patient must score less than 3.

In general: A score of 2 or 3 indicates a need for further screening and diagnostic testing.

Did patient correctly repeat all three words?	Yes	No
	Correct	Incorrect
1. What year is this?	0	1
2. What month is this?	0	1
3. What is the day of the week?	0	1
What were the three objects I asked you to remember?		
4. *Apple* =	0	1
5. *Table* =	0	1
6. *Penny* =	0	1
TOTAL		

REFERENCE

1. Callahan CM, Unverzagt FW, Hui SL, Perkins AJ, Hendrie HC. Six-item screener to identify cognitive impairment among potential subjects for clinical research. *Med Care.* 2002;40(9):771–781.

Short Portable Mental Status Questionnaire (SPMSQ)

In administering the SPMSQ, the interviewer should read the introduction printed at the top: "Sometimes people have trouble remembering things. If you do not know the answers to some of the next questions, that's okay. If you do know the answers, the questions may seem obvious." Each of the 10 questions should be asked as printed, without prompting or cues.

SCORING:*
0–2 errors: normal mental functioning
3–4 errors: mild cognitive impairment
5–7 errors: moderate cognitive impairment
8 or more errors: severe cognitive impairment
*One more error is allowed in the scoring if a patient has had a grade school education or less.
*One less error is allowed if the patient has had education beyond the high school level.

Question	Response	Incorrect Responses
1. What are the date, month, and year?		
2. What is the day of the week?		
3. What is the name of this place?[A]		
4. What is your phone number?[B]		
5. How old are you?		
6. When were you born?[C]		
7. Who is the current president?[D]		
8. Who was the president before him?[E]		
9. What was your mother's maiden name?[F]		
10. Can you count backward from 20 by 3s?[G]		

[A] Can be home, institution, town, or city
[B] If no telephone, can substitute street address
[C] Must give day, month, and year
[D and E] May substitute prime minister
[F] Her first name and last (maiden) name
[G] May repeat or offer probe: "Can you subtract 3 from 20? And 3 from that?"

REFERENCE

1. Pfeiffer E. A short portable mental status questionnaire for the assessment of organic brain deficits in the elderly. *J Am Geriatr Soc.* 1975;23:433–441.

Short Test of Mental Status

Name: _____

Date: _____

Subtest	Ideal Score
Orientation (name, address, building, city, state/ province, day [of the month or the week], month, year)	8
Attention (up to seven digits forward)	7
Learning (apple, Mr. Johnson, charity, tunnel) number of trials for acquisition _____	4
Calculation (5 x 13, 65 – 7, 58 ÷ 2, 29 + 11)	4
Abstraction (orange-banana, horse-dog, table-bookcase)	3
Construction (draw a clock showing a quarter after 11, copy a cube)	4
Information* (president, first president, number of weeks/year, and definition of an island)	4
Recall	4
Total Score*	38 Total

*May need to modify depending on patient, e.g., asking for prime minister instead of president.

Total Score = raw score − (number of trials on learning task − 1).

REFERENCE

1. Kokmen E, Naessens JM, Offord KP. A short test of mental status: description and preliminary results. *Mayo Clin Proc.* 1987;62(4):281–288.

Mini-Mental State Examination

PROCEDURE FOR INTERPRETING THE MINI-MENTAL STATE EXAMINATION*			
Items	Instruction	Scoring	Max
Orientation • Time • Place	What is Year? Season? Date? Day? Month? Where are we: State/Province? County? City/Town? Hospital/Building? Clinic/Floor?	1 for each correct item 1 for each correct item	5 5
Registration	The instructor names 3 unrelated items (e.g., "cook, blue, horse") and asks the patient to repeat back all three. Examiner repeats them until learned.	Score only the first repetition; 1 per item.	3
Mental Control \ Attention	"Count backward from 100 by sevens." OR "Spell WORLD backwards,"	93-86-79-72-65, etc. OR "D-L-R-O-W"	5
Memory	"Earlier I told you the names of 3 items. Please tell me what those were?"	1 for each correct item -spontaneous, uncued	3
Language • Naming	Examiner shows two simple objects (e.g., watch, pen) and ask patient to name them.	1 for each correct item	2 1
• Repetition	Repeat the phrase: "No ifs, ands, or buts."	1 for correct repetition	3
• Comprehension	Have them take a piece of paper and instruct: "Take the paper in our right hand, fold it in half, and put it on the floor."	1 for each correct step	1
• Reading	"Please read this and do what it says." Show printed "CLOSE YOUR EYES."	1 for correct response	1
• Writing	"Make up and write a sentence on anything"	1 if "sensible", e.g., verb with written or implied predicate.	1
Visuospatial Skills	"Please copy this picture." Give blank sheet of paper and ask to draw the intersecting pentagons (see below).	All 10 angles must be present and 2 must intersect.	1

*Actual scale presentation is copyright protected. Instructions and procedures are the authors.

CLOSE YOUR EYES

WRITTEN SENTENCE: _____

_____

_____

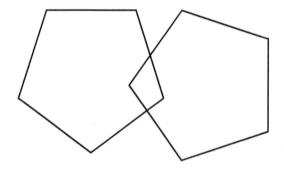

REFERENCE

1. Folstein MF, Folstein SE, McHugh PR. "Mini-mental state." A
   practical method for grading the cognitive state of patients for
   the clinician. *J Psychiatr Res.* 1975;12:189.

MONTREAL COGNITIVE ASSESSMENT (MOCA®)
Version 8.1 English

Name:
Education:
Sex:

Date of birth:
DATE:

VISUOSPATIAL/EXECUTIVE

Copy cube [ ]

Draw CLOCK (Ten past eleven)
(3 points)

[ ] Contour   [ ] Numbers   [ ] Hands

POINTS __ /5

NAMING

[ ]   [ ]   [ ]

__ /3

MEMORY

Read list of words, subject must repeat them. Do 2 trials, even if 1st trial is successful. Do a recall after 5 minutes.

	FACE	VELVET	CHURCH	DAISY	RED	NO POINTS
1ST TRIAL						
2ND TRIAL						

ATTENTION

Read list of digits (1 digit/ sec.).

Subject has to repeat them in the forward order.   [ ]   2 1 8 5 4
Subject has to repeat them in the backward order.   [ ]   7 4 2

__ /2

Read list of letters. The subject must tap with his hand at each letter A. No points if ≥ 2 errors

[ ]   F B A C M N A A J K L B A F A K D E A A A J A M O F A A B

__ /1

Serial 7 subtraction starting at 100.   [ ] 93   [ ] 86   [ ] 79   [ ] 72   [ ] 65

4 or 5 correct subtractions: **3 pts**,   2 or 3 correct: **2 pts**,   1 correct: **1 pt**,   0 correct: **0**

__ /3

LANGUAGE

Repeat: I only know that John is the one to help today. [ ]
The cat always hid under the couch when dogs were in the room.   [ ]

__ /2

Fluency: Name maximum number of words in one minute that begin with the letter F.   [ ] _____ (N ≥ 11 words)

__ /1

ABSTRACTION

Similarity between e.g. orange - banana = fruit   [ ] train - bicycle   [ ] watch - ruler

__ /2

DELAYED RECALL

Memory Index Score (MIS)

(MIS)	Has to recall words WITH NO CUE	FACE	VELVET	CHURCH	DAISY	RED	Points for UNCUED recall only
X3		[ ]	[ ]	[ ]	[ ]	[ ]	
X2	Category cue						MIS = ____ /15
X1	Multiple choice cue						

__ /5

ORIENTATION

[ ] Date   [ ] Month   [ ] Year   [ ] Day   [ ] Place   [ ] City

__ /6

© Z. Nasreddine MD   **www.mocatest.org**

Administered by: _____

Training and Certification are required to ensure accuracy

MIS: /15
(Normal ≥ 26/30)
Add 1 point if ≤ 12 yr edu

TOTAL   __ /30

Interpretation of the MoCA

The formal interpretation of the MoCA has been limited to those who are trained and certified in its administration and scoring (www.mocatest.org).

The MoCA website states that: "A subject who obtains a score below the normal cut-off score of 26 does not necessarily present a cognitive impairment. A subject who obtains a score above the normal cut-off score does not necessarily present intact cognitive functions."

They add that different conditions commonly affect distinct sets of tasks on the MoCA. These include stress, fatigue, educational level, emotional state, and others. The test may be less sensitive to mild cognitive impairment if the examinee is highly educated. An examinee may lose points due to limited cognitive capacities rather than cognitive dysfunction.

For scoring, 18–25 is often considered mildly impaired, 10–17 moderate, and <10 severely impaired. The test can be augmented with a Memory Index Score (MIS) calculated from the following table:

MIS scoring				Total
Number of words recalled spontaneously		multiplied by	3	
Number of words recalled with a category cue		multiplied by	2	
Number of words recalled with a multiple choice cue		multiplied by	1	
		Total MIS (add all points)		__/15

REFERENCES

1. Nasreddine ZS, Phillips NA, Bédirian V, Charbonneau S, Whitehead V, Collin I, Cummings JL, Chertkow H. The Montreal Cognitive Assessment, MoCA: a brief screening tool for mild cognitive impairment. *J Am Geriatr Soc.* 2005 Apr;53(4):695–9.

2. Julayanont P, Brousseau M, Chertkow H, Phillips N, Nasreddine ZS. Montreal Cognitive Assessment Memory Index Score (MoCA-MIS) as a predictor of conversion from mild cognitive impairment to Alzheimer's disease. *J Am Geriatr Soc.* 2014 Apr;62(4):679–84.

RUDAS

The Rowland Universal Dementia Assessment Scale.

Date: _____   Patient Name: _____

Item		Max Score
Memory		
1. (Instructions) I want you to imagine that we are going shopping. Here is a list of grocery items. I would like you to remember the following items, which we need to get from the shop. When we get to the shop in about 5 mins. time, I will ask you what it is that we have to buy. You must remember the list for me. **Tea, Cooking Oil, Eggs, Soap.** Please repeat this list for me (ask person to repeat the list three times). If person did not repeat all four words, repeat the list until the person has learned them and can repeat them, or, up to a maximum of five times.		
Visuospatial Orientation		
2. I am going to ask you to identify/show me different parts of the body. *(Correct = 1)*. Once the person correctly answers 5 parts of this question, do not continue as the maximum score is 5.		
(1) Show me your right foot	____1	
(2) Show me your left hand	____1	
(3) With your right hand, touch your left shoulder	____1	
(4) With your left hand, touch your right ear	____1	
(5) Which is (indicate/point to) my left knee	____1	
(6) Which is (indicate/point to) my right elbow	____1	
(7) With your right hand (indicate/point to) my left eye	____1	
(8) With your left hand (indicate or point to) my left foot	____1	
Praxis		____/5
3. I am going to show you an action/exercise with my hands. I want you to watch me and copy what I do. Copy me when I do this... (One hand in fist, the other palm down on table—alternate simultaneously.) Now do it with me: Now I would like you to keep doing this action at this pace until I tell you to stop— approximately 10 seconds. (Demonstrate at moderate walking pace). Score as:		
Normal = 2 (very few if any errors; self-corrected, progressively better; good maintenance; only very slight lack of synchrony between hands)		
Partially Adequate = 1 (noticeable errors with some attempt to self-correct; some attempt at maintenance; poor synchrony)		
Failed = 0 (cannot do the task; no maintenance; no attempt whatsoever)		
Visuoconstructional Drawing		____/2
4. Please draw this picture exactly as it looks to you (Show cube on back of page). *(Yes = 1)* Score as:		

Item		Max Score
(1) Has person drawn a picture based on a square?	____1	
(2) Do all internal lines appear in person's drawing?	____1	
(3) Do all external lines appear in person's drawing?	____1	
Judgment		____/3
5. You are standing on the side of a busy street. There is no pedestrian crossing and no traffic lights. Tell me what you would do to get across to the other side of the road safely. (If person gives incomplete response that does not address both parts of the answer, use prompt: "Is there anything else you would do?") Record exactly what patient says and circle all parts of response that were prompted. Score as:		
Did person indicate that they would look for traffic *(YES = 2;YES PROMPTED = 1; NO = 0)*	____/2	
Did person make any additional safety proposals? *(YES = 2;YES PROMPTED = 1; NO = 0)*	____/2	
		____/4
Memory Recall		
6. (Recall) We have just arrived at the shop. Can you remember the list of groceries we need to buy? (Prompt: If person cannot recall any of the list, say "The first one was 'tea'." *(Score 2 points each for any item recalled that was not prompted—use only 'tea' as a prompt.)*		
Tea	____2	
Cooking Oil	____2	
Eggs	____2	
Soap	____2	
		____/8
Language		
7. I am going to time you for 1 minute. I would like you to tell me the names of as many different animals as you can. We will see how many different animals you can name in 1 minute. (Repeat instructions if necessary). Maximum score for this item is 8. If person names 8 new animals in less than 1 minute there is no need to continue.		
(1) (5)		
(2) (6)		
(3) (7)		
(4) (8)		
		____/8
TOTAL SCORE =		____/30

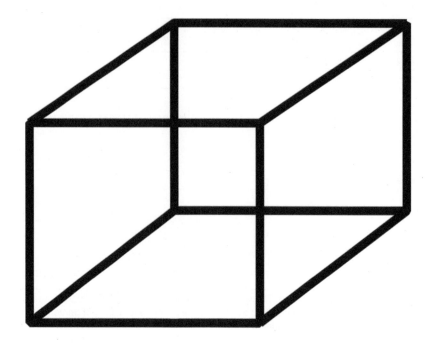

REFERENCE

1. Storey JE, Rowland JT, Basic D, Conforti DA, Dickson HG. The Rowland Universal Dementia Assessment Scale (RUDAS): a multicultural cognitive assessment scale. *Int Psychogeriatr.* 2004;16(1):13–31.

VAMC
Saint Louis University Mental Status Examination

Questions about this assessment tool? E-mail aging@slu.edu

Name_____ Age_____

Is the patient alert?_____ Level of education_____

__/1	**1** 1. What day of the week is it?
__/1	**1** 2. What is the year?
__/1	**1** 3. What state are we in?

4. Please remember these five objects. I will ask you what they are later.

    Apple   Pen   Tie   House   Car

5. You have $100 and you go to the store and buy a dozen apples for $3 and a tricycle for $20.
  1 How much did you spend?
__/3 **2** How much do you have left?

6. Please name as many animals as you can in one minute.
__/3   **0** 0-4 animals   **1** 5-9 animals   **2** 10-14 animals   **3** 15+ animals

__/5 7. What were the five objects I asked you to remember? 1 point for each one correct.

8. I am going to give you a series of numbers and I would like you to give them to me
    backwards. For example, if I say 42, you would say 24.
__/2   **0** 87   **1** 648   **1** 8537

9. This is a clock face. Please put in the hour markers and the time at
    ten minutes to eleven o'clock.
  2 Hour markers okay
__/4 **2** Time correct

1 10. Please place an X in the triangle.

__/2 **1** Which of the above figures is largest?

11. I am going to tell you a story. Please listen carefully because afterwards, I'm going to ask
    you some questions about it.
    Jill was a very successful stockbroker. She made a lot of money on the stock market. She then
    met Jack, a devastatingly handsome man. She married him and had three children. They lived
    in Chicago. She then stopped work and stayed at home to bring up her children. When they were
    teenagers, she went back to work. She and Jack lived happily ever after.

__/8 **2** What was the female's name?   **2** What work did she do?
  2 When did she go back to work?   **2** What state did she live in?

_____ **TOTAL SCORE**

SCORING		
HIGH SCHOOL EDUCATION		**LESS THAN HIGH SCHOOL EDUCATION**
27-30 ----------------------------------	NORMAL	---------------------------------- 25-30
21-26 ----------------------------------	MILD NEUROCOGNITIVE DISORDER	---------------------------------- 20-24
1-20 ----------------------------------	DEMENTIA	---------------------------------- 1-19

_____   _____   _____
CLINICIAN'S SIGNATURE   DATE   TIME

REFERENCE

1. SH Tariq, N Tumosa, JT Chibnall, HM Perry III, and JE Morley. The Saint Louis University Mental Status (SLUMS) Examination for detecting mild cognitive impairment and dementia is more sensitive than the Mini-Mental Status Examination (MMSE) - A pilot study. *Am J Geriatr Psych* 14:900-10, 2006.

Mini-Addenbrooke's Cognitive Examination. American Version A (2014)

Name:					Date of Testing:		
Date of Birth:					Tester's Name:		
Place of Testing:					Education:		
					Occupation:		
					Handedness:		

ATTENTION

Ask: What is the	Day	Date	Month	Year	Attention [Score 0–4]
	_____	_____	_____	_____	_____

MEMORY

Tell: "I'm going to give you a name and address and I'd like you to repeat the name and address after me. So you have a chance to learn, we'll be doing that 3 times. I'll ask you the name and address later."
Score only the third trial

	1st Trial	2nd Trial	3rd Trial		**Memory** [Score 0–7] _____
Harry Barnes					
73 Orchard St.					
Springfield					
Minnesota					

FLUENCY–ANIMALS

Animals

Say: "Now can you name as many animals as possible. It can begin with any letter. You have one minute. Go ahead."

						Fluency. [Score 0–7]
					≥22	7
					17–21	6
					14–16	5
					11–13	4
					9–10	3
					7–8	2
					5–6	1
					<5	0
					Total	Correct

CLOCK DRAWING

Clock: Ask the subject to draw a clock face with numbers and the hands at 10 past 5. (For scoring: circle = 1, numbers = 2, hands = 2 if all correct.)

					Visuospatial. [Score 0–5] _____

MEMORY RECALL

Ask "Now tell me what you remember about that name and address we were repeating at the beginning"

Harry Barnes					**Memory.** [Score 0–7]
73 Orchard St.					_____
Springfield					
Minnesota					
TOTAL SCORE					_____ /30

REFERENCES

1. Frontier Frontotemporal Dementia Research Group, frontierftd.org

2. Hsieh S, McGrory S, Leslie F, Dawson K, Ahmed S, Butler CR, Rowe JB, Mioshi E, Hodges JR. The Mini-Addenbrooke's Cognitive Examination: a new assessment tool for dementia. Dement Geriatr Cogn Disord 2015;39:1–11.

Key Select References

Basic Principles of Mental Status Testing (Chapters 1–6)

Ahmadian N, van Baarsen K, van Zandvoort M, Robe PA. The cerebellar cognitive affective syndrome—a meta-analysis. *Cerebellum.* 2019;18(5):941–950.

Clark DL, Boutros NN, Mendez MF. *The Brain and Behavior.* 4th ed. New York, NY: Cambridge University Press; 2018.

Finney GR, Minagar A, Heilman KM. Assessment of mental status. *Neurol Clin.* 2016;34(1):1–16.

Genetti Gatfield M, Colombo F, Annoni JM. The introduction of emotions and behavior in the assessment of neurological patients. *Front Neurol Neurosci.* 2019;44:15–22.

Grossman M, Irwin DJ. The mental status examination in patients with suspected dementia. *Continuum (Minneap Minn).* 2016;22(2 Dementia):385–403.

Janssen J, Koekkoek PS, Moll van Charante EP, Jaap Kappelle L, Biessels GJ, Rutten G. How to choose the most appropriate cognitive test to evaluate cognitive complaints in primary care. *BMC Fam Pract.* 2017;18(1):101.

Kaufer DI. Neurobehavioral assessment. *Continuum (Minneap Minn).* 2015;21(3 Behavioral Neurology and Neuropsychiatry):597–612.

Kirshner HS. Determination of mental competency, a neurological perspective. *Curr Neurol Neurosci Rep.* 2013;13(6):356.

Mendez MF, Van Gorp W, Cummings JL. Neuropsychiatry, neuropsychology, and behavioral neurology: a critical comparison. *Neuropsychiatry Neuropsychol Beh Neurol.* 1995;8:297–302.

Snyderman D, Rovner B. Mental status exam in primary care: a review. *Am Fam Physician.* 2009;80(8):809–814.

Tang-Wai DF, Freedman M. Bedside approach to the mental status assessment. *Continuum (Minneap Minn).* 2018;24(3 Behavioral Neurology and Psychiatry):672–703.

Tieges Z, Evans JJ, Neufeld KJ, MacLullich AMJ. The neuropsychology of delirium: advancing the science of delirium assessment. *Int J Geriatr Psychiatry.* 2018;33(11):1501–1511.

Arousal, Attention, and Other Fundamental Functions (Chapter 7)

Adamis D, Meagher D, Murray O, et al. Evaluating attention in delirium: a comparison of bedside tests of attention. *Geriatr Gerontol Int.* 2016;16(9):1028–1035.

Leonard M, O'Connell H, Williams O, et al. Attention, vigilance and visuospatial function in hospitalized elderly medical patients: relationship to neurocognitive diagnosis. *J Psychosom Res.* 2016;90:84–90.

Meagher J, Leonard M, Donoghue L, et al. Months backward test: a review of its use in clinical studies. *World J Psychiatr.* 2015;5(3):305.

Schroeder RW, Twumasi-Ankrah P, Baade LE, et al. Reliable digit span: a systematic review and cross-validation study. *Assessment.* 2012;19(1):21–30.

Shimoyama I, Ninchoji T, Uemura K. The finger-tapping test: a quantitative analysis. *Arch Neurol.* 1990;47(6):681–684.

Tieges Z, Brown LJ, MacLullich AM. Objective assessment of attention in delirium: a narrative review. *Int J Geriatr Psychiatry.* 2014;29(12):1185–1197.

Language and Speech (Chapter 8)

Barton JJ, Hanif HM, Eklinder Bjornstrom L, Hills C. The word-length effect in reading: a review. *Cogn Neuropsychol.* 2014;31(5–6):378–412.

Binder JR. Current controversies on Wernicke's area and its role in language. *Curr Neurol Neurosci Rep.* 2017;17(8):58.

Bunton K. Speech versus nonspeech: different tasks, different neural organization. *Sem Speech Lang.* 2008;29:267–275.

Gleichgerrcht E, Fridriksson J, Bonilha L. Neuroanatomical foundations of naming impairments across different neurologic conditions. *Neurology.* 2015;85(3):284–292.

Goodglass H, Kaplan E, Barresi B. Boston Diagnostic Aphasia Examination. Third Edition. Austin, TX: *Psychological Assessment Resources,* 2001.

Lorch MP. The long view of language localization. *Front Neuroanat.* 2019;13:52.

Morin A, Teichmann M. Jargonaphasia: a systematic overview and characterization in primary progressive aphasia. *Eur Neurol.* 2018;80(1-2):55–62.

Strand EA, Duffy JR, Clark HM, et al. The Apraxia of Speech Rating Scale: a tool for diagnosis and description of apraxia of speech. *J Commun Disord.* 2014;51:43–50.

Tosto G, Gasparini M, Lenzi GL, et al. Prosodic impairment in Alzheimer's disease: assessment and clinical relevance. *J Neuropsychiatry Clin Neurosci.* 2011;23(2):E21–E23.

Wilson SM, Eriksson DK, Schneck SM, Lucanie JM. A quick aphasia battery for efficient, reliable, and multidimensional assessment of language function. *PLoS One.* 2018;13(2):e0192773.

Ziegler W. Speech motor control is task-specific: evidence from dysarthria and apraxia of speech. *Aphasiology.* 2003;17(1):3–6.

Memory and Semantic Knowledge (Chapter 9)

Binder JR, Desai RH. The neurobiology of semantic memory. *Trends Cogn Sci.* 2011;15(11):527–536.

Cepeda NJ, Pashler H, Vul E, et al. Distributed practice in verbal recall tasks: a review and quantitative synthesis. *Psychol Bull.* 2006;132(3):354.

Chapman CA, Hasan O, Schulz PE, Martin RC. Evaluating the distinction between semantic knowledge and semantic access: evidence from semantic dementia and comprehension-impaired stroke aphasia. *Psychon Bull Rev.* 2020;27(4):607–639.

Gifford KA, Liu D, Damon SM, et al. Subjective memory complaint only relates to verbal episodic memory performance in mild cognitive impairment. *J Alzheimers Dis.* 2015;44(1):309–318.

Gliebus GP. Memory dysfunction. *Continuum (Minneap Minn).* 2018;24(3 Behavioral Neurology and Psychiatry):727–744.

Hawkins KA, Dean D, Pearlson GD. Alternative forms of the Rey Auditory Verbal Learning Test: a review. *Behav Neurol.* 2004;15(3–4):99–107.

Matthews BR. Memory dysfunction. *Continuum (Minneap Minn).* 2015;21(3 Behavioral Neurology and Neuropsychiatry):613–626.

Rosenbaum RS, Murphy KJ, Rich JB. The amnesias. *Wiley Interdiscip Rev Cogn Sci.* 2012;3(1):47–63.

Scalzo SJ, Bowden SC, Ambrose ML, Whelan G, Cook MJ. Wernicke-Korsakoff syndrome not related to alcohol use: a systematic review. *J Neurol Neurosurg Psychiatry.* 2015;86(12):1362–1368.

Szabo K. Transient global amnesia. *Front Neurol Neurosci.* 2014;34:143–149.

Xu Y, Chen K, Zhao Q, et al. Short-term delayed recall of auditory verbal learning test provides equivalent value to long-term delayed recall in predicting MCI clinical outcomes: a longitudinal follow-up study. *Appl Neuropsych Adult.* 2020;27(1):73–81.

Yang Q, Guo QH, Bi YC. The brain connectivity basis of semantic dementia: a selective review. *CNS Neurosci Ther.* 2015;21(10):784–792.

Constructional, Perceptual, and Spatial Abilities (Chapter 10)

Adair JC, Barrett AM. Spatial neglect clinical and neuroscience review: a wealth of information on the poverty of attention. *Ann NY Acad Sci.* 2008;1142:21.

Amodeo S, Mainland BJ, Herrmann N, et al. The times they are a-changin' clock drawing and prediction of dementia. *J Geriatric Psychiatr Neurol.* 2015;28(2):145–155.

Barton JJ. Disorder of higher visual function. *Curr Opin Neurol.* 2011;24(1):1–5.

Corrow SL, Dalrymple KA, Barton JJ. Prosopagnosia: current perspectives. *Eye Brain.* 2016;8:165–175.

Coslett HB. Apraxia, neglect, and agnosia. *Continuum (Minneap Minn).* 2018;24(3 Behavioral Neurology and Psychiatry):768–782.

De Vries SM, Heutink J, Melis-Dankers BJ, et al. Screening of visual perceptual disorders following acquired brain injury: a Delphi study. *App Neuropsychol Adult.* 2018;25(3):197–209.

Gainotti G, Trojano L. Constructional apraxia. *Handb Clin Neurol.* 2018;151:331–348.

Goll JC, Crutch SJ, Warren JD. Central auditory disorders: toward a neuropsychology of auditory objects. *Curr Opin Neurol.* 2010;23(6):617–627.

Haque S, Vaphiades MS, Lueck CJ. The visual agnosias and related disorders. *J Neuroophthalmol.* 2018;38(3):379–392.

Stewart L, von Kriegstein K, Warren JD, Griffiths TD. Griffiths, Music and the brain: disorders of musical listening. *Brain.* 2006;129:2533–2553.

Lopez A, Caffò AO, Bosco A. Topographical disorientation in aging. Familiarity with the environment does matter. *Neurol Sci.* 2018;39(9):1519–1528.

Mendez MF, Ringman JM, Shapira JS. Impairments in the face-processing network in developmental prosopagnosia and semantic dementia. *Cogn Behav Neurol.* 2015;28(4):188.

Moreaud O. Balint syndrome. *Arch Neurol.* 2003;60(9):1329–1331.

Parton A, Malhotra P, Husain M. Hemispatial neglect. *J Neurol Neurosurg Psychiatry.* 2004;75(1):13–21.

Shell AR. Auditory agnosia. *Handb Clin Neurol.* 2015;129:573–587.

Siuda-Krzywicka K, Bartolomeo P. What cognitive neurology teaches us about our experience of color. *Neuroscientist.* 2020;26(3):252–265.

Unzueta-Arce J, García-García R, Ladera-Fernández V, et al. Visual form-processing deficits: a global clinical classification. *Neurología.* 2014;29(8):482–489.

Van der Ham IJM, Martens MAG, Claessen MHG, van den Berg E. Landmark agnosia: evaluating the definition of landmark-based navigation impairment. *Arch Clin Neuropsychol.* 2017;32(4):472–482.

Verhallen RJ, Bosten JM, Goodbourn PT, et al. General and specific factors in the processing of faces. *Vision Res.* 2017;141:217–227.

Wolfe J, Horowitz TS. Visual search. *Scholarpedia.* 2008;3(7):3325.

Praxis and Related Cortical Movements Abnormalities (Chapter 11)

Canzano L, Scandola M, Gobbetto V, et al. The representation of objects in apraxia: from action execution to error awareness. *Front Hum Neurosci.* 2016;10:39.

Ellenstein A, Kranick SM, Hallett M. An update on psychogenic movement disorders. *Curr Neurol Neurosci Rep.* 2011;11(4):396–403.

Goldenberg G. Apraxia. *Wiley Interdiscip Rev Cogn Sci.* 2013;4(5):453–462.

Park JE. Apraxia: review and update. *J Clin Neurol.* 2017;13(4):317–324.

Petreska B, Adriani M, Blanke O, et al. Apraxia: a review. *Prog Brain Res.* 2007;164:61–83.

Watson CE, Chatterjee A. The functional neuroanatomy of actions. *Neurology.* 2011;76(16):1428–1434.

Calculations and Related Functions (Chapter 12)

Ardila A, Rosselli M. Acalculia and dyscalculia. *Neuropsychol Rev.* 2002;12(4):179–231.

Deloche G, Seron X, Larroque C, I, et al. https://pubmed.ncbi.nlm.nih.gov/8021307/ Calculation and number processing: assessment battery; role of demographic factors. *J Clin Exp Neuropsychol.* 1994;16(2):195–208.

Dobato JL, Hernández-Laín A, Acalculia Caminero AB. Neurological bases, evaluation and disorders. *Rev Neurol.* 2000;30(5):483–486.

Goodglass H, Kaplan E, Barresi B. Boston Diagnostic Aphasia Examination. Third Edition. Austin, TX: *Psychological Assessment Resources,* 2001.

Rusconi E. Gerstmann syndrome: historic and current perspectives. *Handb Clin Neurol.* 2018;151:395–411.

Sixtus E, Lindemann O, Fischer MH. Incidental counting: speeded number naming through finger movements. *J Cogn.* 2018;1(1):44.

Zamarian L, Scherfler C, Kremser C, et al. Arithmetic learning in advanced age. *PLoS One.* 2018;13(2):e0193529.

Executive Operations and Abilities (Chapter 13)

Archibald SJ, Mateer CA, Kerns KA. Utilization behavior: clinical manifestations and neurological mechanisms. *Neuropsychol Rev.* 2001;11(3):117–130.

Chan RC, Shum D, Toulopoulou T, et al. Assessment of executive functions: review of instruments and identification of critical issues. *Arch Clin Neuropsych.* 2008;23(2):201–216.

Conway AR, Kane MJ, Bunting MF, et al. Working memory span tasks: a methodological review and user's guide. *Psychon Bull Rev.* 2005;12(5):769–786.

Dai M, Li Y, Gan S, et al. The reliability of estimating visual working memory capacity. *Sci Rep.* 2019;9(1):1–8.

Duffau H. The "frontal syndrome" revisited: lessons from electro-stimulation mapping studies. *Cortex.* 2012;48(1):120–131.

Hellmuth J, Mirsky J, Heuer HW, et al. Multicenter validation of a bedside antisaccade task as a measure of executive function. *Neurology.* 2012;78(23):1824–1831.

Hurtado-Pomares M, Carmen Terol-Cantero M, Sánchez-Pérez A, et al. The frontal assessment battery in clinical practice: a systematic review. *Int J Geriatr Psych.* 2018;33(2):237–251.

Leyhe T, Saur R, Eschweiler GW, et al. Impairment in proverb interpretation as an executive function deficit in patients with amnestic mild cognitive impairment and early Alzheimer's disease. *Dement Geriatric Cogn Disord.* 2011;1(1):51–61.

Reber J, Tranel D. Frontal lobe syndromes. *Handb Clin Neurol.* 2019;163:147–164.

The Neurological Behavioral Examination (Chapter 14)

Aboulafia-Brakha T, Christe B, Martory MD, et al. Theory of mind tasks and executive functions: a systematic review of group studies in neurology. *J Neuropsychol.* 2011;5(1):39–55.

Byom LJ, Mutlu B. Theory of mind: mechanisms, methods, and new directions. *Front Hum Neurosci.* 2013;7:413.

Carota A, Bogousslavsky J. Neurology versus psychiatry? Hallucinations, delusions, and confabulations. *Front Neurol Neurosci.* 2019;44:127–140.

Feinberg TE, Venneri A. Somatoparaphrenia: evolving theories and concepts. *Cortex.* 2014;61:74–80.

First MB. Desire for amputation of a limb: paraphilia, psychosis, or a new type of identity disorder. *Psychol Med.* 2005;35(6):919–928.

Flanagan EC, Lagarde J, Hahn V, et al. Executive and social-cognitive determinants of environmental dependency syndrome in behavioral frontotemporal dementia. *Neuropsychology.* 2018;32(4):377.

Kranick SM, Hallett M. Neurology of volition. *Exp Brain Res.* 2013;229(3):313–327.

Meinhardt-Injac B, Daum MM, Meinhardt G, et al. The two-systems account of theory of mind: testing the links to social-perceptual and cognitive abilities. *Front Hum Neurosci.* 2018;12:25.

Stanton BR, Carson A. Apathy: a practical guide for neurologists. *Pract Neurol.* 2016;16(1):42–47.

Stone J, Pal S, Blackburn D, Reuber M, Thekkumpurath P, Carson A. Functional (psychogenic) cognitive disorders: a perspective from the neurology clinic. *J Alzheimers Dis.* 2015;48(Suppl 1):S5–S17.

Strikwerda-Brown C, Ramanan S, Irish M. Neurocognitive mechanisms of theory of mind impairment in neurodegeneration: a transdiagnostic approach. *Neuropsychiatr Dis Treat.* 2019;15:557.

Overview of Scales and Inventories (Chapter 15) and General Mental Status Scales, Rating Instruments, and Behavior Inventories (Chapter 16)

References included, primarily in Chapter 16.

Overview of Neuropsychological Testing (Chapter 17)

Casaletto KB, Heaton RK. Neuropsychological assessment: past and future. *J Int Neuropsychol Soc.* 2017;23(9-10):778–790.

Lezak MD, Howieson DB, Bigler ED, Tranel D. *Neuropsychological Assessment.* 5th ed. New York, NY: Oxford University Press; 2012.

Zucchella C, Federico A, Martini A, Tinazzi M, Bartolo M, Tamburin S. Neuropsychological testing. *Pract Neurol.* 2018;18(3):227–237.

Tele-Neurobehavior and Computerized Cognitive Tests (Chapter 18)

Bauer RM, Iverson GL, Cernich AN, Binder LM, Ruff RM, Naugle RI. Computerized neuropsychological assessment devices: joint position paper of the American Academy of Clinical Neuropsychology and the National Academy of Neuropsychology. *Arch Clin Neuropsychol.* 2012;27(3):362–373.

Bloem BR, Dorsey ER, Okun MS. The coronavirus disease 2019 crisis as catalyst for telemedicine for chronic neurological disorders. *JAMA Neurol.* 2020;77(8):927–928.

Carlozzi NE, Goodnight S, Casaletto KB, et al. Validation of the NIH toolbox in individuals with neurologic disorders. *Arch Clin Neuropsychol.* 2017;32(5):555–573.

Castanho TC, Amorim L, Zihl J, Palha JA, Sousa N, Santos NC. Telephone-based screening tools for mild cognitive impairment and dementia in aging studies: a review of validated instruments. *Front Aging Neurosci.* 2014;6:16.

Loh PK, Ramesh P, Maher S, Saligari J, Flicker L, Goldswain P. Can patients with dementia be assessed at a distance? The use of telehealth and standardised assessments. *Intern Med J.* 2004;34(5):239–242.

Martin-Khan M, Flicker L, Wootton R, et al. The diagnostic accuracy of telegeriatrics for the diagnosis of dementia via video conferencing. *J Am Med Dir Assoc.* 2012;13(5):487 .e19–24.

Patel UK, Malik P, DeMasi M, Lunagariya A, Jani VB. Multidisciplinary approach and outcomes of tele-neurology: a review. *Cureus.* 2019;11(4):e4410.

Sternin A, Burns A, Owen AM. Thirty-five years of computerized cognitive assessment of aging—where are we now?. *Diagnostics (Basel).* 2019;9(3):114.

Zygouris S, Tsolaki M. Computerized cognitive testing for older adults: a review. *Am J Alzheimers Dis Other Demen.* 2015;30(1):13–28.

Index

Note: Page numbers followed by 't' indicate tables, 'f' figures, and 'b' boxes.